Immunomic Discovery of Adjuvants and Candidate Subunit Vaccines

Immunomics Reviews
An Official Publication of the International Immunomics Society

---

This peer-reviewed book series offers insight on immunology for the 21st century. The technological revolution has borne advances in high-throughput instrumentation and information technology, initiating a renaissance for biomathematics, and biostatistics. Cross-fertilization between genomics and immunology has led to a new field called immunomics, transforming the way in which theoretical, clinical and applied immunology are practiced. Immunomics Reviews will cover integrative approaches and applications to the theory and practice of immunology and explore synergistic effects resulting from a combination of technological advances and the latest analytical tools with the traditional fields of basic and clinical immunology.

For further volumes:
http://www.springer.com/series/7528

Darren R. Flower • Yvonne Perrie
Editors

Immunomic Discovery of Adjuvants and Candidate Subunit Vaccines

Springer

Editors
Darren R. Flower
University of Aston
Aston Pharmacy School
School of Life and Health
Sciences
Birmingham, UK

Yvonne Perrie
University of Aston
Aston Pharmacy School
School of Life and Health
Sciences
Birmingham, UK

ISBN 978-1-4614-5069-6 ISBN 978-1-4614-5070-2 (eBook)
DOI 10.1007/978-1-4614-5070-2
Springer New York Heidelberg Dordrecht London

Library of Congress Control Number: 2012949423

Printed on acid-free paper

Springer is part of Springer Science+Business Media (www.springer.com)

Preface

Within the wider context of immunovaccinology and vaccine discovery, this book will address and explore a range of new strategies and technologies, both informatics-based and experimental, which support and complement both traditional and emerging approaches to vaccine design and discovery. This book looks in turn at reverse vaccinology and the identification of putative candidate antigens, at the discovery of a wide range of different types of adjuvants, and finally at the development of sophisticated new delivery mechanisms, such as liposomes and other applications of nanotechnology. The expectation of this book is very straightforward: to foster and foment interest in those areas of vaccinology, which have thus far not received the level of interest that they perhaps deserve. We have tried to balance the optimism of which we are all guilty with some rationality. Not all of the approaches described will ultimately bear fruit, but each should nonetheless be investigated with the same diligence.

When writing a book, it is usual to acknowledge the contributions made by a whole tranche of people, and acknowledge this sooner rather than later.

First, we would like to thank all the authors for their contributions and for their patience and forbearance. Without their help none of what follows would have been possible.

We would also like to thank many colleagues for their help. Most notable are the following: Prof Peter Beverley, Dr Persephone Borrow, Dr David Tough, Dr Elma Tchillian, and Dr Jagadeesh Bayry.

Lastly, we would like to extend our thanks to everyone at Springer for their efforts in bringing this work to fruition.

Birmingham, UK

Darren R. Flower
Yvonne Perrie

Contents

Contributors

Hifzur Rahman Ansari Bioinformatics Centre, Institute of Microbial Technology, Chandigarh, India

Fiona S. L. Brinkman Department of Molecular Biology and Biochemistry, Simon Fraser University, Burnaby, BC, Canada

Valeria Cafardi Microbial Molecular Biology, Novartis Vaccines and Diagnostics, Siena, Italy

Matthew N. Davies Institute of Psychiatry, King's College London, London, UK

Bhavjinder K. Dhillon Department of Molecular Biology and Biochemistry, Simon Fraser University, Burnaby, BC, Canada

Irini A. Doytchinova Medical University of Sofia, Sofia, Bulgaria

Alexander D. Edwards Reading School of Pharmacy, Reading, UK

Darren R. Flower School of Life and Health Sciences, University of Aston, Birmingham, UK

Stephen V. Gordon School of Veterinary Medicine, University College Dublin, Dublin, Ireland

Yongqun He Unit for Laboratory Animal Medicine, Department of Microbiology and Immunology and Center for Computational Medicine and Bioinformatics, University of Michigan Medical School, Ann Arbor, MI, USA

Malou Henriksen-Lacey CICbiomaGUNE, Guipúzcoa, Spain

S. Hook New Zealand's National School of Pharmacy, University of Otago, Dunedin, New Zealand

Tom Jin Aeras, Rockville, MD, USA

Gareth J. Jones TB Research Group, Animal Health and Veterinary Laboratories Agency—Weybridge, Surrey, UK

Randip Kaur School of Life and Health Sciences, Aston University, Birmingham, UK

Daniel J. Kirby School of Life and Health Sciences, Aston University, Birmingham, UK

Afzal R. Mohammed School of Life and Health Sciences, Aston University, Birmingham, UK

Yvonne Perrie School of Life and Health Sciences, University of Aston, Birmingham, UK

T. Rades New Zealand's National School of Pharmacy, University of Otago, Dunedin, New Zealand

Gajendra P. S. Raghava Bioinformatics Centre, Institute of Microbial Technology, Chandigarh, India

Samantha Sampson Centre for Respiratory Infection, Imperial College London, London, UK

Davide Serruto Microbial Molecular Biology, Novartis Vaccines and Diagnostics, Siena, Italy

John L. Telford Microbial Molecular Biology, Novartis Vaccines and Diagnostics, Siena, Italy

Eric Tsao Aeras, Rockville, MD, USA

Anil Vangala School of Pharmacy and Chemistry, Kingston University, London, UK

Martin Vordermeier TB Research Group, Animal Health and Veterinary Laboratories Agency—Weybridge, Surrey, UK

Jitinder Wilkhu School of Life and Health Sciences, Aston University, Birmingham, UK

Nancy Y. Yu Department of Molecular Biology and Biochemistry, Simon Fraser University, Burnaby, BC, Canada

Chapter 1
Immunomic Discovery of Adjuvants, Delivery Systems, and Candidate Subunit Vaccines: A Brief Introduction

Darren R. Flower and Yvonne Perrie

Abstract Mass vaccination, when coupled to profound improvements in general sanitation, has given rise to the most remarkable transformation in public health in human history. Yet the development of vaccines remains largely trapped in the past, a hostage to the methodology of Pasteur. Infectious disease continues to threaten humanity, with new and renascent diseases emerging continually. The last two decades have seen a breath-taking revival in the commercial market for vaccines and the simultaneous emergence of a whole tranche of new technologies that promise to free vaccine development from the muddle of empirical thinking. In this short introduction, we set the scene for this renaissance, and explore how the combination of computational and experimental techniques promise so much for the future development of vaccines and the science of vaccinology.

The following statement long ago became a truism: that the development of mass vaccination coupled to profound improvements in general sanitation have engendered the most startlingly and amazing transformation in public health. If we travel backwards about hundred years, to the years directly preceding the First World War, human mortality was caused, in the main, by influenza, pneumonia, diarrhoea, and enteritis: totalling about 30 % of fatalities. At the same time, the great killers of today, cancer and heart disease, brought about no more than 12 % of deaths. Journey back another two hundred years—to the dying days of the seventeenth century—and average life expectancy seldom exceeded four decades. The main causes of death were again contagious disease: tuberculosis, smallpox, yellow fever, malaria, and dysentery, affecting infants, children, and adults, all alike. In the early years of the twenty-first century, things are radically different. Infectious disease is responsible for less than 2 % of deaths in the developed world, while chronic disease causes over 60 % of deaths.

D.R. Flower (✉)
School of Life and Health Sciences, University of Aston, Aston Triangle, Birmingham, UK
e-mail: d.r.flower@aston.ac.uk

D.R. Flower and Y. Perrie (eds.), *Immunomic Discovery of Adjuvants and Candidate Subunit Vaccines*, Immunomics Reviews: 5, DOI 10.1007/978-1-4614-5070-2_1,

Vaccination and sanitation are indisputably the most efficient, and thus cost-effective, prophylactic treatments for infectious disease. Together they are the firm bedrock upon which the modern world resides. The truth of this is often ignored by those intoxicated by the many distractions of life in the early twenty-first century, from burgeoning social media to the recondite discoveries of the Large Hadron Collider. People say that the Internet or the iPad or even Facebook have transformed the world. If there is any truth in such assertions, then such transformations are at best shallow and superficial compared to the extraordinary reworking of lives that has transpired over hundreds rather than tens of years. The source of such change can be traced back, in part at least, to the discovery and exploitation of vaccines, vaccination, and vaccinology.

For around the first 100 years of the vaccine story, the story was solely that of smallpox. As recently as the late 1960s, some 10–12 million cases of smallpox were recorded in 31 countries, with annual deaths of 2 million. Yet today smallpox has, with the exception of a few well-guarded stockpiles, been completely eradicated: there have been no new cases for 30 years. The story of smallpox is thus the high point of the vaccination story; no other disease has been eradicated. Polio or poliomyelitis is the next nearest to full eradication, having long been targeted by a systematic, coordinated, worldwide eradication campaign. In 1991, one such programme run by the Pan American Health Organization effected a partial eradication of polio in the western hemisphere. Subsequently, the Global Polio Eradication Program has radically reduced polio throughout the rest of the world, so that today we can count cases worldwide in the tens or hundreds instead of the hundreds-of-thousands or millions.

Yet, vaccine-preventable disease still kills millions. Infectious and contagious disease cause approximately 25 % of world mortality, particularly in children under five. While in developed countries, mortality for diseases such as diphtheria, polio, or measles is less than 0.1 %, in other parts of the world deaths from such infectious diseases is significant. Pertussis, tetanus, influenza, Hib, hepatitis B are all responsible for deaths that number in the hundreds-of-thousands. Perhaps the most execrable situation is measles, which accounts for 70,000 (over 5) and 540,000 (under 5) deaths. However, the leading global causes of death worldwide remain tuberculosis; diarrhoeal illnesses, especially rotaviruses; HIV/AIDS; and malaria. In 2010, 8.8 million contracted TB and 1.4 million died. Disturbing though these numbers may seem, they nonetheless represent a significant reversal of a once ever-escalating trend. The number with latent TB peaked in 2005 at 9 million, while deaths from TB reached their peak at 1.8 million in 2003.

However, these bald numbers are likely to be significant underestimates. Let us also look at malaria. Murray et al. have recently provided evidence that deaths from malaria over the thirty-year span to 2010 are much higher than previously believed [1]. Their epidemiological figures show a peaked distribution over this period, increasing from around a million in 1980, peaking at approximately 1,820,000 in 2004, and then reducing to about 1,240,000 in 2010, with the greatest number dying in Africa. These figures are roughly twice the values published by the WHO. It seems unlikely that the WHO's estimates for other major diseases are uniformly more accurate.

Why are these numbers so high? A principal reason is that there are no effective vaccines for either malaria or HIV, two of the WHO's big three diseases; nor is there expectation that such vaccines will appear in the near future, irrespective of the optimism of those working in the area. And as for tuberculosis—which is carried by around 2 billion people worldwide—the only licensed vaccine has limited efficacy. Many viral infections remain recalcitrant threats of the first order. About 350 million people are infected with hepatitis B, 170 million by hepatitis C, and 40 million by human immunodeficiency virus type 1 (HIV-1). This dire situation is further compounded by the threat from the 35 new or previously unknown infectious diseases identified in the past 30 years: HIV, West Nile fever, Ebola, dengue fever, SARS, and the potentially pandemic H5N1 influenza. Every year, between 5 and 15 % of the global population becomes infected with a new influenza strain, causing upwards of half-a-million deaths. It is widely thought that there will be a continual emergence of new infectious diseases during the present century: emerging zoonotic infections and antibiotic-resistant bacteria prominent amongst them.

In the face of declining birth rates, coupled to decades of ever-enhancing nutrition, advances in treatment regimens and medicines are leading the population of most developed and developing countries figuratively to age: that is for larger and larger proportions of the population to live to maturity and beyond. Growth in life expectancy is matched by growth in the diseases of old age. These include neurodegenerative diseases, principally Parkinson's or Alzheimer's disease; cardiovascular diseases; and stroke. Disease has altered significantly in the preceding century. It will continue to alter during the century to come. Some alterations we can predict; others will escape the forecaster's eye. Disease, particularly infectious disease, has been beaten, or, at least, severely restrained. Many factors have conspired to effect this—improved water quality, better precautionary hygiene, improved nutrition, decreased overcrowding—as well as many interventionary measures, principally antibiotic therapy and vaccines.

Hitherto, vaccines have been an uncompromising success, yet, as we see, so much more needs to be done if the full potential of vaccines is to be achieved. Although the licensing and use of vaccines varies between countries, 25–30 commonly licensed vaccines target a range of viral or bacterial infectious diseases, with approximately 14 paediatric diseases targeted during the first few years of life. Other than paediatric vaccination, most vaccines are used by travellers to tropical or subtropical regions; a significant minority fight infection in the developing world.

Vaccination also works to greatly reduce the morbidity of disease, often imbuing lifetime protection; this is particularly important for benign yet economically important infections, such as the so-called common cold. Diverse sporadic or epidemic infections of the human respiratory track—as caused by an excess of 200 distinct viruses, such as RSV or, more properly, respiratory syncytial virus, coronaviruses, influenza A and B, rhinoviruses, parainfluenza virus, and cytomegalovirus—remain a principal cause of hospitalisation and community morbidity with an estimated 60 % of GP referrals associated with such infections, and cause the loss of enormous numbers of working days in developed countries.

Given the recalcitrance, and the immense investment in treatment and prophylaxis, it may be that many of the diseases alluded to above will never be eradicated, as smallpox was, and that vaccines alone will not be enough. We may instead need a complex network of prophylactic and therapeutic measures at least as complex as the diseases themselves in order to effectively reduce the prevalence of the disease and to treat those who become infected. Whatever other countermeasures we may have recourse to—artemisinin-based drugs, genetically manipulated vectors, or insecticide-treated bednets—the clinical and cost effectiveness of vaccines means they remain the must-have component in the ongoing search for better means of combating endemic infectious disease.

Beyond infectious disease lies what is possibly the most underexplored area within the ever burgeoning field of vaccinology and vaccination: vaccines against allergy and allergic disease; vaccines that target so-called lifestyle diseases, such as those deriving from addiction; and vaccines that target chronic diseases, the most important of which is cancer. Therapeutic vaccines against cancer are probably the best studied amongst the more novel, innovative, and underexplored areas at the forefront of vaccine discovery. The present overall whole-life risk from cancer, at least in developed countries, runs at or about 40 %. The figure is currently rising. There are approximately 3·2 million new cancer cases in Europe each year, resulting in around 1·7 million deaths. In the USA, over one and half million new cases are reported annually. Clearly, this is an important disease burden, and thus a key target for the pharmaceutical and biotechnology industries.

Lifestyle vaccines are another innovation, of which much is expected in certain quarters. They target all kinds of medical problems, ranging from drug addiction through dental caries, all the way to major genetic and multifactorial diseases, including obesity. Versatility and flexibility are major hallmarks of the vaccination concept. Vaccines take many forms and work in many ways. This facet has been exploited in the development of life-style vaccines. Let us look at serious addiction. During 2009, the United Nations Office on Drugs and Crime estimated 3.3–6.1 % of the global population abused so-called illicit substances—a serious problem indeed with an enormous implicit health, economic, and behavioural burden, with the worst excesses coming from cannabis abuse and the abuse of amphetamine, cocaine, and opiates. Anti-drug vaccines generate antibodies able to bind particular drugs; the drug–antibody complexes thus generated should have too high a molecular weight to penetrate the blood–brain barrier effectively, thus reducing the amount and rate of drug egress into the brain and so inhibiting psychoactive effects at the system level. Anti-addiction vaccines have been with us for some time, beginning over 40 years ago, when two proof-of-principle studies [2, 3] demonstrated in rats and in rhesus monkeys that morphine could be used as a hapten in order to create an antibody against morphine addiction. Today, addiction vaccines are being developed to target a range of major abused drugs, such as nicotine, cocaine, various amphetamines, and heroin.

Anti-allergy vaccination also offers great potential for successful commercial exploitation. The prophylaxis and treatment of allergy can now be addressed in many ways, including, notably, recombinant proteins and DNA vaccines. Vaccines against the common cold or anti-allergy vaccines are similar in mechanism to many lifestyle vaccines. These do not save lives directly but do help to greatly reduce the vast economic burden of disease morbidity.

An array of interconnecting factors that have made the pharmaceutical and biotechnology industries re-evaluate the potential of vaccines as a commercially viable product. Prior to 1980, there were relatively few vaccines, most targeting major pandemic diseases of the developed or developing worlds. Subsequently, partly as a result of enhanced technology as discussed at length in the current book, many vaccines have become available, most recently the cervical papillomavirus vaccine. Likewise, there are hundreds upon hundreds of vaccines in trials. The growth rate in the sales of vaccines reflects this feverish and febrile activity: $5 billion in 2000, $6 billion in 2003, $11 billion in 2006, rising to $19 billion in 2009 and $22 billion in 2010; projected sales for 2015 are about $35 billion. The rate of sales growth for vaccines is something like 16 %, compared to the sluggish drugs market, meandering its desultory way at 4 % per annum. There is profit in vaccines, clearly; what remains problematic for the profit-driven decision-making processes of big pharma is the haphazard and probabilistic nature of vaccine discovery. What the pharmaceutical industry needs is the capacity to apply the same systematic, automated, high-technology approaches used to identify new small-molecule drugs to the discovery and development of vaccines.

No right-minded scientist, looking back across the last 200 years, would wish to argue seriously with the contention that the design and development of vaccines is an innately labour-intensive process. The processes deployed to meet the objective of creating new and better vaccines are in desperate need of change. This change must be radical if we hope to simplify such processes. Simple processes are hopefully also fast and efficient processes. In the search for subunit vaccine antigens, one technical development—reverse vaccinology—has proved the most profound and hopeful.

Just over a decade ago, Rino Rappuoli used the expression "reverse vaccinology" to describe development of vaccines using a genomic-based approach, rather than the ponderous empirical methods favoured then, and still in use today. Reverse vaccinology seems about to deliver on its early potential: the European Medicines Agency is in the process of evaluating Novartis's Bexsero, the first commercial vaccine developed using the reverse vaccinology approach. The vaccine may become the first vaccine effectively to combat meningococcus B, a disease causing over 50 % of global meningococcal meningitis. A decision on Bexsero is expected shortly.

During the development of Bexsero, new protective protein antigens were identified using genomics: initially over 600 surface-exposed proteins were predicted from the *N. meningitidis* proteome as molecules liable to host immune surveillance, of which about 350 were then expressed in *E. coli*. This number was reduced by using these proteins to immunize 350 sets of mice, identifying 91 that could induce antibodies in vivo, 29 of which killed *N. meningitidis* in vitro. By comparing the genomes of 31 clinical strains, a further subset of proteins offering broad protection could be identified.

Reverse vaccinology has become perhaps the most famous well-developed approach amongst many advanced approaches now available within the discipline of vaccinology. Indeed, a whole range of other, high-technology methods and techniques have been and are being developed to complement and optimise reverse vaccinology. Capitalising on its success, these offer new hope in our constant struggle with infection; all we need is for this technology to be fostered, developed, and utilised.

This book is intended to fill a gap, if not a void, in current thinking within vaccine design and development by attempting to draw together several disparate strands; and, by doing so, also identify and illuminate some important areas replete with potential. Science, in much the same way that all human activities, from the most profound to the most trivial, follows fashion and progresses by tracking trends. Whether we think of publically funded science or the pharmaceutical industry, similar phenomena are observed. Science follows the money, and money follows consensus. The decision-making process underpinning the strategic direction that policy in both publically funded science and the pharmaceutical industry takes is only in part influenced by science. It is also regrettably in thrall to many, sometimes contradictory, voices: the fickleness of public opinion, vested interests of many hues and flavours, and the myopia of the profit margin, amongst many others. This is because the decision-makers in such organisations are seldom if ever scientists engaged in doing science directly; management and policy, at both the strategic and tactical levels, are often swayed by the prevalence of opinion.

In the pharmaceutical industry, for instance, this is manifest as the next big thing: combinatorial libraries, genomics, high-throughput screening, antisense, even molecular modelling; all were hailed as transformative saviours that would remove happenstance and unpredictability from drug discovery—yet as the current parlous state of the pharmaceutical industry readily attests, while all promised much, none really delivered. No single technique can achieve everything, which is why we should always develop a large range of alternatives, both informatics-based and experimental, all running in parallel.

Central to computational immunology is the capacity to make accurate predictions. Yet, obtaining routes to prediction that are accurate, robust, and dependable continually eludes us. Immunoinformatics deals with empirical, data-dependent methods. The success and utility of such methods depends very much on the data used to propagate and parameterise them; they cannot escape the severe limitations imposed by the data used to create them. The data from which we build models forms a complex phase space of structural and property variation, which can be extremely multidimensional, with a high degree of interdimensional correlation. When the data we work with is reliable and our knowledge of it is complete, then we can create useful models by applying standard methods from computer science to build accurate and predictive models relating observed biological activity to underlying measurable or predictable properties. Usually, such approaches are also much superior when used to interpolate than they are when used to extrapolate. We need complete and thorough data sets effectively and efficiently able to explore the complex relationships between structure and function, necessitating continuous improvement in all aspects of data quality.

Within the wider context of vaccine design and discovery, we shall in this book describe and explore a range of key alternative strategies and technologies, both informatics-based and experimental, which are, by degrees, both supportive and complementary to reverse vaccinology and more traditional approaches to vaccine discovery. This book looks in turn at reverse vaccinology and the identification of putative candidate antigens, at the discovery of a wide range of different types of adjuvants, and finally at the development of sophisticated new delivery mechanisms, such as liposomes and other applications of nanotechnology.

In Chap. 2, Cafardi et al. review the present state of play with respect to reverse vaccinology, with particular emphasis on how completion of bacterial genomes impinges upon the vaccine discovery. They show how this approach allows the development vaccines that are difficult or near impossible to address with conventional approaches. They also highlight how advances in genome-based techniques and in so-called next-generation sequencing approaches and technologies will help to enhance reverse vaccinology, enabling timely identification of novel candidate antigens for new, emerging, or recrudescent infectious diseases.

In Chap. 3, Flower et al. review the discovery of candidate vaccine antigens in more detail. Placing their analysis in the context of emerging ideas about the possible nature of immunogenicity and how it may be propagated by elements of the immune response at the system level, the authors discuss the three main approaches to the identification of novel immunogenic antigens: sequence similarity-based approaches, whereby the antigen nature of a protein is inherited from similar sequences; methods based on identifying the subcellular location of microbial proteins, on the basis that proteins with only certain locations would be accessible to immune surveillance; and the use of empirical alignment-independent approaches to the prediction of antigens. Usefully, the chapter also includes discussion of expert systems for antigen discovery.

In Chap. 4, Vordermeier et al. review how genomics and the development of bioinformatics have radically transformed the cattle vaccinology of bovine tuberculosis. Within the context of a generalised infrastructure of bioinformatic analytical techniques, the authors describe in detail how the application of comparative *in silico* transcriptome and genome analysis is able to undertake prospective prioritisation of immunogenic antigens for experimental testing, leading to the identification of candidate subunit vaccines.

In Chap. 5, He explores the use of epitope-focused immunoinformatic analysis in the prediction of optimal vaccine candidates when undertaking a genome-wide reverse vaccinology exercise. Specifically, He describes the web-server Vaxign, concentrating on a case study: vaccine design against the virulent bacterium *Francisella tularensis*, where 12 candidates were chosen using a combination of pertinent selection criteria.

In Chap. 6, Dhillon et al. offer us a wide-ranging review of methods and strategies for two important areas of immunoinformatic analysis within the domain of vaccine discovery: predicting the immunogenic subcellular location of microbial proteins and identifying proteins encoded by so-called genomic islands. While in Chap. 7, Ansari et al. describe a variety of database systems that facilitate immunoinformatics and antigen selection.

Chapters 8 and 9 look at adjuvants and their discovery. In Chap. 8, Edwards describes the basis of adjuvant action, and the role played by macromolecular adjuvants. In Chap. 9, Flower explores and examines different varieties of molecular adjuvant and their discovery, concentrating on small molecule adjuvants, and their systematic identification using virtual screening technology. This topic is put into context by a thorough review of extant adjuvants, molecular mechanisms of adjuvant action, as well as macromolecular adjuvants and how various adjuvants engage pattern recognition receptors of the innate immune system.

In addition to the characteristics of the antigen and the adjuvant independently, how the antigen and adjuvant are presented to the immune system has a major impact on the biological output of the vaccine. Indeed, the co-delivery and continued association of antigen and adjuvant may be a prerequisite in effective immunisation. This is not a new idea; the ability of alum to promote an antigen depot effect at the site of action has been ascribed as one of its main mechanisms of action for several years. For example, since 1977 the WHO has recommended that over 80 % of diphtheria toxoid needs to be adsorbed to alum for its effective use [4]. Whilst this does not ensure that the antigen remains adsorbed to alum after injection and exposure to interstitial fluid, it is thought to at least initially promote co-location of the antigen with the alum adjuvant. However, alum is not the only adjuvant able to promote the co-delivery of antigens and adjuvants in one system; a range of particulate delivery systems can offer this. Examples of such delivery systems include lipid-based systems (e.g., liposomes, niosomes, ISCOMs) and microparticles. Each of these systems offer a suite of advantages and disadvantages and when considering the choice of delivery system attributes including antigen-loading capacity, antigen retention and protection both on storage and within the biological milieu, and the ability to incorporate adjuvants within the delivery system all require optimisation and this is without consideration of the ability of the delivery system to act as an adjuvant in its own right. In this book we aim to address these issues by considering several of the most commonly employed particulate vaccine delivery systems.

Out of these particulate delivery systems liposomes are one of the most established systems; liposomes were first reported as an effective immunological adjuvant for diphtheria toxoids by Allison and Gregoriadis in 1974 [5]. Since then, a large array of understanding on their design has been gathered and strong links between their formulation and function identified. Of these parameters, the composition of the liposomes will play a pivotal role. For example, the surface charge of liposomes used for vaccine delivery can influence the interactions between liposomes and protein antigens, and affect how liposomes interact with cells. This manipulation of surface charge can range from the inclusion of anionic lipids such as phosphatidylserine, which may facilitate the targeting of antigen presenting cells through interaction with phosphatidylserine receptors. Alternatively, the use of cationic lipids can improve the loading of anionic antigens to the liposomes and upon injection promote a depot effect at the site of injection, promoting the co-delivery of antigen and adjuvant to dendritic cells (e.g., [6, 7]). However, this depot effect is more than electrostatically driven, with the choice of cationic lipids used in the formulation having an impact as explored in Chap. 10.

In addition to liposomes, there are a range of alternative surfactant-based delivery systems, such as niosomes. These are similar in many ways to liposomes; however, non-ionic surfactants form the main component of their bilayers. The most common composition of niosomes investigated for vaccine delivery is 1-monopalmitoyl glycerol, cholesterol, and dicetyl phosphate. One might argue this is not a niosome formulation due to the inclusion of anionic dicetyl phosphate. However, the addition of charged surfactants has proven to enhance the stability of these vesicles and their inclusion in these vesicles is common practice. Generally, niosomes exhibit many similarities to liposomes; however, potential advantages cited include their lack of predisposition to oxidative degradation, as well potential lower cost of components and reduced variability compared to natural phospholipids. Whilst with current manufacturing methods, the cost and reproducibility of phospholipids is less of an issue, niosomes still offer a useful alternative to liposome formulations. In particular, niosomes appear an attractive option for oral delivery of vaccines due to their ability to withstand the harsh gastrointestinal environment as outlined in Chap. 11.

With both liposomes and niosomes, immunostimulatory agents can be easily incorporated within the system and in some cases this can result in restructuring of the particulate delivery system as is the case with ISCOMs (Chap. 12). ISCOMs are prepared from a mixture of phospholipid, cholesterol, and a saponin (often Quil A). Whilst a phospholipid/cholesterol mixture would normally form liposomes, the addition of appropriate concentrations of saponin to the mixture can result in restructuring of the system to form spherical, open, cage-like structures around 40 nm in size, as nicely shown in Chap. 12. Given that their structures are open, ISCOMs cannot incorporate hydrophilic antigens, and antigens need to display a degree of lipophilicity for inclusion into ISCOMs. If required, antigens can be modified through a range of methods to incorporate lipophilic regions within their structure, thereby promoting their incorporation into the structure. Alternatively, similar to cationic liposomes, cationic ISCOMs (where cationic components are used to build their structure) can electrostatically bind a range of anionic antigens and enhance their delivery. In Chap. 12 the formulation, preparation, and application of ISCOMs as vaccine adjuvants is considered.

However, lipid-based systems are only one group of particulate delivery systems, and polymeric systems have also been extensively studied. In particular the use of biodegradable polymers to formulate nano- and microparticulate delivery systems for vaccines has been widely investigated. Much like the lipid-based systems, there is a wide selection of options to consider in the formulation of polymeric nanoparticles and microspheres for vaccine delivery, with polyester polymers offering advantages due to their clinical approved use in a range of medical products. As with the other systems considered, immunostimulatory agents can be incorporated within these polymer constructs and thus these systems can act as delivery systems and adjuvants for antigens. Within Chap. 13, the design of polymeric microspheres as vaccine adjuvants is considered from the choice of base polymer, through to optimisation of process parameters, and finally to considerations of their stability as a product.

Whilst much of current research into the development of vaccines has focused on the design of vaccines for administration of a particulate suspension, dry powder vaccines may hold considerable advantages. In Chap. 14, the authors consider the design of dry powder vaccines. Such vaccines may offer low-cost, temperature-stable products suitable for pulmonary delivery, with the added advantage that the pulmonary route avoids the use of needles (and their associated risks). Furthermore, it can allow for the effective delivery of antigens to target cells of the immune system without the harsh conditions faced by orally delivered vaccines. The development of spray-drying methods outlined in Chap. 14 supports the ability of such powder vaccines to be delivered using conventional dry powder inhalers already clinically licensed for pulmonary delivery.

Therefore, by considering these vaccine delivery platforms in conjunction with the appropriate choices for antigen and adjuvant it is hoped that the threefold multi-component nature of a vaccine can be considered more completely than before. When viewed conceptually, vaccines comprise an important triad. The first part of the vaccine, and in a sense the most important, is the biological component. This is the whole protein, or whole organism, or epitope-based part which confers the ability to be recognised by the immune system. It is this part which differentiates one vaccine from another, an anti-flu vaccine from an anti-TB vaccine. The second part of the vaccine is the adjuvant, which is one of many alternatives, that confers an immunogenicity to many vaccines that they would otherwise not possess. It often does this in a generic fashion, such as via agonising the innate immune system, so that the same adjuvant is quite capable of functioning in many different vaccine formulations. The final and third part of the vaccine is the delivery vehicle, as opposed to the delivery mechanism, such as oral vaccines versus injectable. The vehicle can be things as different as a viral vector or a liposome. An attenuated or heat-treated whole-organism vaccine can be thought of as combining all three parts of this triad in one supra-molecular moiety. Of course, this is a gross simplification, and many other things go into deployable vaccine formulations, such as preservatives, contaminants, and other chemical or biological components that so exercise the anti-vaccine lobby. Hopefully, this book will encourage us to think of vaccines in these terms, and provides the background necessary to engage with each of the three components of the vaccine triad.

With this in mind, the anticipation inherent with this work is indeed simple and straightforward: to foster and foment interest in those areas of vaccinology that this far have not received the level of intense work that they richly deserve. To help achieve this, we have sought to balance optimistic positivity and cold, hard rationality. Not all of the approaches described will ultimately bear fruit, but each should, nonetheless, be examined with equal diligence, sedulousness, and assiduity.

References

1. Murray CJ, Rosenfeld LC, Lim SS, Andrews KG, Foreman KJ, Haring D, Fullman N, Naghavi M, Lozano R, Lopez AD (2012) Global malaria mortality between 1980 and 2010: a systematic analysis. Lancet 379:413–431
2. Berkowitz B, Spector S (1972) Evidence for active immunity to morphine in mice. Science 178:1290–1292
3. Bonese KF, Wainer BH, Fitch FW, Rothberg RM, Schuster CR (1974) Changes in heroin self-administration by a rhesus monkey after morphine immunisation. Nature 252:708–710
4. World Health Organization. Manual for the production and control of vaccines—tetanus toxoid. blg/undp/77.2 Rev.1, 1977 [ref type: serial (book, monograph)].
5. Allison AG, Gregoriadis G (1974) Liposomes as immunological adjuvants. Nature 252:252
6. Henriksen-Lacey M, Bramwell VW, Christensen D, Agger E-M, Andersen P, Perrie Y (2010) Liposomes based on dimethyldioctadecylammonium promote a depot effect and enhance immunogenicity of soluble antigen. J Control Release 142(2):180–186
7. Kamath AT, Rochat A-F, Christensen D, Agger EM, Andersen P, Lambert P-H, Siegrist C-A (2009) A liposome-based mycobacterial vaccine induces potent adult and neonatal multifunctional T cells through the exquisite targeting of dendritic cells. PLoS One 4:e5771

Chapter 2
Bacterial Genomes and Vaccine Design

Valeria Cafardi, John L. Telford, and Davide Serruto

Abstract Since its introduction, vaccinology has been very effective in controlling and eliminating life-threatening infectious diseases. However, in several cases, the conventional approach to identifying protective antigens, based on biochemical, immunological, and microbiological methods, has failed to deliver successful vaccine candidates against major human pathogens. The availability of complete bacterial genome sequences has allowed scientists to change the paradigm and approach vaccine development starting from genomic information, a process named reverse vaccinology. This can be considered as one of the most powerful examples of how genomic information can be used to develop vaccines that were difficult or impossible to tackle with conventional approaches. The ever-growing genomic data, the new genome-based approaches and high-throughput sequencing technologies will help to complement reverse vaccinology to enable timely development of new vaccine antigens against emerging infectious diseases.

2.1 Introduction

Vaccines are currently available for infectious diseases caused by various viruses and bacteria and the prevention of disease and death by vaccination has profoundly improved the public health of many populations globally. Louis Pasteur, who developed the first vaccine against rabies, established in 1881 the basic paradigm for vaccine development, which included the isolation, inactivation, and injection of the causative microorganism. These basic principles have guided vaccine development during the twentieth century. All existing vaccines are based on killed or live-attenuated microorganisms or subunits purified from the microorganism such as toxins detoxified by chemical treatment, purified antigens or polysaccharide

J.L. Telford (✉)
Microbial Molecular Biology, Novartis Vaccines and Diagnostics, Siena, Italy
e-mail: john.telford@novartis.com

D.R. Flower and Y. Perrie (eds.), *Immunomic Discovery of Adjuvants and Candidate Subunit Vaccines*, Immunomics Reviews: 5, DOI 10.1007/978-1-4614-5070-2_2,

conjugated to proteins. At the end of the twentieth century, most of the vaccines that could be developed by these traditional technologies had been developed and they allowed the control and, in some cases, the eradication of many important infectious diseases [78]. Although very successful, in several instances these approaches were not able to deliver vaccines against certain pathogens and on other occasions the vaccines obtained with these classical approaches were no longer adequate due to safety concerns and low efficacy. Killed and attenuated vaccines, based on the whole organisms, may contain several factors that may have reactogenic activity and may induce undesirable inflammatory response. The attenuated vaccines could also revert to the virulent status and chemicals used for inactivating pathogens could be present as traces in the final composition. In addition, classical biochemical and microbiological methods used to identify protective subunits were hampered by the limited number of candidate antigens that could be identified as well as the time required for their identification. Remarkable progresses were recently made by the introduction of new technologies such as recombinant DNA and chemical conjugation of proteins to polysaccharides, as well as advances in the identification of novel adjuvants.

The genome era, initiated with the completion of the first bacterial genome, that of *Haemophilus influenzae* in 1995 [1], catalyzed a new revolution in vaccine development. Advances in sequencing technology and bioinformatics have resulted in an exponential growth of genome sequence information. The study of genomes by both computational and experimental approaches has significantly advanced our understanding of the physiology and pathogenicity of many microbes and has provided insights into the mechanisms of genome evolution as well as microbial population structures [2, 3].

Genomes and genome-based technologies have also the potential to help in the development of therapeutics and vaccines. The availability of whole-genome sequences has entirely changed the approach to vaccine development. The genome represents a list of virtually all the protein antigens that the pathogen can express at any time. It becomes possible to choose potentially surface-exposed proteins in a reverse manner, starting from the genome rather than from the microorganism with an approach called reverse vaccinology [4]. In this review we will describe how genomic information has been successful in the identification of novel protein antigens against various human pathogens. We will also focus on recent reports that have contributed to the discovery of novel vaccine candidates providing the proof of concept of genome-based approaches such as pan-genome investigation, subtractive reverse vaccinology, and DNA microarray analysis. A future view of how high-throughput sequencing methods might positively influence vaccine design will also be discussed.

2.2 Reverse Vaccinology: A Novel Genomic Approach to Antigen Identification

The recent genome revolution has extended the confines in vaccine research. Genome mining has revolutionized the approach to vaccine development and provided a new innovation to antigen selection and design. The approach starting from the genomic information leading to the identification of potential vaccine candidates is termed reverse vaccinology [4]. The availability of complete bacterial genome sequences offers a comprehensive catalogue of genes encoding all the potential proteins of a pathogen, with the potential to rationally select vaccine candidates rather than empirically test them one at a time. Furthermore, the prediction of antigens is independent of the need to culture the pathogen in vitro. On the basis of the concept that surface-exposed proteins are susceptible to antibody recognition and are therefore the most suitable vaccine antigens, a complete genome sequence can be screened using bioinformatics algorithms to select open reading frames (ORFs) encoding putative surface-exposed or secreted proteins. Putative surface proteins can be readily identified based on the combination of several features including the presence of signal peptide sequences, membrane spanning regions, lipoprotein signature, and motifs such as sortase attachment sites (LPTXG sites). Moreover, proteins with homology to known virulence factors or protective antigens from other pathogens can be selected based on homology. Several computational methods are available to search for surface-associated or secreted proteins: PSORT is used for the prediction of protein sorting signals and localization sites in amino acid sequences; SignalP predicts the presence and location of signal peptide cleavage sites in amino acid sequences from different organisms, Gram-positive and Gram-negative prokaryotes; TMpred program makes a prediction of membrane spanning regions and their orientation. Although much progress can be made in silico, the experimental approach is necessary to establish unambiguously the localization of the protein in living bacteria. Furthermore, screening for sequence homologies to human proteins for their exclusion in the selection process can help to avoid problems of autoimmunity.

After candidate surface antigens are identified in silico, they are produced as recombinant proteins and their immunogenicity is assayed to measure their potential as vaccine candidates. The feasibility of the reverse vaccinology approach relies on the availability of a high-throughput system for protective immunity screening and also on good correlate of protection. In the paragraphs below, we will describe how genomic information has been successful in the identification of novel potential vaccine candidates against various human pathogens, such as *Neisseria meningitidis* serogroup B, *Streptococcus agalactiae*, and pathogenic *Escherichia coli*.

2.2.1 The First Vaccine Obtained Through Reverse Vaccinology: The Serogroup B Meningococcus Vaccine

The concept of reverse vaccinology was applied for the first time to serogroup B *N. meningitidis* (MenB). *N. meningitidis* is the major cause of meningitis and sepsis, two devastating diseases that can kill children and young adults within hours, despite the availability of effective antibiotics. It is a Gram-negative bacterium that colonizes asymptomatically the upper nasopharynx tract of about 5–15 % of the human population. However, in a significant number of cases, the bacterium can traverse the epithelium and reach the bloodstream causing septicemia. From the blood meningococcus is able to cross the blood–brain barrier and infect the meninges, causing meningitis [5, 6].

N. meningitidis can be classified in 13 serogroups on the basis of the chemical composition of the capsule polysaccharide. However, more than 95 % of total cases of invasive disease are caused by five major serogroups: A, B, C, Y, and W135. Vaccines against serogroups A, C, Y, and W135 were developed in the 1960s by using the purified capsular polysaccharide as antigen. Second-generation, conjugated vaccines have now been introduced. The chemical composition of the polysaccharide of serogroup B, which resembles a molecule present in human tissues, makes a polysaccharide-based vaccine poorly immunogenic and a possible cause of autoimmunity.

In the last 40 years a lot of efforts have been directed to the identification of meningococcus B antigens as the basis of new vaccines. However, the high variability of these proteins among the different MenB strains represents a serious obstacle to the production of a globally effective anti-MenB vaccine [5]. As a consequence there are no effective vaccines available for the prevention of MenB disease, which is responsible for one third of meningococcal disease in the United States, and up to 80 % of cases in Europe.

In 1998, the research team at Novartis Vaccines embarked on a large-scale genome project. To develop a universal vaccine against serogroup B, the genome of a MenB isolate (MC58 strain) has been sequenced and used to discover novel antigens [7, 8].

The identification of new previously unidentified antigens was a process that took the research team 18 months to achieve. The sequence of the virulent strain was determined by the shotgun strategy and in order to identify novel vaccine antigens a strategy has been aimed to select, among the more than 2,000 predicted proteins, those that were predicted to be surface-exposed or secreted and their potential to induce protection against disease was tested. *N. meningitidis* is essentially an extracellular pathogen and the major protective response relies on circulating antibodies: complement-mediated bactericidal activity is, in fact, the accepted correlate for in vivo protection and as such is the surrogate endpoint in clinical trials of potential meningococcal vaccines. On the basis of this evidence, the group worked on the assumption that protective antigens are more likely to be found among surface-exposed or secreted proteins. Hence the initial selection of candidates is based on computer predictions of secretion or surface location. Of the 2,158 predicted ORFs in the *N. meningitidis* genome, 570 were selected by these criteria and could therefore represent new potential vaccine candidates. The selected ORFs were amplified, cloned and analyzed for expression in a heterologous system as either C-terminal His-tag or N-terminal glutathione *S*-transferase fusion proteins. These two expression systems were chosen to achieve the highest level of expression and the easiest purification procedure by a single chromatography step. Of the 570, 350 ORFs were successfully cloned in *E. coli* and purified in a sufficient amount for mice immunizations. Most of the failures, both in cloning and in expression, were related to proteins with more than one transmembrane spanning region. This is likely to be due to toxicity for *E. coli* or to their intrinsic insolubility.

Each purified recombinant protein was used to immunize mice. Immune response was analyzed by Western blot analysis on total cell extracts to verify whether the protein was expressed and by enzyme-linked immunosorbent assay and flow cytometry on whole cells to verify whether the antigen was surface-exposed in meningococcus. Finally, the bactericidal assay was used to evaluate the complement-mediated killing activity of the antibodies (serum bactericidal activity), since this property correlates with vaccine efficacy in humans [9, 10].

Of the 91 proteins found to be positive in at least one of these assays, 28 were able to induce antibodies with bactericidal activity [8]. Several of the antigens previously identified using conventional approaches showed strain variability or were only expressed in some strains, and most of them are effective only against the homologous strains. Therefore, the potential vaccine candidates identified were evaluated for degree of sequence variability among multiple isolates and serogroups of *N. meningitidis*. Many of the newly identified serogroup B antigens included surface-exposed proteins or lipoproteins with a globular structure and without membrane spanning domains and many of them are not abundant on the bacterial surface. Reverse vaccinology has therefore proven to be a rapid and reliable approach to identifying vaccine candidates. In the case of serogroup B, these potential vaccine candidates, able to induce broad strain coverage, were subjected to further evaluation and characterization. The candidates were gradually funneled down, a process that took a further 24 months. Finally, the three most immunogenic antigens on the basis of their ability to induce bactericidal activity or in vivo passive protection were selected to be used in a multicomponent vaccine. They were NHBA [11], fHbp [12, 13], and NadA [14, 15]. Other two antigens (named GNA2091 and GNA1030) were also selected. To further enhance their immunogenicity and facilitate large-scale manufacturing of the vaccine, four of the selected antigens were combined into two fusion proteins so that the resulting protein vaccine contained three recombinant proteins. The antigen NHBA was fused to GNA1030 while GNA2091 was fused to fHbp. NadA was included as a single antigen as it did not perform well when fused to a partner. It is thought that this may be due to the fact that the protein may loose its native trimeric organization. Results showed that the two fusion proteins formulated with aluminum hydroxide induced immunes in both FACS and bactericidal assays. These antibodies were more potent than those induced by the individual antigens. Twenty micrograms of each of the two fusion proteins and of the NadA antigen were adsorbed to an adjuvant suitable for human use aluminum hydroxide to make the vaccine formulation that was used in subsequent studies. The rationale behind combining antigen was to increase the spectrum of vaccine coverage, minimizing the possibility of bacterial evasion and development of selection mutants [16].

After successful preclinical studies, the MenB vaccine entered the long path of vaccine development that included testing safety and immunogenicity in adult volunteers [17], initial testing in infants [18, 19], and finally, a large-scale, phase III clinical trial that is the basis for a European license application (Fig. 2.1).

2.2.2 From One to Multiple Genomes: Pan-Genome Reverse Vaccinology

While the genome sequence of a single strain reveals many aspects of the biology of a species, it fails to address how genetic variability drives pathogenesis within a bacterial species and also limits genome-wide screens for vaccine candidates or for antimicrobial targets to a single strain. The availability of genome sequences for different isolates of a single species enables quantitative analyses of their genomic diversity through comparative genomic analyses. The higher the number of isolates and the broader the selection of strains, the better the estimate of whole species heterogeneity.

The advantage of multiple genome analysis in vaccine design is highlighted by the discovery of universal vaccine candidates against *S. agalactiae*, the group B *Streptococcus* (GBS). GBS is the leading cause of illness and death among newborn infants. Nine distinct capsular serotypes of GBS have been described; however, the major disease-causing isolates in Europe and the United States belong to only five serotypes: Ia, Ib, II, III, and V [20]. A comparative genomic hybridization analysis revealed that there was significant variation in gene content among different clinical isolates of GBS [21], supporting the idea that one genome sequence was not enough to fully capture the diversity of the species and to enable the identification of broadly protective vaccine candidates. For this reason, additional GBS strains belonging to the five major serotypes were sequenced and compared allowing the definition of the species pan-genome [22]. The pan-genome can be defined as the global gene repertoire pertaining to a species. In general, it can be divided in three parts: the core genome, which includes the set of genes invariably present and conserved in all the isolates; the "dispensable genome," comprising genes present in some but not all the strains, and the strain-specific genes, which are present only in one single isolate.

Maione et al. have applied the pan-genome concept to GBS vaccine discovery. Bioinformatic algorithms were used to select from the pan-genome genes that encode putative surface-associated and secreted proteins. After testing a consistent number of selected proteins in a mouse model of infection, four antigens were

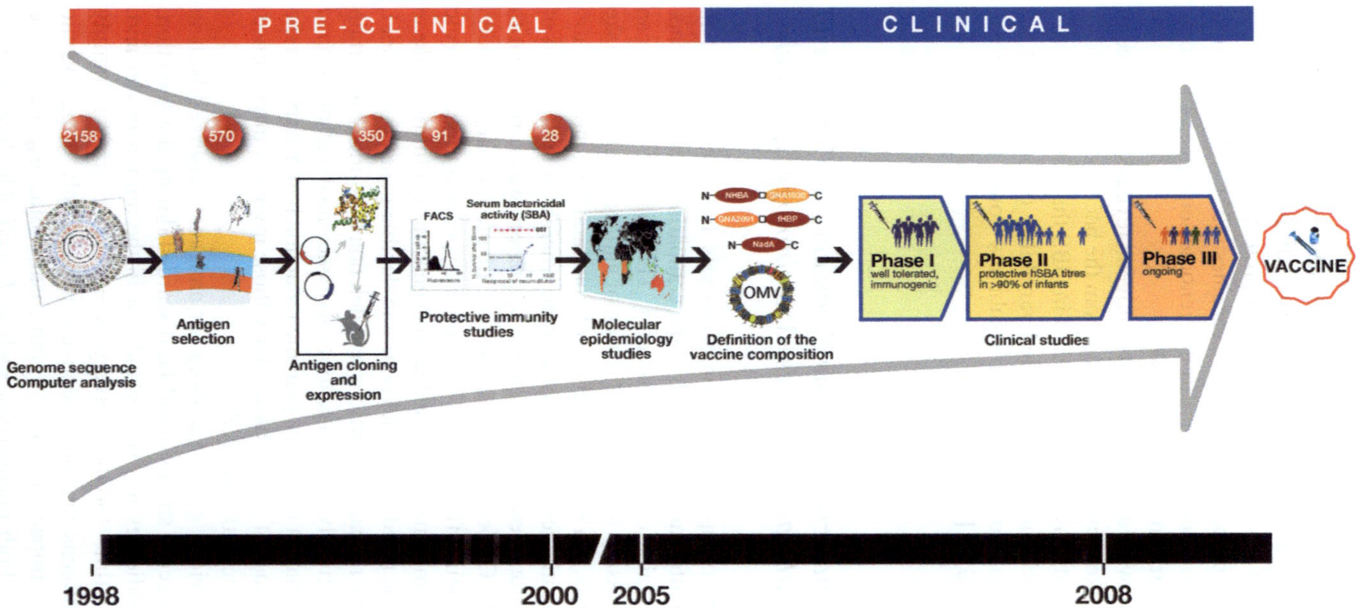

Fig. 2.1 Reverse vaccinology approach applied to *Neisseria meningitidis*. Based on the complete genome sequence of *N. meningitidis* strain MC58 (2158 ORFs), genetic sequences potentially encoding for novel surface exposed proteins were identified. DNA sequences encoding 570 potential surface-exposed antigens were amplified by PCR and cloned into an *Escherichia coli* expression vector. 350 recombinant proteins were successfully produced, purified, and used to immunize mice. The optimal recombinant protein candidates were then selected based on their surface expression and the ability to induce serum bactericidal antibodies: 91 new surface-exposed proteins and 28 novel protein antigens that were able to induce antibodies with bactericidal activity were identified. The antigens selected by reverse vaccinology were prioritized based on these criteria: (i) the protein has to be surface-exposed; (ii) the protein has to be conserved in sequence across a range of different MenB strains; (iii) the protein must induce a broad bactericidal antibody response. The three top antigens that met the prioritization criteria were NadA, fHBP, and NHBA; they gave high bactericidal titers and were bactericidal against most of the strains tested. The recombinant antigens were formulated with outer membrane vesicles and tested in preclinical studies and clinical trials in adults, adolescents, and infants.

identified that were capable of significantly increasing the survival rate among challenged mice. Unexpectedly, only one of these antigens was part of the core genome, the remaining three belonging to the dispensable genome. The final vaccine formulation comprises a combination of the four antigens, which provide overall almost universal strain coverage, with levels of protection similar to those seen when using capsular carbohydrate-based vaccines [23]. This example demonstrates the importance of having access to the genome sequence of multiple strains and performing upfront genome comparisons.

Characterization of the newly identified vaccine antigens revealed that three of them are able to form pilus-like structures extending from the bacterial surface [24]. Furthermore, three pilus islands have been discovered in GBS that encode structurally distinct pilus types [25]. Because of the limited variability of GBS pili, it has been suggested that a combination of three pilin subunits could lead to broad protective immunity against GBS [26].

2.2.3 The Utility of Analyzing Genome Sequences of Commensal Bacteria: The Subtractive Reverse Vaccinology Approach

While in the case of GBS, comparative genome analysis has been applied to disease-causing isolates, an alternative approach is the comparison between pathogenic and nonpathogenic strains of the same species. This kind of analysis can provide the information necessary for the identification of antigens that really make the difference in pathogenesis. An elegant example of comparative genome analysis is that described for uropathogenic strains of *E. coli*, whereby a comparison of UPEC genomes with other complete *E. coli* genome sequences was carried out to help identifying sets of "UPEC-specific" and strain-specific proteins, respectively, that may form the basis of their different individual phenotypes and uropathogenic potential. Comparative genome analysis revealed that genome evolution in these bacteria cannot be simply described by a "backbone and flexible gene pool" model, but must also be described by repeated insertions and deletions occurring in certain parts of the genome [27]. Similarly, whole-genome sequence analyses of *Listeria* and *Neisseria* spp. revealed that an extensive genome reduction had occurred in the nonpathogenic species with loss of genes, particularly those involved in virulence, host interaction, and metabolic pathways [28–30].

From a vaccine point of view, genes encoding for antigens conserved both in pathogenic and in nonpathogenic strains could be discarded during the selection, reducing the number of candidates to express and test in the animal model and, consequently, reducing the time for the delivery of a vaccine. This is mainly because the selection of antigens that are selectively present only in pathogenic strains might reduce the impact on the commensal flora, especially for microorganisms that possess both phenotypes, such as *E. coli*. The first example of a subtractive reverse vaccinology approach has been recently published.

Gomes Moriel et al. performed a comparative genome analysis between pathogenic extraintestinal *E. coli* (ExPEC) and commensal *E. coli* strains with the aim of identifying genes specific for pathogenic strains and therefore an ideal target for a vaccine that will not interfere with the natural commensal gut flora of the human host. Authors have selected 230 antigens that have been tested for protection in vivo. Nine antigens were protective in a mouse model of sepsis and the molecular epidemiology analysis showed that these nine antigens are conserved among several pathogenic *E. coli* strains suggesting that by combining some of these antigens a broadly cross-protective vaccine may be developed [31]. A protective antigen (named ECOK1_3385) was identified and active immunization with the antigen or passive protection with sera raised against it provided nearly complete protection from bacteremia and mortality. It is interesting to notice that this antigen was expressed by nonpathogenic strains but not secreted due to the absence of a type II secretion system involved in the surface localization of this antigen [31].

2.2.4 Reverse Vaccinology Explains Biology: Characterization of the Vaccine Antigens Identified

In addition to the discovery of many previously unknown antigens, which have led to successful vaccine development in several instances, reverse vaccinology has made possible studies on antigen function, leading to an understanding of the biology of the pathogen. The two most notable examples are the discovery of factor H binding protein in meningococcus and the discovery of pili in Gram-positive pathogens. In the case of meningococcus, following the publication of the protective antigen GNA1870, two independent laboratories found that this antigen binds the human complement regulator factor H (fH) [32, 33]. This discovery led to an understanding that meningococcus can grow in human blood by downregulating the alternative pathway of complement activation [13]. However, because the same protein was unable to bind Factor H from animal species such as mice and rats [79], the discovery also allowed the understanding of the species specificity of meningococcus and that failure to develop an animal model for meningococcus was because of the fact that the bacterium is unable to grow in the blood of mice and rats. Transgenic animals expressing human factor H may likely be the solution for a meningococcus animal model.

In the second case, while pili had been known for decades to be an essential component for the pathogenesis of Gram-negative bacteria, they were not known to be present in Gram-positive pathogens before the sequencing and analysis of the genomes of *Streptococcus pyogenes*, *S. agalactiae*, and *Streptococcus pneumoniae* [34]. Following screening for protective antigens by reverse vaccinology, it was found that a protective antigen of GBS was a component of a high molecular weight pilus [24]. This new line of research soon led to the identification of similar surface protrusions in *S. pyogenes* and in *S. pneumoniae* [35, 36], revealing a unique mechanism of pathogenesis for these three important Gram-positive human pathogens.

2.3 Lessons Learned While Exploiting Reverse Vaccinology Approaches

The reverse vaccinology approach has been applied to other pathogenic bacteria including *Bacillus anthracis*, *Porphyromonas gingivalis*, *S. pneumoniae*, *Chlamydia pneumoniae*, and *Brucella melitensis* [37]. All the results obtained so far showed that genome mining allowed to increase the number of candidate vaccine antigens by several orders of magnitude. However, during the development of new vaccine antigens through reverse vaccinology, we understood that parallel genome-based studies can be applied in order to better characterize the candidates and understand their potentials.

In the development of a universal vaccine capable of inducing protection against virtually all circulating strains, accurate characterization of the selected vaccine candidates is highly recommended. The analysis of the sequence conservation of a given antigen is a fundamental aspect in its evaluation as vaccine candidate. Bacterial pathogens use a broad range of microevolutionary tools (like phase variation and antigenic variability) to escape the human immune response.

The analysis should be performed on a strain collection representing globally diverse geographic regions that take into account the target population of the vaccine. In the era of genomics, the availability of multiple genome sequences greatly facilitates the analysis of sequence conservation. However, the number of genomes available is usually not sufficient to cover the diversity of a species or its global geographic representation. Hence, large molecular epidemiology studies on a restricted number of genes encoding the best vaccine antigens are necessary. For example, in the case of MenB, a panel of strains was selected as representative of the meningococcus diversity. In order to evaluate the sequence variability the genes encoding vaccine antigens were sequenced and compared [38]. Performing these studies we learnt that the discovery of previously unknown protein antigens has generated new challenges because the presence and sequence variability of these antigens are not completely aligned with classical typing systems used to characterize the population structures of bacterial pathogens [38]. New antigens usually segregate in the bacterial population in a manner that is independent of conventional markers, such as those used to define serotypes, and genetic markers, such as those used in MLST (multilocus sequence typing), and so we need to identify new ways to type bacteria in order to evaluate the efficacy of new vaccines. In the case of MenB a new typing system, named MATS (meningococcal antigen typing system), has been developed as a basis for molecular epidemiology studies and evaluation of vaccine coverage [39]. Another critical aspect that must be considered during the development of a widely protective vaccine is the expression profile of the antigens identified. Bacteria have different and complex mechanisms to regulate gene expression [40]. For vaccine discovery programs, it is of key importance to know what genes are expressed during host infection and also to understand the mechanism of regulation of the genes encoding the vaccine antigens. These notions will help to understand (i) whether these genes are expressed during infection so gene products can be the target of the antibodies generated by vaccination and (ii) whether they are expressed in the laboratory conditions used to evaluate antigen immunogenicity (e.g., serum bactericidal assay or opsonophagocitosis).

These lessons suggest that genome mining can be complemented by functional genomics approaches in order to obtain a comprehensive characterization of the antigens identified. For example an upfront comparison of whole-genome sequences from strains representative of the genetic diversity of a bacterial species can be a powerful tool for the selection of the most conserved antigens. Global genome profiling of gene expression in different conditions resembling infection or even better in infected hosts can be an approach to advance the study of genes involved in the pathogenesis and select those expressed in vivo.

2.4 Applications of Functional Genomics and High-Throughput Sequencing in Vaccine Design

Functional genomics methods, linking genotype to phenotype, empower the use of highly parallel methodologies that allow investigators to study all the genes or all the proteins of a pathogen in the context of a host or under various physiological states of interest [3]. These approaches are complementary to in silico antigen identification. These include the large-scale analysis of gene transcription by DNA microarray, the identification of the whole set of proteins encoded by a microorganism by two-dimensional gel electrophoresis and mass spectrometry, as well as the use of protein chips to analyze immunological responses in human sera. All these approaches have been widely applied to vaccine design, with the purpose of identifying sets of genes expressed during infection and involved in pathogenesis (Table 2.1).

In the past few years, unprecedented efforts have been made to develop and deploy new sequencing technologies [2, 41, 42]. The advent of new sequencing technologies that can produce sequence data much more cheaply and speedily than traditional methods has recently transformed the study of many fields of microbiology, from epidemiology to functional genomics.

With respect to traditional sequencers, new sequencing platforms can perform highly parallel sequencing of amplified DNA fragments without the need for cloning, thus generating, in the form of short reads, an output having a much higher order of magnitude. Three technologies have undergone a wide spread on the market: Roche 454 (Roche) [43], Genome Analyzer (Solexa/Illumina) [44], and SOLiDTM (Applied Biosystems) [45]. Their technical features are significantly different and have been described in several recent reviews [46, 47].

Table 2.1 Examples of bacterial genomes that have been explored for vaccine components using functional genomic approaches

Pathogen	Disease	Brief description of the approaches	References
Neisseria meningitidis B	Major cause of bacterial septicemia and meningitis	Reverse vaccinology, see text for details	[8]
		Microarray—Analysis of the MenB transcriptome during adhesion to host epithelial cells led to the identification of 189 genes with increased expression under conditions that mimicked in vivo host–pathogen interactions. Twelve of these genes were confirmed by FACS analysis to express surface proteins accessible to the immune system (with four of these being detected only after adhesion to epithelial cells), five of which induced bactericidal protective antibodies in mice	[50]
Streptococcus pneumoniae	Most common cause of fatal community-acquired pneumonia in the elderly and is also one of the most common causes of middle ear infections and meningitis in children	Reverse vaccinology: all the ORFs of the genome sequence of a clinical isolate of *S. pneumoniae* were evaluated to determine whether the gene products contained sequence motifs predictive of their localization on the surface of the bacterium. This led to the identification of 130 ORFs. Mice were immunized with 108 of these proteins and 6 were shown to confer protection against disseminated *S. pneumoniae* infection. All the six protective antigens were broadly distributed among several pneumococcus strains and showed immunogenicity during human infection	[51]
		Comparative genomics: the genome of an avirulent strain (R6) of *S. pneumoniae* has been sequenced. Comparative genome hybridization using DNA arrays revealed differences between the genomes of avirulent and virulent *S. pneumoniae*, which could contribute to differences in virulence and antigenicity. This comparison might lead to the	[52]

		identification of some specific proteins as potential target for vaccine development	
Staphylococcus aureus	Infects wounds and causes severe infections. Following acquisition of resistance to most available antibiotics has emerged as an important opportunistic pathogen	Genomic peptide libraries: *S. aureus* peptides were displayed on the surface of *Escherichia coli* via fusion to one or two outer membrane proteins (LamB and FhuA) and probed with sera selected for high antibody titers and opsonic activity. The exhaustive screening of these libraries by magnetic cell sorting determines the profile of antigens, which are expressed in vivo and elicit an immune response in humans. A total of 60 antigenic proteins were identified	[53]
		Serological proteome analysis: A surface protein preparation from *S. aureus* was resolved by 2D electrophoresis and analyzed by immunoblotting using two pools, each consisting of five sera coming from healthy donors or patients. Twenty-one spots were isolated and analyzed by mass spectrometry allowing the identification of 15 proteins including known and new vaccine candidates	[54]
Porphyromonas gingivalis	Periodontal pathogen that has been implicated in the etiology of chronic adult periodontitis	Reverse vaccinology: applying a series of bioinformatics tools 120 putative new antigens have been identified from the genome of *P. gingivalis*. The selected genes were cloned and expressed in *E. coli* and screened by Western blot using sera from human periodontitis patients. These candidates were reduced to a set of 40 proteins, which were purified and used to immunize mice that were subsequently challenged with live bacteria in a subcutaneous abscess model. Two antigens demonstrated protection in this model of infection and therefore could represent potential vaccine candidates	[55]

(continued)

Table 2.1 (continued)

Pathogen	Disease	Brief description of the approaches	References
Streptococcus agalactiae (Group B streptococcus)	Leading cause of bacterial sepsis, pneumonia, and meningitis in neonates in the United States and Europe	Proteomics: Proteome analysis of the outer surface proteins of this pathogen allowed the discovery of novel surface proteins. Sera raised against some of these proteins were protective in a neonatal animal model against a lethal dose of the pathogen	[56]
		Pan genome reverse vaccinology—see text for details	[23]
Streptococcus pyogenes (Group A streptococcus)	Causes many human infections ranging from mild pharyngitis to severe diseases, including toxic shock syndrome, necrotizing fasciitis, and rheumatic fever	Comparative genomics: Analysis of the genome of four GAS strains led to the discovery of four new extracellular proteins. These proteins are very well conserved as observed applying sequencing and genetic population analysis. Western immunoblot confirmed that all four proteins are made during the course of distinct GAS infections and immunization with the purified form of one of these can confer protection in a murine model of infection	[57]
		Surface proteome—Surface digestion of live bacteria with different proteases allowed fast and consistent identification of proteins that are expressed on the bacteria surface and thus exposed to the immune system. The cell-surface peptide fragments generated after protease treatment of GAS strain SF370 were recovered, concentrated, and analyzed by tandem mass spectrometry and identified using bioinformatic examination. Seventy-two proteins were identified, of which only four were predicted by the PSORT algorithm to be cytoplasmic proteins indicating that the method was highly specific for surface-exposed proteins. Among the surface proteins identified it was proven that some induce protection in an animal model of infection	[58]

Chlamydia pneumoniae	Causes pneumonia and is also associated with atherosclerotic and cardiovascular disease	Reverse vaccinology, proteomic: As a result of in silico analysis of *C. pneumoniae* genome, 157 putative surface-exposed proteins have been identified. Recombinant forms were expressed in *E. coli*, purfied and used to immunize mice. Antisera were used to detect cell-surface localization by FACS analysis. 2D gel electrophoresis and mass spectrometry were used to confirm the expression of the FACS-positive antigens in the elementary body phase of development. The result of these systematic genome–proteome combined approach allowed the identification of 28 new vaccine candidate antigens	[59]
ExPEC	Extraintestinal pathogenic *E. coli* (ExPEC) are the cause of a diverse spectrum of invasive infections in humans and animals, leading to urinary tract infections, meningitis, or septicemia	Subtractive reverse vaccinology—see text for details	[31]
		Surface proteome of OMV: outer membrane vesicles (OMVs) produced by a tolR mutant of the pathogenic IHE3034 strain were analyzed by 2D electrophoresis coupled to mass spectrometry. The analysis led to the identification of 100 proteins, most of which are localized to the outer membrane and periplasmic spaces. Interestingly, seven of the identified proteins appear to be specific for pathogenic *E. coli* and therefore are potential targets for vaccine and drug development	[60]

The high amount of information that can result from high-throughput sequencing applications, thanks also to the development of computational tools able to manage so much sequence data, is improving our understanding of the complexity of bacterial genomes. One of the next challenges of vaccinology is to apply these technologies to help and improve the identification and characterization of vaccine antigens in the reverse vaccinology approach.

2.4.1 Studies on Antigen Variability and Population Structures

In the reverse vaccinology approaches conducted thus far, molecular epidemiology studies on antigen presence and variability have been conducted on a small number of antigens when they have been already selected and tested for expression and immunogenicity. On the contrary, it would be useful to start new reverse vaccinology projects by sequencing the genomes of a collection of strains representing globally diverse geographic areas that take into account the target population of the vaccine. The application of the new sequencing technologies will make this approach feasible. The large collection of genomic data generated will help upfront in the identification of the most conserved protein antigens. Moreover, genomic information will help to define the dimension of the pan-genome and to characterize the population structure, shedding light on the complexity of bacterial species. It will be possible to identify the major lineages inside the population and their geographical distribution and also evaluate how genetic exchange occurs between lineages, leading to a better understanding of the mechanisms involved in the evolutionary process of a bacterial species against which a vaccine has to be designed (Fig. 2.2a).

Recent works have demonstrated that new sequencing technologies have the potential to study the dynamics of bacterial pathogens. For example, studying a single strain of methicillin-resistant *Staphylococcus aureus*, Harris et al. demonstrated the potential of this approach in tracing transmission events over a short timescale, within a hospital environment or between hospitals, and in identifying the sources of outbreaks [48]. By comparing whole-genome sequences of many isolates of the same antibiotic-resistant strain of *S. pneumoniae*, Croucher et al. reconstructed its evolution and global spread. Moreover, they shed light on the effects that clinical practices as antibiotic use and vaccination can have on the evolution of this pathogen [49].

New sequencing technologies will also open up opportunities for monitoring pathogen vaccine escape by screening for evidence of immune selection in the genomes of pathogen populations before and after vaccination. By deep sequencing of microbial populations it will be possible to identify antigens under immune selection by monitoring the clustering of single nucleotide polymorphisms and other mutations that affect protein sequence.

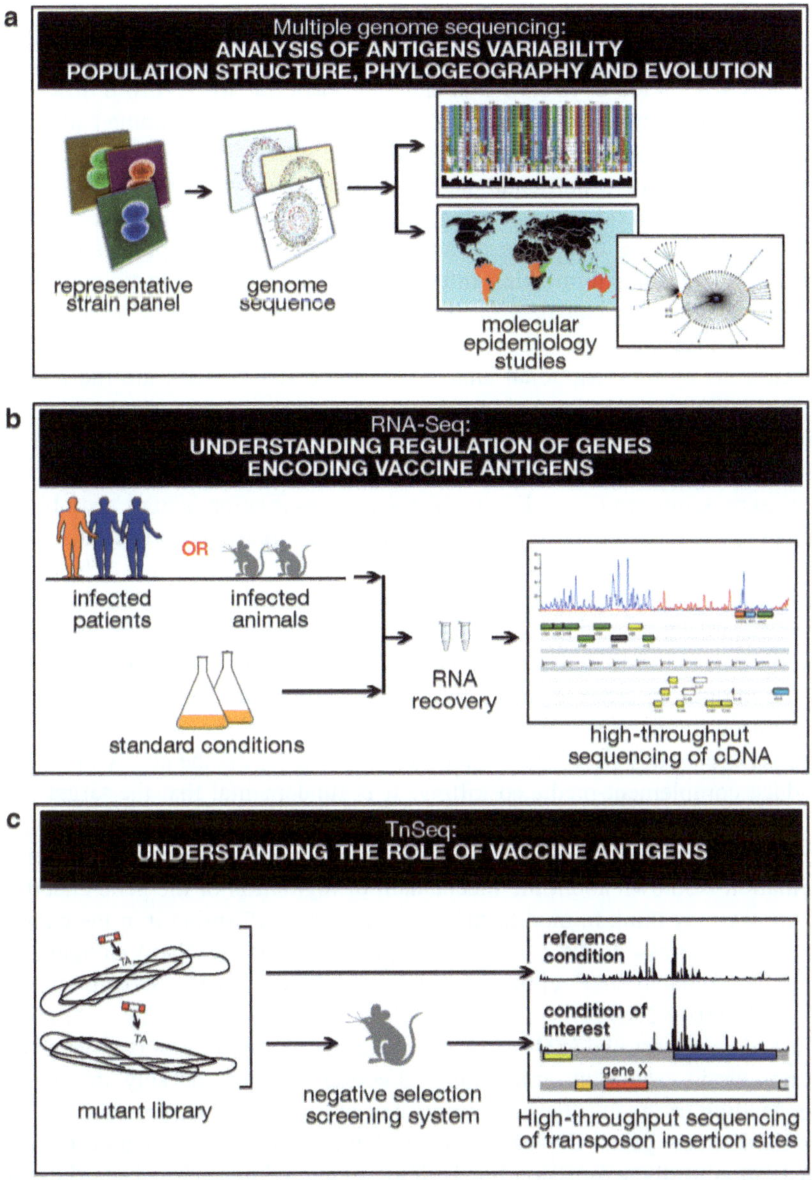

Fig. 2.2 Application of novel sequencing approaches to vaccine antigens identification. Three applications of next-generation sequencing technologies and their impact on vaccine design are schematically represented. (**a**) Analysis of antigen variability, distribution, and evolution by high-throughput sequencing of different isolates. (**b**) High-throughput transcriptional profiling of antigens by RNA-Seq in different in vitro, ex vivo, and in vivo conditions. (**c**) High-throughput functional characterization of vaccine antigens in different conditions mimicking infection by TnSeq.

2.4.2 Transcriptomics

To rapidly respond to environmental changes, bacteria have evolved different and complex mechanisms to regulate gene expression. While the genome carries all the necessary genes, bacteria can save considerable energy by expressing only those that are required in a particular stage of their life cycle [40]. Transcriptional regulation is an important aspect that needs to be considered when designing a new vaccine. During the phase of antigen selection, transcriptional profiling of bacteria in conditions mimicking infection can lead to the identification of novel virulence factors that can be considered as vaccine antigens. Moreover, once a panel of candidates has been selected, antigens of interest can be better characterized by transcriptional analysis, to understand which are the conditions influencing their expression.

From a vaccine coverage point of view, an important aspect to take into consideration is that discrepancy between the sequence conservation of an antigen and its expression can occur. Even when gene conservation is high, variability can occur in terms of expression. There may be several reasons for such discrepancy. First, the genomic organization can vary from strain to strain thus affecting gene expression. Second, activity of transcriptional regulators can also vary, and this is not predictable from the nucleotide sequence of the selected antigens. Therefore transcriptional studies must be carried out, as an approach complementary to genome mining, in order to select antigens that are expressed in the conditions of interest used to assess the functionality of an antigen. For example, in the case of MenB we use an in vitro serum bactericidal assay to assess the ability of antibodies to induce complement-mediated killing. It is fundamental that the target antigen under evaluation be expressed in the particular in vitro condition otherwise we might underestimate the role of the antigen as a vaccine candidate. If sufficient information is known about the mechanism of regulation of the gene encoding an antigen, we may think to modify the in vitro assay performing it in the conditions where it is expressed. An example is represented by the NadA antigen, which is highly regulated and repressed during standard in vitro growth conditions {[15] #642;[80] #29037}.

Last but not least, the analysis of the transcriptional profile of pathogens during infection or in conditions mimicking infection has considerably improved our understanding of the mechanisms implicated in host–pathogen interaction.

In the last few years, DNA microarrays have been extensively used to simultaneously monitor the expression levels of all annotated genes in a bacterial population (Table 2.1). Gene expression can be studied by growing pathogens in an appropriate in vivo or ex vivo model of infection (e.g., cell and tissue cultures, animal models) and, after recovering the bacteria for RNA preparation and labeling, the gene activity is analyzed and compared to the expression of the genes under in vitro conditions [61].

The need for a more precise and comprehensive identification of microbial transcriptomes, independently of any annotated sequence feature, recently led to the development of tiling microarrays, which generally represent both strands and the intergenic regions of the genome. These new arrays have revealed an unexpectedly high degree of transcriptome complexity in bacterial species, allowing detection of unannotated genes, noncoding RNAs, alternative and antisense transcripts, and untranslated regions [62]. However, hybridization-based approaches present several limitations. In particular, they rely upon existing knowledge about genome sequence and the dynamic range of detection is limited by cross-hybridization and saturation signals.

Following progress in DNA sequencing and development of new computational tools, genome-wide studies on bacterial gene expression have begun to shift from microarray technology to a new method termed RNA sequencing (RNA-seq), in which high-throughput sequencing of cDNA is carried out.

Over preexisting approaches, RNA-Seq presents several advantages. Following sequencing, the resulting reads are either aligned to a reference genome or assembled de novo to produce a transcription map. This also means that transcripts that do not correspond to existing genomic sequences can be detected. RNA-Seq provides a far more precise measurement of the levels of transcripts than other methods, having very low if any background signal and no upper limit for quantification, which correlates with the number of sequences obtained. Transcripts can be precisely located to a single-base resolution. Moreover, it can help genome sequencing in revealing sequence variations in the transcribed regions [63].

In the last few years, RNA-seq has been applied to the transcriptome analysis of several pathogens. Yoder-Himes and coworkers used RNA-Seq to examine the transcriptional response of two closely related strains of *Burkholderia cenocepacia*, one isolated from a cystic fibrosis patient and the other from soil, in conditions mimicking human sputum and soil. Despite the high degree of DNA sequence similarity of the two strains, the authors were able to detect a large number of regulatory differences between them, which may represent specific adaptations to the niches from which they were isolated [64]. Similarly, the RNA-seq approach has been successfully applied to the transcriptome analysis of other species, such as *Salmonella enterica* serovar Typhi [65], *Listeria monocytogenes* [66], *B. anthracis* [67], *Acinetobacter baumannii* [68], *Chlamydia thracomatis* [69], and *Helicobacter pylori* [70].

We can predict that in the near future this technique, enabling the simultaneous transcriptomic analysis of all the antigens of interest more speedily and precisely than it was previously possible, will become a helpful tool for antigen identification and characterization. Moreover, without any need to accurately design probed arrays, RNA-Seq will allow comparison of the expression profiles of multiple strains. We can also imagine that RNA-seq will be used in some applications that aim to characterize host–pathogen interactions without any need to separate the two RNA populations and allowing to understand not only how the pathogen adapts to cause an infection but also how the host (or an animal model) responds to the infection. For example, RNA could be isolated from infected patients and both the pathogen and the host transcriptional responses analyzed (Fig. 2.2b).

Knowledge of strains and conditions in which an antigen of interest is expressed can provide fundamental complementary information regarding the potential protective capability of each antigen that will help in the prioritization of the antigens. Moreover, analyzing expression levels on a whole-transcriptome scale and in a high-throughput fashion can lead in a short time to the identification of in vitro and in vivo conditions in which an antigen is expressed. These will be the conditions in which that antigen can be immunologically characterized and its function investigated in depth.

2.4.3 *Identification of Genes Involved in Pathogenesis*

While RNA expression can provide indication on the expression of an antigen in a certain condition related to pathogenesis, other approaches are needed to demonstrate its role in the establishment of the disease or the survival of the pathogen in the host. In order to identify bacterial genes involved in survival and pathogenesis, a variety of methods have been set up in the past few years. All these approaches rely on random mutagenesis and require a detection system that allows simultaneous screening of a pool of mutants.

A strategy that has been extensively used to evaluate gene expression in vivo is IVET (in vivo expression technology), which identifies promoters that are active in vivo but not in vitro using a library of random genomic fragments ligated to a promoterless reporter gene [71]. Another methodology that has been used is STM (signature-tagged mutagenesis). In STM, unique hybridization tags are introduced into each mutant by transposon mutagenesis [72]. All the mutants are pooled and used to infect an animal or alternatively are exposed to a selected condition mimicking a stage of infection. "Negative selection" of the clones unable to survive is then carried out by comparing hybridization of the input pool (the entire mutant library) with that of the output pool (a subset of the library containing all the survived mutants). This approach allowed the identification of *Salmonella typhimurium* mutants showing an attenuated virulence in a murine model of typhoid fever [72]; similarly, *N. meningitidis* genes involved in the establishment of systemic infection could be selected in an infant rat model [73] (Table 2.1).

These methods allow selection of virulence factors on a large scale, providing useful information for both identification of new vaccine candidates and their prioritization.

Taking advantage of next-generation sequencing technology, a new method has recently been developed. In this method, called Tn-Seq, a saturated transposon insertion library is generated. Upon growth under a test condition of interest (in vitro or in vivo) insertion mutants with a lower fitness decrease in the population, while other mutants remain the same or increase in frequency. Changes in frequency are determined by high-throughput sequencing of the transposon flanking regions [74, 75].

Using a saturated mariner transposon insertion library, van Opijnen et al. have been able to evaluate fitness of *S. pneumoniae* genes in standard laboratory conditions [74]. Langridge et al. have used a similar approach, named TraDIS (transposon-directed insertion-site sequencing), to assay simultaneously every gene of *S. enterica* serovar Typhi for both essentiality in standard laboratory growth conditions and contribution toward bile tolerance. They clearly show how the possibility to sequence at high resolution large numbers of mutants allows the screening of very rich libraries. Moreover, the semi-quantitative nature of the assay allows the identification not only of essential and dispensable genes, but also advantageous and disadvantageous genes during growth [76]. Using mouse as a model of pulmonary infection Gawronski et al have identified genes required by *H. influenzae* to resist host defenses during lung pathogenesis [77]. This study shows the potential of this Tn-seq approach to provide new vaccine targets for prevention of *H. influenzae* pulmonary infection.

Providing a link between genotype and phenotype in a high-throughput fashion, Tn-Seq is likely to become the tool of choice for the characterization of bacterial pathogenesis (Fig. 2.2c). Given a selected condition, the entire gene content of a pathogen can be screened speedily and at unprecedented resolution. Moreover, negative selection can be carried out in multiple conditions, mimicking different stages of infection, thus revealing which genes are most important to establish successful infection. Tn-Seq can thus become very helpful in screening vaccine candidates on a whole-genome scale on the basis of their role in vivo.

2.5 Conclusions

Genomics has introduced a new paradigm to bacterial pathogenesis. Instead of dissecting bacterial components in vitro, the new approach starts with the complete information on the genome sequence and then identifies the important factors in virulence. Moreover, the availability of complete genome sequence information of many pathogens has led to a new paradigm in vaccine development. If a suitable assay is available, every protein synthesized by the pathogen can be tested as a vaccine candidate without any prior selection based on incomplete knowledge of the pathogenicity and immunogenicity of the organism. Several years into the reverse vaccinology approach, we have a previously unbelievable insight into a pathogen's genome and its use to identify new vaccine candidates. However, the approaches used for vaccine development are continually being refined based on improved understanding of microbial molecular epidemiology, evolution, virulence, host–pathogen interactions and increased understanding of the complexity of microbial communities as well as improved genome-based technologies. One, or a combination, of the approaches described in this chapter typically drives vaccine discovery projects, with the approach used being heavily dependent on the characteristics of the target pathogen and the vaccine antigens to be identified.

Finally, the progress made in the genomic era has finally put the realization of vaccines for many pathogens within reach as demonstrated by the new MenB vaccine recently developed. Many diseases still cannot be controlled by vaccination and more infectious diseases are expected to emerge or reemerge. In this new era of vaccine development, we would expect the evolution of genome-based approaches that will provide a number of candidate antigens for new vaccines to control and eradicate microbial infections.

References

1. Fleischmann RD et al (1995) Whole-genome random sequencing and assembly of Haemophilus influenzae Rd. Science 269(5223):496–512
2. Medini D et al (2008) Microbiology in the post-genomic era. Nat Rev Microbiol 6(6):419–430
3. Raskin DM et al (2006) Bacterial genomics and pathogen evolution. Cell 124(4):703–714
4. Rappuoli R (2001) Reverse vaccinology, a genome-based approach to vaccine development. Vaccine 19(17–19):2688–2691
5. Stephens DS, Greenwood B, Brandtzaeg P (2007) Epidemic meningitis, meningococcaemia, and Neisseria meningitidis. Lancet 369(9580):2196–2210
6. Caugant DA, Maiden MC (2009) Meningococcal carriage and disease—population biology and evolution. Vaccine 27(suppl 2):B64–B70
7. Tettelin H et al (2000) Complete genome sequence of Neisseria meningitidis serogroup B strain MC58. Science 287(5459):1809–1815
8. Pizza M et al (2000) Identification of vaccine candidates against serogroup B meningococcus by whole-genome sequencing. Science 287(5459):1816–1820
9. Borrow R, Balmer P, Miller E (2005) Meningococcal surrogates of protection–serum bactericidal antibody activity. Vaccine 23(17–18):2222–2227
10. Goldschneider I, Gotschlich EC, Artenstein MS (1969) *Human immunity to the meningococcus*. I. The role of humoral antibodies. J Exp Med 129(6):1307–1326
11. Serruto D et al (2010) Neisseria meningitidis GNA2132, a heparin-binding protein that induces protective immunity in humans. Proc Natl Acad Sci USA 107(8):3770–3775
12. Masignani V et al (2003) Vaccination against Neisseria meningitidis using three variants of the lipoprotein GNA1870. J Exp Med 197(6):789–799
13. Seib KL et al (2009) Factor H-binding protein is important for meningococcal survival in human whole blood and serum and in the presence of the antimicrobial peptide LL-37. Infect Immun 77(1):292–299
14. Capecchi B et al (2005) Neisseria meningitidis NadA is a new invasin which promotes bacterial adhesion to and penetration into human epithelial cells. Mol Microbiol 55 (3):687–698
15. Comanducci M et al (2002) NadA, a novel vaccine candidate of Neisseria meningitidis. J Exp Med 195(11):1445–1454
16. Giuliani MM et al (2006) A universal vaccine for serogroup B meningococcus. Proc Natl Acad Sci USA 103(29):10834–10839
17. Kimura A et al (2011) Immunogenicity and safety of a multicomponent meningococcal serogroup B vaccine and a quadrivalent meningococcal CRM197 conjugate vaccine against serogroups A, C, W-135, and Y in adults who are at increased risk for occupational exposure to meningococcal isolates. Clin Vaccine Immunol 18(3):483–486
18. Findlow J et al (2010) Multicenter, open-label, randomized phase II controlled trial of an investigational recombinant Meningococcal serogroup B vaccine with and without outer membrane vesicles, administered in infancy. Clin Infect Dis 51(10):1127–1137

19. Snape MD et al (2010) Immunogenicity and reactogenicity of a 13-valent-pneumococcal conjugate vaccine administered at 2, 4, and 12 months of age: a double-blind randomized active-controlled trial. Pediatr Infect Dis J 29(12):e80–e90
20. Johri AK et al (2006) Group B Streptococcus: global incidence and vaccine development. Nat Rev Microbiol 4(12):932–942
21. Tettelin H et al (2002) Complete genome sequence and comparative genomic analysis of an emerging human pathogen, serotype V Streptococcus agalactiae. Proc Natl Acad Sci USA 99 (19):12391–12396
22. Tettelin H et al (2005) Genome analysis of multiple pathogenic isolates of Streptococcus agalactiae: implications for the microbial "pan-genome". Proc Natl Acad Sci USA 102 (39):13950–13955
23. Maione D et al (2005) Identification of a universal Group B streptococcus vaccine by multiple genome screen. Science 309(5731):148–150
24. Lauer P et al (2005) Genome analysis reveals pili in Group B Streptococcus. Science 309 (5731):105
25. Rosini R et al (2006) Identification of novel genomic islands coding for antigenic pilus-like structures in Streptococcus agalactiae. Mol Microbiol 61(1):126–141
26. Margarit I et al (2009) Preventing bacterial infections with pilus-based vaccines: the group B streptococcus paradigm. J Infect Dis 199(1):108–115
27. Brzuszkiewicz E et al (2006) How to become a uropathogen: comparative genomic analysis of extraintestinal pathogenic Escherichia coli strains. Proc Natl Acad Sci USA 103 (34):12879–12884
28. Hain T et al (2007) Pathogenomics of Listeria spp. Int J Med Microbiol 297(7–8):541–557
29. Perrin A et al (2002) Comparative genomics identifies the genetic islands that distinguish Neisseria meningitidis, the agent of cerebrospinal meningitis, from other Neisseria species. Infect Immun 70(12):7063–7072
30. Perrin A, Nassif X, Tinsley C (1999) Identification of regions of the chromosome of Neisseria meningitidis and Neisseria gonorrhoeae which are specific to the pathogenic Neisseria species. Infect Immun 67(11):6119–6129
31. Moriel DG et al (2010) Identification of protective and broadly conserved vaccine antigens from the genome of extraintestinal pathogenic Escherichia coli. Proc Natl Acad Sci USA 107 (20):9072–9077
32. Madico G et al (2007) Factor H binding and function in sialylated pathogenic neisseriae is influenced by gonococcal, but not meningococcal, porin. J Immunol 178(7):4489–4497
33. Schneider MC et al (2007) Interactions between Neisseria meningitidis and the complement system. Trends Microbiol 15(5):233–240
34. Telford JL et al (2006) Pili in gram-positive pathogens. Nat Rev Microbiol 4(7):509–519
35. Barocchi MA et al (2006) A pneumococcal pilus influences virulence and host inflammatory responses. Proc Natl Acad Sci USA 103(8):2857–2862
36. Mora M et al (2005) Group A Streptococcus produce pilus-like structures containing protective antigens and Lancefield T antigens. Proc Natl Acad Sci USA 102(43):15641–15646
37. Adu-Bobie J et al (2003) Two years into reverse vaccinology. Vaccine 21(7–8):605–610
38. Bambini S et al (2009) Distribution and genetic variability of three vaccine components in a panel of strains representative of the diversity of serogroup B meningococcus. Vaccine 27 (21):2794–2803
39. Donnelly J et al (2010) Qualitative and quantitative assessment of meningococcal antigens to evaluate the potential strain coverage of protein-based vaccines. Proc Natl Acad Sci USA 107 (45):19490–19495
40. Telford JL (2008) Bacterial genome variability and its impact on vaccine design. Cell Host Microbe 3(6):408–416
41. Hall N (2007) Advanced sequencing technologies and their wider impact in microbiology. J Exp Biol 210(Pt 9):1518–1525

42. Schuster SC (2008) Next-generation sequencing transforms today's biology. Nat Methods 5 (1):16–18
43. Margulies M et al (2005) Genome sequencing in microfabricated high-density picolitre reactors. Nature 437(7057):376–380
44. Bennett ST et al (2005) Toward the 1,000 dollars human genome. Pharmacogenomics 6 (4):373–382
45. Shendure J et al (2005) Accurate multiplex polony sequencing of an evolved bacterial genome. Science 309(5741):1728–1732
46. Ansorge WJ (2009) Next-generation DNA sequencing techniques. N Biotechnol 25 (4):195–203
47. Metzker ML (2010) Sequencing technologies—the next generation. Nat Rev Genet 11 (1):31–46
48. Harris SR et al (2010) Evolution of MRSA during hospital transmission and intercontinental spread. Science 327(5964):469–474
49. Croucher NJ et al (2011) Rapid pneumococcal evolution in response to clinical interventions. Science 331(6016):430–434
50. Grifantini R et al (2002) Previously unrecognized vaccine candidates against group B meningococcus identified by DNA microarrays. Nat Biotechnol 20(9):914–921
51. Wizemann TM et al (2001) Use of a whole genome approach to identify vaccine molecules affording protection against Streptococcus pneumoniae infection. Infect Immun 69 (3):1593–1598
52. Hoskins J et al (2001) Genome of the bacterium Streptococcus pneumoniae strain R6. J Bacteriol 183(19):5709–5717
53. Etz H et al (2002) Identification of in vivo expressed vaccine candidate antigens from Staphylococcus aureus. Proc Natl Acad Sci USA 99(10):6573–6578
54. Vytvytska O et al (2002) Identification of vaccine candidate antigens of Staphylococcus aureus by serological proteome analysis. Proteomics 2(5):580–590
55. Ross BC et al (2001) Identification of vaccine candidate antigens from a genomic analysis of Porphyromonas gingivalis. Vaccine 19(30):4135–4142
56. Hughes MJ et al (2002) Identification of major outer surface proteins of Streptococcus agalactiae. Infect Immun 70(3):1254–1259
57. Reid SD et al (2002) Postgenomic analysis of four novel antigens of group a streptococcus: growth phase-dependent gene transcription and human serologic response. J Bacteriol 184 (22):6316–6324
58. Rodriguez-Ortega MJ et al (2006) Characterization and identification of vaccine candidate proteins through analysis of the group A Streptococcus surface proteome. Nat Biotechnol 24 (2):191–197
59. Montigiani S et al (2002) Genomic approach for analysis of surface proteins in Chlamydia pneumoniae. Infect Immun 70(1):368–379
60. Berlanda Scorza F et al (2008) Proteomics characterization of outer membrane vesicles from the extraintestinal pathogenic Escherichia coli DeltatolR IHE3034 mutant. Mol Cell Proteomics 7(3):473–485
61. Serruto D et al (2004) Biotechnology and vaccines: application of functional genomics to Neisseria meningitidis and other bacterial pathogens. J Biotechnol 113(1–3):15–32
62. Sorek R, Cossart P (2010) Prokaryotic transcriptomics: a new view on regulation, physiology and pathogenicity. Nat Rev Genet 11(1):9–16
63. Croucher NJ, Thomson NR (2010) Studying bacterial transcriptomes using RNA-seq. Curr Opin Microbiol 13(5):619–624
64. Yoder-Himes DR et al (2009) Mapping the Burkholderia cenocepacia niche response via high-throughput sequencing. Proc Natl Acad Sci USA 106(10):3976–3981
65. Perkins TT et al (2009) A strand-specific RNA-Seq analysis of the transcriptome of the typhoid bacillus Salmonella typhi. PLoS Genet 5(7):e1000569

66. Mraheil MA et al (2011) The intracellular sRNA transcriptome of Listeria monocytogenes during growth in macrophages. Nucleic Acids Res 39(10):4235–4248
67. Passalacqua KD et al (2009) Structure and complexity of a bacterial transcriptome. J Bacteriol 191(10):3203–3211
68. Camarena L et al (2010) Molecular mechanisms of ethanol-induced pathogenesis revealed by RNA-sequencing. PLoS Pathog 6(4):e1000834
69. Albrecht M et al (2010) Deep sequencing-based discovery of the Chlamydia trachomatis transcriptome. Nucleic Acids Res 38(3):868–877
70. Sharma CM et al (2010) The primary transcriptome of the major human pathogen Helicobacter pylori. Nature 464(7286):250–255
71. Mahan MJ, Slauch JM, Mekalanos JJ (1993) Selection of bacterial virulence genes that are specifically induced in host tissues. Science 259(5095):686–688
72. Hensel M et al (1995) Simultaneous identification of bacterial virulence genes by negative selection. Science 269(5222):400–403
73. Sun YH et al (2000) Functional genomics of Neisseria meningitidis pathogenesis. Nat Med 6 (11):1269–1273
74. van Opijnen T, Bodi KL, Camilli A (2009) Tn-seq: high-throughput parallel sequencing for fitness and genetic interaction studies in microorganisms. Nat Methods 6(10):767–772
75. van Opijnen, T. and A. Camilli, Genome-wide fitness and genetic interactions determined by Tn-seq, a high-throughput massively parallel sequencing method for microorganisms. Curr Protoc Microbiol, 2010. Chapter 1: p. Unit1E 3.
76. Langridge GC et al (2009) Simultaneous assay of every Salmonella Typhi gene using one million transposon mutants. Genome Res 19(12):2308–2316
77. Gawronski JD et al (2009) Tracking insertion mutants within libraries by deep sequencing and a genome-wide screen for Haemophilus genes required in the lung. Proc Natl Acad Sci USA 106(38):16422–16427
78. Rappuoli R (2004) From Pasteur to genomics: progress and challenges in infectious diseases. Nat Med 10(11): 1177–85
79. Granoff DM et al. (2009) Binding of complement factor H (fH) to Neisseria meningitidis is specific for human fH and inhibits complement activation by rat and rabbit sera. Infect Immun 77(2): 764–9
80. Metruccio MM et al (2009) A novel phase variation mechanism in the meningococcus driven by a ligand-responsive repressor and differential spacing of distal promoter elements. PLoS Pathog 5(12): e1000710

Chapter 3
Identification of Candidate Vaccine Antigens In Silico

Darren R. Flower, Matthew N. Davies, and Irini A. Doytchinova

Abstract The identification of immunogenic whole-protein antigens is fundamental to the successful discovery of candidate subunit vaccines and their rapid, effective, and efficient transformation into clinically useful, commercially successful vaccine formulations. In the wider context of the experimental discovery of vaccine antigens, with particular reference to reverse vaccinology, this chapter adumbrates the principal computational approaches currently deployed in the hunt for novel antigens: genome-level prediction of antigens, antigen identification through the use of protein sequence alignment-based approaches, antigen detection through the use of subcellular location prediction, and the use of alignment-independent approaches to antigen discovery. Reference is also made to the recent emergence of various expert systems for protein antigen identification.

3.1 Introduction

The overwhelming case for vaccines and vaccination was long ago proven, yet vaccines remain stubbornly underused. Controversy continues to surround vaccines: it took over 10 years for a contentious connection between autism and the MMR vaccine 1998 to be finally and ambiguously discredited [1]. Yet, for all the prevalence of misinformation and muddled thinking, mass vaccination represents—by far and away—the most efficient, efficacious, and effective form of prophylactic medical intervention currently available to combat disease.

During most of the last century, in the developed world, over 600,000 people died on average annually from a combination of smallpox, diphtheria, polio, measles, and rubella; today this figure has fallen below 100. Smallpox in particular was always a dreaded killer. Indeed, even during the 1960s, at least 10 million cases

D.R. Flower (✉)
School of Life and Health Sciences, University of Aston, Aston Triangle, Birmingham, UK
e-mail: d.r.flower@aston.ac.uk

D.R. Flower and Y. Perrie (eds.), *Immunomic Discovery of Adjuvants and Candidate Subunit Vaccines*, Immunomics Reviews: 5, DOI 10.1007/978-1-4614-5070-2_3,

of smallpox were reported annually from across the globe, leading to about 2 million deaths a year. Yet, today, the disease has been completely eradicated. In the last 30 years, there have been no known cases. Poliomyelitis or polio is the other large-scale disease which has come closest to eradication. Its success too has been formidable: in 1991, the Pan American Health Organization effectively eradicated polio from the Western Hemisphere, since when the Global Polio Eradication Programme has significantly decreased the overall incidence of Poliomyelitis through the rest of the world. In 1988, there were approximately 350,000 cases spread through 125 countries; in the past years, global figures amounted to less than 2,000 annually.

Yet, in spite of such remarkable success, death from vaccine-preventable diseases remains unacceptably high [2]. There are over 70 common infectious diseases responsible for one in four deaths globally. Rotavirus and Pneumococcus are pathogens causing diarrhoea and pneumonia, the leading causes of infant deaths in underdeveloped countries. In the next decade, effective, widespread vaccination programs against such pathogenic microbes could save the lives of 7.6 million children under 5 years of age. Hepatitis B causes 600,000 deaths in adults and children aged over 5. Seasonal, non-pandemic influenza kills upwards of half a million globally each year. For those aged under 5 in particular, a series of diseases causes an extraordinary and largely preventable death toll. For example, tetanus accounts every year for 198,000 deaths, pertussis is responsible for over 290,000 deaths, Hib gives rise to in excess of 386,000 deaths, diphtheria accounts for 4,000 deaths, and yellow fever over 15,000 deaths. Arguably, the most regrettable, the most lamentable situation is that of measles. Measles accounts for the unneeded deaths of 540,000 under-fives and over 70,000 adults and older children.

Despite this, the situation is by no means bleak. By the close of 2008, approximately 42 million had been vaccinated against Hib and 192 million children against hepatitis B. During its first decade, vaccinations against polio, Hep B, Hib, measles, pertussis, and yellow fever funded by GAVI had prevented the unnecessary loss of over 5 million lives. There are approximately 50 vaccines licensed for use in humans, around half of these are widely prescribed. Yet, most of these vaccines target the prevention of common childhood infections, with the remainder addressing tropical diseases encountered by travellers to the tropics; only a relatively minor proportion combat endemic disease in under-developed countries. Balancing the persisting need against the proven success and anticipated potential, vaccines remain an area of remarkable opportunity for medical advance, leading directly to unprecedented levels of saved and improved lives.

From a commercial perspective, the vaccine arena has long been neglected, in part because of the quite astonishing success limned above; today, and in comparative terms at least, activity within vaccine discovery is feverish [3, 4]. During the last 15 years, tens of vaccines and vaccine candidates have moved successfully through clinical trials, and vaccines in late development number in the hundreds. In stark contrast to antibiotics, vaccine resistance is negligible and nugatory.

Despite the egregious and outrageous success enjoyed by vaccines, many major issues persist. The World Health Organisation long ago identified tuberculosis

(TB), HIV, and malaria as the three most significant life-threatening infectious diseases globally. No vaccine has been licensed for malaria or HIV, and there seems little realistic hope for such vaccines appearing in the immediate future. Bacille Calmette Guérin (BCG), the key anti-TB vaccine, is of limited efficacy [5]. Levels of morbidity and mortality generated by diseases already targeted by vaccines remain high. Influenza is the key example, with a global annual estimated death toll in the region of half a million.

In the twenty-first century, the world continues to be threatened by infectious and contagious diseases of many kinds: visceral leishmaniasis, Marburg's disease, West Nile, dengue, as well as SARS potentially pandemic H5N1 influenza, and over 190 human and emerging zoonotic infections, as well as the persisting threat from HIV, TB, and malaria mentioned above. All this is further compounded by the additional risk arising from antibiotic-resistant bacteria and bioterrorism, not to mention major quasi-incidental issues, such climate change, an accelerating growth in the world's population, increased travel, and the overcrowding seen within the burgeoning populations concentrated into major cities [6].

For reasons we shall touch on below, the discovery of vaccines is both more urgent and more difficult than it has ever been. In an era where conventional drug discovery has been seen to fail—or at least as seen by cupiditous investors, for whom the current model of pharmaceutical drug discovery is broken—vaccines are one of a number of biologically derived therapies upon which the future economic health of the pharmaceutical industry is thought to rest. The medical need, as stated above, is clear. Set against this is the unfortunate realisation that vaccines exist for most easily targeted diseases, those mediated by neutralising antibodies, and so outstanding vaccine-targets are those of more intractable diseases mediated primarily by cellular immunity. To address those properly requires what all discoveries required: hard work and investment; but they also need new ideas, new thinking, and new vaccine discovery technology. Amongst, these are computational techniques, the most promising of which are those targeting the discovery of novel vaccine antigens: the candidate subunit vaccines of tomorrow see Fig. 3.1.

3.2 Vaccines

Vaccines are agents—either molecular (epitope- or antigen-based vaccines) or supramolecular (attenuated or inactivated whole pathogen vaccines)—which are able to create protective immunity against specific pathogenic infectious microorganisms and any diseases to which they might give rise. Protective immunity can be characterised as an enhanced but highly specific response to consequent re-infection—or infection by an evolutionarily closely related micro-organisms—made by the adaptive immune system. Such increased or enhanced immunity is facilitated by the quantitative and qualitative augmentation of immune memory, which is able to militate against the pernicious effects of infectious disease. Vaccines synergise with the herd immunity they help engender, leading to reduced transmission rates as well as prophylaxis against infection.

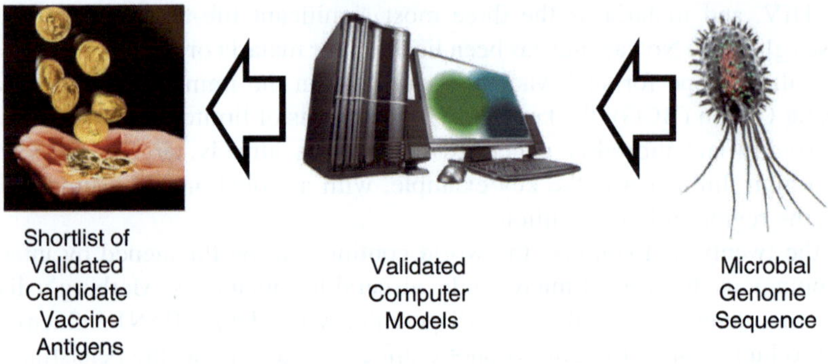

Fig. 3.1 Whole antigen discovery. When looking at a reverse vaccinology process, the discovery of candidate subunit vaccines begins with a microbial genome, perhaps newly sequence, progresses through an extensive computational stage, ultimately to deliver a shortlist of antigens which can be validated through subsequent laboratory examination. The computational stage can be empirical in nature; this is typified by the statistical approach embodied in vaxijen [115]. Or this stage can be bioinformatic; this involves predicting subcellular location and expression levels and the like. Or, this stage can take the form of a complex mathematical model which uses immunoinformatic models combined with mathematical methods, such as metabolic control theory [153], to predict cell-surface epitope populations

The term “vaccine” derives from vacca (Latin for cow). The words vaccine and vaccination were coined specifically for anti-smallpox immunization by the discoverer of the technique, Edward Jenner (1749–1823). These terms were later extended by Louis Pasteur (1822–1895) to include a far more extensive orbit or remit, including the entire notion of immunisation against any disease [2, 3, 6].

Several fundamentally distinct varieties of vaccine exist. These include *inter alia* inactivated or attenuated whole pathogen-based vaccines; subunit vaccines are based on one or more protein antigens, vaccines based upon one or more individual epitopes, carbohydrate-based vaccines, and combinations thereof. Hitherto, the best-used and, thus, the most successful types of vaccine were built from attenuated—“weakened” or non-infective or otherwise inactivated—pathogenic whole organisms, be they bacterial or viral in nature. Well-known examples include the following: the BCG vaccine which acts prophylactically against tuberculosis and Albert Sabin’s anti-poliomyelitis vaccine based on attenuated poliovirus. The vast majority of subunit vaccines are immunogenic protein molecules, and are typically discovered using a somewhat haphazard search process.

Concerns over the safety of whole-organism vaccines long ago prompted the development of other kinds of vaccine strategy, including those based upon antigens as the innate or immanent active biological constituent of either single or composite vaccines. The vaccine which targets Hepatitis B is a good exemplar of a so-called subunit vaccine as it is based on a protein antigen: the viral envelope hepatitis B surface antigen. Other types of as-yet-unproven vaccines include those based on epitopes and others based on antigen-presenting cells; many have entered clinical trials, but none have fulfilled their medical or commercial potential.

It is often difficult to capture the proper scientific meaning and use of recondite terms, often borrowed from common usage or archaic language. So, let us be more specific. An immunogen—a molecular moiety exhibiting the property of immunogenicity—is any material or substance capable of eliciting a specific immune response. An antigen, on the other hand, is a molecular moiety exhibiting the property of antigenicity. It is a substance or material recognised by a primed immune system. Such a persisting state of immune readiness may be mediated by humoral immunity (principally via the action of soluble antibodies) or by cellular immunity (as mediated by T-cells, antigen presenting cells (APCs), or other phagocytic cells), or a combination of both, in what is often referred to as a "recall" response.

Immunogenicity is vital: it is the signature characteristic or property that prompts a certain molecular moiety to evoke a significant immune response. Here, we shall strictly limit use of "immunogen" and "antigen" to a sole meaning. Here, an "antigen" or an "immunogen" will mean a protein that is capable of educing some kind of discernible response from the host immune system. Specifically, and for practical reasons, we will almost exclusively be referring to proteins derived from a pathogenic micro-organism.

At present, the prophylaxis engendered by all current effective vaccines—all except BCG—is primarily mediated by the humoral immune system, via soluble antibodies. However, the disease mechanisms of most serious diseases for which vaccines are not available are usually mediated by cellular immunity. Thus, for untreated disease, we seek to identify immunogenicity generated principally by cellular responses or by a combination of cellular and humoral responses, rather than by humoral immunity alone.

To some extent, subunit vaccines can be thought to represent something of a compromise between vaccines based on attenuated or otherwise inactivated whole-organisms and the many more recent and more innovative vaccine strategies typified by epitope or poly-epitope vaccines. Vaccines based around whole pathogens have long engendered safety concerns [7–9]. From the Lubeck disaster and the cutter incident [10–12] to the recent MMR debacle, issues over safety, real or imagined, have always dogged the development of vaccines [1, 9]. Indeed, during the eighteenth century the pre-vaccination practice of variolation against Smallpox prefigured much of the current debate over the perceived danger of vaccines [13].

While the case for vaccines is unanswerable, we should not be complacent. Any live vaccine, however extensively attenuated, can revert to a pathogenic, disease-inducing form. This is currently an on-going issue for polio vaccination [14]. Other issues, particularly the chemical or biological contamination of vaccines during manufacture, remain enduring and persistent problems. Undesired immunogenicity, the type leading to severe and pathological immune responses, rather than enduring immune memory, is a concern for both whole-organism and subunit-based vaccines, as well as putative biologics [15]. Immunologists and vaccinologists have thus long sought alternatives to the use of whole organisms as vaccines. Subunit vaccines and conjugate vaccines are one such. Vaccines based on epitopes, singly or in combination, are another. The diversity of innovations in vaccine design holds much potential for success, but, thus far at least, has proved spectacularly unsuccessful in a clinical context.

Logically, a vaccine that relies solely on, at most, a few well-chosen epitopes, should be effective, efficacious, and, above-all, safe. Epitopes, as peptides, may be cytotoxic and might possibly prompt some kind of inopportune immune response but cannot be infective or revert to infectivity. In many ways, epitopes are closer in size and share many properties with synthetic small molecules; possibly dealing with their pharmacokinetics as such may be better than thinking of them as biologic drugs. In practice, of course, epitope-based vaccines, like subunit vaccines, suffer from poor immunogenicity, necessitating the use of a complex combination of adjuvants and complicated delivery systems.

For diverse reasons, including immunogenicity, stimulating protective immune responses against intracellular pathogens remains problematic when using non-replicating vaccines. Why should this be? First, the immune response is very complex, involving both the innate and adaptive immunity, and significant interaction between them. In all probability, and particularly when viewed in the context of the whole population, many epitopes and danger signals are involved; likewise, the many different immune actors, be they acting at the cellular or molecular levels, interact with each other and are subject to complex mechanisms of genetic, epigenetic, and system-level control and regulation. It may be that only the large and complex organism-sized vaccines can induce the range of immune responses necessary across the population to induce protection, since they comprise a potential host of immunogenic molecular moieties, not just a single immunodominant epitope See Fig. 3.2.

In that which follows, we shall seek to explore the availability and accessibility of informatic techniques and informatic tools used to identify candidate subunit vaccines of microbial origin. Yet, we shall start by adding context with an examination of experimental approaches to antigen discovery: so-called reverse vaccinology. Reverse vaccinology already relies on informatics, but, in a sense at least, what we would like to do using informatics is to reproduce as much as is possible the steps inherent in successful reverse vaccinology in silico rather than in vitro.

3.3 Reverse Vaccinology and the Experimental Identification of Antigens

Reverse vaccinology, and the necessary computational support, is a much more prevalent means of identifying subunit vaccines [16]. See Fig. 3.1. Even today, many experimentalists retain a deep and atavistic distrust of all computation. Experimentalists seldom trust the reliability and dependability of computational methodology, choosing to trust instead in what they believe to be infallible, if actually rather elusive, empirical reliability of observations, experiments, and the whole paraphernalia of laboratory experimentation. Yet, things are in the process of

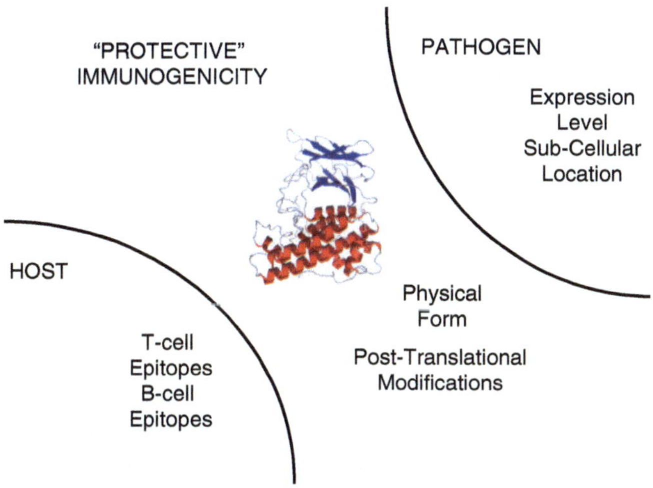

Fig. 3.2 Factors underlying immunogenicity. As elaborated in the text, the phenomenon of immunogenicity can be explored through the diversity of underlying factors contributing to the instigation of the immune response. The can be assigned to the host (epitope recognition), the pathogen (location and expression level), and also factors intrinsic to the protein antigen itself, such as the possession of post-translational danger signals

changing, and this change is likely to accelerate as we move forward into a future that looks more parsimonious and uncertain by the day.

Vaccines have come a long way from the days when they were prepared directly from the fluids of smallpox pustules or extracts of infected spinal cords. Yet vaccine discovery and development remains firmly empirical. Many modern vaccines still comprise entire inactivated pathogens. While vaccines targeting papillomavirus, tetanus, hepatitis B, and diphtheria are subunit vaccines, few are recombinant proteins devoid of contaminants. Some would argue that the only molecular vaccines are glycoconjugates: oligosaccharides conjugated to immunogenic carrier proteins.

Conventional empirical, experimental, laboratory-based microbiological ways to identify putative candidate antigens require cultivation of target pathogenic micro-organisms, followed by teasing out their component proteins, analysis in a series of in-vitro and in-vivo assays, animal models and with the ultimate objective of isolating one or two proteins displaying protective immunity.

Unfortunately, in reality, the process is more complex, and more confusing, and much more confounding as this brief synopsis might suggest. Cultivating pathogens outside the environment offered by their host organism can be difficult, even impossible. Not every protein is readily expressed in adequate quantities in vitro, and many proteins are only expressed in an intermittent basis during the time course of infection. Thus, a considerable number of potential, putative, and possible vaccine candidate antigens could be missed by conventional experimental approaches.

Reverse vaccinology [16–19] has the potential to analyse genomes for potential antigens, initially scanning "open reading frames" (ORFs), then selecting proteins because they are open to surveillance by the host immune system. This usually involves some complex combination of informatic-based prediction methodologies. Recombinant expression of the resulting set of identified molecules can overcome their reduced natural abundance, which has often prevented us recognising their true potential. By enlarging the repertoire of native antigens, this technology can help to foster the development of a new cohort of vaccines.

Reverse vaccinology was originally established and has been established by studying *Neisseria meningitidis*, which is responsible for meningococcal meningitis and sepsis. Vaccines are currently available for all serotypes, except that serogroup B. *N. meningitidis* ORFs were found initially [20, 21]; 570 proteins were then identified, 350 expressed in vitro and 85 found to be surface exposed. Seven proteins elicited immunity over many strains. The culmination of this work was a "universal" vaccine for serogroup B based on five antigens [22]. This proto-vaccine, when used with Alum as adjuvant, induced murine bactericidal antibodies versus 78 % of 85 meningococcal strains drawn from the world population of *N. meningitidis*. Strain coverage increases to over 90 % when used with CpG or MF59 as adjuvant.

Another key illustration is *Porphyromonas gingivalis*, an anaerobic gram-negative bacterium found in the chronic adult inflammatory gum disease periodontitis. Initially, 370 ORFS were identified [23]; of these, 120 protein sequences were open to immune surveillance and 40 were positive for several sera. Two antigens were found to be protective in mice.

Yet another fascinating instance is provided by *Streptococcus pneumoniae*, a prime cause of meningitis, pneumonia, and sepsis [24, 25]. In this study, 130 potential ORFs were initially identified, with 108 of these proteins being readily expressed. Finally, six proteins were seen to induce protection against the pathogen.

More recently, other and more advanced experimental techniques, such as microarrays, are beginning to come on-stream, opening up a gallimaufry of possible technologies to the new but maturing field of reverse vaccinology. The following gives but a taste of what is to come.

Using ribosome display to undertake in-vitro protein selection, Weichart et al. [26] identified within the methicillin-resistant COL strain of the virulent human pathogen *Staphylococcus aureus* 75 genes, the majority of which were secreted or surface-localized proteins; of these, 25 % had cell envelope function, 24 % were transporter proteins, and 9 % were virulence factors or toxins.

Using an ingenious combination of advanced proteomics techniques and in-vitro assays, Giefing et al. [27] identified 18 novel vaccine candidates which prevented infections in children and in the elderly caused by a variety of pneumococcus serotypes; four demonstrating major protection versus sepsis in animals. Two leads—StkP (a serine/threonine protein kinase) and PcsB (a structural protein with a role in cell wall separation of group B *Streptococcus*)—showed clear cross-protection as potential candidate vaccines against four separate pneumococcal serotypes.

Using a whole proteome microarray, and in order to identify protein antigens, Eyles et al. [28] probed serum from BALB/c mice previously immunized with a vaccine comprising: killed *Francisella tularensis* and two immunomodulatory adjuvants. Eleven out of the top twelve immunogenic antigens were known already as immunoreactive, although 31 further proteins were discovered using this experimental approach. In further work from this consortium, Titball and co-workers [29] constructed a protein microarray of 1,205 *Burkholderia pseudomallei* proteins, treated it with 88 patient samples, identifying 170 antigens. This smaller set was treated with a further 747 distinct sera from 10 groups of patients, identifying 49 putative candidate antigens.

This survey, brief though it is, helps to highlight the potential power of reverse vaccinology for vaccine discovery. However, since the number of antigens is high, given all the potential difficulties in characterising and expressing them, it is important to note that both computational and experimental techniques and methodologies will doubtlessly omit important and interesting proteins from further analysis, though not necessarily for the same or similar reasons. Thus, with the burgeoning discipline of reverse vaccinology, both computational and experimental techniques are in need of constant development and improvement.

3.4 Immunoinformatics

Compared to its role to drug discovery, genomics, and a host of other bioscience sub-disciplines, bioinformatics support for the preclinical discovery and development of vaccine is in its infancy; yet, as interest in vaccine discovery increases, the situation changes. There are two key types of bioinformatics support for vaccine design, discovery, and development. At the technical level, the first of these cannot be properly or meaningfully distinguished from general support for target discovery. It includes the annotation of pathogen genomes, more conventional host genome annotation, and the statistical analysis of immunological microarray experiments. The second form of support concentrates on immunoinformatics, that is, the informatics analysis of immunological problems, principally epitope prediction.

B-cell epitope prediction remains defiantly basic or is largely dependent on a sometimes unavailable knowledge of three-dimensional protein structure. Both structure- [30] and data-driven [31] prediction of antibody-mediated epitopes evince poor results. However, methods developed to predict T-cell epitopes now possess considerable algorithmic sophistication. Moreover, they continue to develop and evolve, as well as extend their scope and remit to address new and ever larger and more challenging epitope prediction problems. Presently, accurate and reliable T-cell epitope prediction is restricted to predicting the binding of peptides to the major histocompatibility complex (MHC). Class I peptide-MHC prediction can be reasonably accurate, or is for properly characterised, well-understood alleles [32]. Yet a number of key studies have demonstrated that class

II MHC binding prediction is almost universally inaccurate, and is thus erratic and unreliable [33–35]. A similar situation persists for structure-driven prediction of MHC epitopes [36, 37].

Irrespective of poor predictive performance, several other problems exist for epitope prediction. For T cell prediction in particular, a prime concern is with the availability or rather lack of availability of relevant data. It is now known that immunogenic T cell epitopes, thought previously to be peptides no more than 10 amino acids in length, can be 16 or more residues long. Longmer epitopes now greatly expand the number of possible peptides open to inspection by T cells [38–41]. The inadequate results generated by B cell epitope prediction algorithms may indicate that a fundamental reinterpretation of extant B cell epitope data is necessary before improved methods become feasible.

These factors, when taken together, are consistent with the notion that methods relying only on the possession of certain epitopes will not be fully effective when tasked with antigen or immunogen identification. This is supported by information indicating a lack of correspondence between selected antigens and experimentally verified protective proteins.

3.5 Genomic-Level Identification of Antigens

There are many means of identifying antigenic proteins. Most focus on the properties of protein sequence and structure, but arguably one of the most insightful is instead to examine properties, both local and global, of the underlying nucleic acid. One notable way is to look for evidence of the horizontal or lateral transfer of so-called pathogenicity islands or PAIs. Horizontal transfer, such as transformation, conjugation, or transduction, is distinct from the vertical transfer of genetic material from an ancestor within its lineage. It typically involves an organism incorporating genetic material from an evolutionarily distant organism without being its offspring.

PAIs are a specific type of genomic island; that is, part of a genome acquired through direct transfer between microbes. A genomic island can occur in distantly related species and may be mono- or multi-functional; there are many sub-classes classified by function. Other examples include antibiotic resistance islands, metal resistance, and secretion system islands. The gene products of PAIs are crucial to the propagation of disease pathogenesis, much as the PAIs themselves are key to the evolution of pathogenesis. Pathogen-associated type III and type IV secretion systems are, for example, often found together in the same PAI.

Detecting such large (>10 Kb) and discrete clusters of genes clusters, habitually possessing a characteristically atypical G/C content, at least when compared with the remainder of the genome, leads, in turn, to the individual identification within clusters of virulence-associated protein antigens. Prokaryotic PAIs are frequently associated with tRNA-encoding genes, many are flanked by repeat structures, and many contain fragments of mobile genetic elements such as plasmids and phages.

PAIs can be identified by combining analysis of nucleotide composition and phylogeny, amongst others. Composition-based approaches rely on the natural variation between genome sequences from different species. Regions of the genome with abnormal composition, as demonstrated by nucleotide or codon bias, may be potentially transferred horizontally. Such methods are prone to inaccuracies; these result from inherent genomic sequence variation, such as is seen in highly expressed genes, and the observation that over time the sequences of genomic islands alter to mirror the composition of host genomes.

Evolution-based approaches seek regions that may have been transferred horizontally by comparing related species. Put at its simplest: a putative genomic island present in one species, but absent from several related species, is consistent with horizontal transfer. Of course, the island may have been present in the last common ancestor shared by the species compared and subsequently been lost from the other species. A less likely explanation would be that the island arose by mutation and selection in this species and no other. To decide, a body of extra evidence would need to be explored, such as the size of the PAI, the mechanistic ease of deletion, the consistent presence of the island in more distantly related species, the relative pathogenicity of island-less species, and the divergence of the genome relative to that of other related species.

Many methods, which seek to quantify and leverage these somewhat vague notions, are now available [42–44]. Such analysis at the nucleic acid level shares many features in common with approaches used to identify CpG islands in eukaryotic genomes [45–48]. Recently, Langille et al. tested six sequence-composition genomic island prediction methods and found that IslandPath-DIMOB and SIGI-HMM had the greatest overall accuracy [49].

Island Path was designed to help identify prokaryotic PAIs, through the visualisation of common PAI characteristics such as mobile element-associated genes or atypical sequence composition [50]. SIGI-HMM is a very accurate sequence composition-based genomic island predictor, which combines a Hidden Markov Model (HMM) and codon usage measurement to identify genomic islands [51].

In another work, Yoon et al. coupled heuristic sequence searching methods, which aimed simultaneously to identify PAIs and individual virulence genes, with composition and codon-usage bias [52]. Exploiting a machine learning approach, Vernikos and Parkhill sampled the structural features of genomic islands using a hypothesis-free, bottom-up search, with the objective of explicitly quantifying the contribution made by each feature to the overall structure of different genomic islands [53]. Arvey et al. sought to identify large chromosomal regions with atypical features using a general divergence measureable to quantify the compositional difference between genomic segments [54]. IslandPick is a comparative genomic island predictor, rather than a composition-based approach, that can identify very probable genomic islands and very probable non-genomic islands within investigated genomes but does require that several phylogentically related genomes are available [49]. Observing PAIs as having a G + C composition closer to their host genome, Wang et al. used so-called genomic barcodes to identify PAIs.

These barcodes are based on the fact that the frequencies of 2-mers to 7-mers, and their reverse complement, are very stable across a whole genome when using a window size of over 1,000 bps and that this constituted a characteristic signature for genomes [55].

The ready detection of PAIs, as a tool in computational reverse vaccinology, has been greatly aided by the deployment of several web-based resources. A key example of a server that successfully integrates several accurate genomic island predictors is IslandViewer [56], which combines the methods: IslandPick [49], IslandPath [50], and SIGI-HMM [51] and is available at the URL: http://www.pathogenomics.sfu.ca/islandviewer/query.php. The GUI facilitates the visualisation of genomic islands and downloading of data at the gene and chromosome levels in a variety of formats.

Another important, web-accessible resource is PAIDB or the PAI database. This is a wide-ranging database of PAIs, containing 112 distinct PAIs and 889 GenBank accessions present in 497 strains of pathogenic bacteria [57]. PAIDB may be accessed via the URL: http://www.gem.re.kr/paidb.

Thus, alternative techniques and methodologies are required in order to select and to rank proteins likely to be protective antigens and thus candidate vaccines. Below, we shall explore three key approaches: subcellular location prediction, alignment-dependent sequence similarity searching, and alignment-independent empirical statistical approaches.

3.6 Identifying Antigens Using Sequence Similarity

In this section, we consider, perhaps, the clearest and cleanest way to identify potential new antigens in any microbial genome to alignment-dependent sequence similarity searching. There are two complimentary but distinct ways of identifying the immunogenicity of a protein from its sequence. One is to look for significant similarity to proteins of known immunogenicity. This idea seems so straightforward as to be almost facile. The other approach is somewhat less obvious conceptually but almost as straightforward logistically and involves seeking to identify antigens as proteins without discernible sequence similarity to any host protein. Let us turn to the first of these two alternatives.

Let us begin by stating or rather reiterating the obvious. If we know the sequence of an existing antigen or antigens, we can use sequence searching to find similar sequences in the target genome [58, 59]. Any candidate antigens selected by this process can then be selected for further verification and validation. The same old, familiar caveats apply here: are chosen thresholds appropriate? Are high-scoring matches an artefact or are they real and meaningful? The litany of such conditions is all too familiar to anyone well versed in sequence similarity searching. Clearly, when a sequence search is run, using BLAST or FASTA3, for example, an enormously long list of nearly identical proteins might ensue, or one that does not get any hits at all, or almost any intervening result might be obtained. As reflective practitioners, we must judge which result can be classified as useful and which cannot, and in so doing, identify sets of suitable thresholds, above which we expect usefulness and below which we might anticipate little or no utility. Thresholds are contingent upon the sequence family studied, as well as being dependent solely on the problem investigated. Thus heuristically identified cut-offs are desirable, but much thinking and empirical investigation are required to select appropriate values.

Of course, the process adumbrated above presupposes that sufficient antigenic protein sequences are known. Compilation of this data is the role of the database. Recently, extensive literature mining, coupled with factory-scale experimentation, has created many functional immunology databases, although databases, such as SYFPEITHI [60, 61], focussing on cellular immunology—primarily MHC processing, presentation, and T cell recognition—have existed for 15–20 years. Arguably, the best extant database is the HIV molecular immunology database [62], although clearly the depth of the database is at the expense of generality and breadth. Other recent databases include MHCBN [63, 64] and EPIMHC [65], amongst many others. Two databases, warrant particular attention: AntiJen [66], formerly known as Jenpep [67, 68]; and IEDB [69].

Implemented as a relational postgreSQL database, AntiJen integrates a wide-ranging set of data items, much of which is not stored by other databases. In addition to the kind of cellular immunological information familiar from SYFPEITHI, such as MHC binding and T cell data, AntiJen additionally archives B cell epitopes and also includes a significant stockpile of quantitative data: kinetic, thermodynamic, as well as functional, including measurements of immunological peptide–protein and protein–protein interactions. The IEDB database is considerably more extensive than other equivalent database systems, benefiting from the input of 13 dedicated epitope sequencing projects. IEDB has come to eclipse other work in this area. Although both AntiJen and IEDB are full of epitope-focussed information of many flavours, they remain incomplete concerning immunogenic antigens. Fortuitously, specific antigen-orientated—rather than epitope-focussed—databases are starting to be available.

Arguably, the most obvious and most unambiguous example of an antigen is virulence factor (VF): proteins, such as toxins, able to induce disease directly by attacking a host. Analysis of known pathogens has allowed recurring VF systems of 40+ distinct proteins. Often, sets of VFs exist as discrete, distinct genome-encoded PAIs, as well as being more widely spread through the genome.

Clearly, antigens do not need to be VFs in order to be immunogenic and thus candidates for subunit vaccines. Instead, they need only be accessible to the immune system. They do not need to directly or indirectly mediate infection. Thus, other databases are needed which capture, collate, and archive the burgeoning plethora of antigen-orientated data. Recently, we have helped developed a very different database: AntigenDB [70]. It contains over 500 antigens collated from the primary scientific literature, as well as other sources. Another related database system has been christened VIOLIN (vaccine investigation and online information network) [71], which allows straightforward curation and the analysis and comparison of research data across diverse pathogens in the context of human medicine, animal models, laboratory model systems, and natural hosts.

As we outline above, in addition to identifying sequence similarity to known antigens, another idea gaining ground is that the immunogenicity of an antigen is solely determined by the absence of similarity to host proteins. Some think this is the prime determinant of potential protein immunogenicity [72, 73]. Such ideas are supported by the belief that immune systems are actively educated to lack reactivity to self-proteins [74], a process—often termed "immune tolerance"—which is generated via epitope-specific mechanisms [75, 76].

What we really want is a meaningful measure of the "foreignness" of a protein correlating with its immunogenicity. Usually, "evolutionary distance" substitutes for "foreignness." Clearly, such an evolutionary distance must be specified in terms of biomacromolecular structures or sequences. But, is this practically useful for selecting candidate vaccines?

Another way to formulate this idea is to say that the probability that a protein is immunogenic is exclusively a product of its dissimilarity, at the whole-sequence or sequence-fragment level, to each and every protein contained within the host proteome. Most search software is well matched to this problem. In terms of fragment length, the typical length of an epitope might seem logical, since the epitope is the molecular moiety typically recognised during the initial phase of an immune response. Yet, even at the epitope level—say a peptide of 8–16 amino acid residues—even a single conservative mutation or mismatch in an otherwise identical match might prove significant. Single sequence alterations may totally abrogate or significantly enhance neutralising antibodies binding or recognition by the machinery of cellular immunology.

We have attempted to benchmark sequence similarity and correlate it with immunogenicity in order to explore the potential of this idea in a quantitative fashion. To that end, we examined the differences between sets of antigens and non-antigen using sequence similarity scores. We looked specifically at sets of 100 known non-antigenic and 100 antigenic protein sequences from six sources: bacteria, viruses, fungi, and parasites, as well as allergens and tumours [77–79], comparing pathogen sequence to those from humans and mice using BLAST [80].

Most non-antigenic and antigenic sequences were non-redundant; implying a lack of homologues between pathogens and host proteomes, although certain parasite antigens, such as catalases and heat shock proteins, had a much greater level of similarity. We were not able to determine a suitable and appropriate threshold based on the hypothesis of non-redundancy to the host's proteome, suggesting that this is not a viable solution to vaccine antigen identification.

However, rather than looking at nucleic acid sequences, or at protein sequences using an alignment-based approach, a new set of techniques, based upon alignment-free techniques, has been and is being developed; as this approach begins to show significant potential, we shall examine it next.

3.7 Identifying Antigens through Subcellular Location Prediction

Proteins accessible to immune system surveillance are assumed to lie external to the microbial organism or be attached to its surface rather than being sequestered and sequestrated within the cell. For bacteria, this means being located on—or in—the outer membrane surface or being secreted. Thus, being able to accurately predict the physical location of a putative antigen can provide considerable insight into the likelihood that a particular protein will prove to be an immunogenic and possibly protective.

There are two basic kinds of prediction method for identifying subcellular location: manual rule construction and the application of data-driven machine learning methods. Data used to discriminate between compartments include sequence-derived features of the protein, such as hydrophobic regions; the amino acid composition of the whole protein; the presence of certain specific motifs; or a combination thereof. Accuracy differs significantly between different methods and different compartments, mostly resulting from the deficiency and inconsistency of data used to derive models. Gross overall sequence similarity is unable to predict protein sub-cellular location reliably or accurately. Even nearly identical protein sequences may be found in distinct locations, while there are many proteins which exist simultaneously at several distinct locations within the cell, often having equally distinct functions at these different sites [81].

Eukaryotes and prokaryotes have quite distinct subcellular compartments. The number of such compartments used in prediction studies varies. A common schema reduces prokaryotic to three compartments (cytoplasmic, periplasmic, and extracellular) and eukaryotic cells to four compartments (nuclear, cytoplasmic, mitochondrial, and extracellular). Other structural classifications evince in excess ten eukaryotic compartments. Ten compartments maybe a conservative estimate, such is the complex richness of sub-cellular structure. Any prediction method must account for permanent, transient, and multiple locations, and, in addition, multi-protein complexes and membrane-bound organelles as possible sites.

Numerous signal sequences exist. Several methods predict lipoproteins. The prediction of proteins translocated via the TAT-dependent pathway is important but has yet to be addressed properly. However, amongst binary, single-outcome approaches, SignalP is probably the most accurate and reliable method available. It uses neural networks to predict the presence and probable cleavage sites of type II or N-terminal Spase-I-cleaved secretion signal peptides [82–84]. This signal is common to both prokaryotic and eukaryotic organisms. SignalP has recently been enhanced with a HMM intended to discriminate cleaved from uncleaved signal anchors. A limitation of SignalP is its proclivity to over-predict: it cannot properly discriminate reliably between a number of very similar yet functionally different signal sequences, regularly predicting lipoproteins and integral membrane proteins as type II signals.

Many methods have been devised capable of dividing a genome or virtual-proteome between the various subcellular locations of a eukaryotic or prokaryotic cell. PSORT is a good example; it is a multicategory prediction procedure, comprising many different programmes [85–88]. PSORT I predicts 17 subcellular compartments, while PSORT II predicts ten different locations. iPSORT deals with several compartments: chloroplast, mitochondrial, and proteins secreted from the cell, while PSORT-B focuses solely on predicting bacterial sub-cellular locations.

Another effective programme is HensBC [89]. HensBC can assign gene products to one of four different types (nuclear, mitochondrial, cytoplasmic, or extracellular) with an accuracy of about eight out of ten for gram-negative bacteria. Another programme, SubLoc [90], predicts prokaryotic subcellular location divided between three compartments. Another programme is Gpos-PLoc [91], which integrates several basic classifiers. Other methods include Phobius [92], LipoP 1.0 [93], and TatP 1.0 [94]. A comparison of several such programmes, using 272 mycobacterial proteins as a gold standard [95], showed subcellular localisation prediction and possessed high predictive specificity.

We have developed a set of methods which predict bacterial subcellular location. Using a set of methods for lipoprotein, TAT secretion, and membrane protein prediction [96–102], three different Bayesian network architectures were implemented as software pipelines able to predict specific subcellular locations, and two serial implementations using a hierarchical decision structure, and a parallel implementation with a confidence-level-based decision engine [103]. The soluble-rooted serial pipeline performed better than the membrane-rooted predictor. The parallel pipeline outperformed the serial pipeline but was significantly less efficient. Genomic test sets proved more ambiguous: the serial implementation identified 22 more of the 74 proteins of known location yet more accurate predictions are made overall by the parallel implementation.

The implications of this work are clear. The complexity of subcellular structures must be integrated fully into sub-cellular location prediction. In extant studies, many important cellular organelles are not considered; different routes by which proteins can reach the same compartment are ignored; and proteins existing simultaneously at several locations are likewise discounted. Clearly, combining high specificity predictors for each compartment appropriately must be the way forward [103].

Many difficulties, problems, and quandaries persist; the most keenly felt is the lack of high-quality, verified, and validated datasets which unambiguously established the location of well-characterised proteins. This dearth is particularly serious for certain types of secreted protein, such as type III secretion. In a similar manner, considerably more work is required to accurately predict the locations for proteins of viral origin; while certain studies are encouraging [104, 105], the complexity of viral interaction with host organisms continues to confound attempts at analysis.

3.8 Identifying Antigens Using Alignment-Independent Methods

Predicting antigens in silico typically utilise bioinformatics tools. Such tools can identify signal peptides or membrane proteins or lipoproteins successfully, yet the majority of algorithms tend to depend on motifs characteristic of antigens or, more generally, sequence alignment as the principal arbiter of definitive and meaningful sequence relationships. This is potentially a problem of some magnitude, particularly given the wide range of evolutionary rates and mechanisms amongst microbial proteins. Certain protein families do not, however, show obvious or significant sequence similarity, despite having common biological properties, functions, and three-dimensional structures [106, 107].

Thus alignment-based approaches may not always produce useful and unequivocal results, since they assume a direct sequence relationship that can be identified by simple sequence search techniques. Immunogenicity, as a signature characteristic, may be encrypted within the structure and/or sequence instead. This may be encoded so cryptically or so subtlety as to completely confound or at least mislead conventional sequence alignment protocols. Discovery of utterly novel and previously unknown antigens will be totally stymied by the absence of similarity to known antigenic proteins.

Alignment-dependent methods tend to dominate bioinformatics and, by extension, immunoinformatics. Several authors have chosen to look at alternative strategies, implementing so-called alignment-independent or alignment-free techniques. The first authors to do so were Mayer et al., who reported that protective antigens had a different amino acid composition compared to control groups of non-antigens [108]. Such a result is unsurprising since it has long been known that the structure and sequence composition of proteins adapted to the different redox environments of different sub-cellular compartments [109].

Mayer's analysis was formulated primarily in terms of univariate comparisons of antigens versus controls for different properties. Subsequently, we explored bivariate comparison in terms of easily comprehensible scatter-plots. See Fig. 3.3 for representative examples. What their results ably demonstrate is the potential for the discrimination of antigens and non-antigens by the appropriate selection of orthogonal descriptors. The challenge, of course, is to identify a robust choice of descriptors which are capable of extrapolating as well interpolating when used predictively.

Progressing beyond this type of analysis, and synergising with our other work on alignment-independent representation [110–114], we have initiated the development of new methods to differentiate antigens—and thus potential vaccine candidates—and non-antigens, using more sophisticated alignment-free approach to sequence representation [115, 116]. Rather than focus on epitope versus non-epitope, our approach utilises data on protective antigens derived from diverse pathogens to create statistical models capable of predicting whole-protein antigenicity.

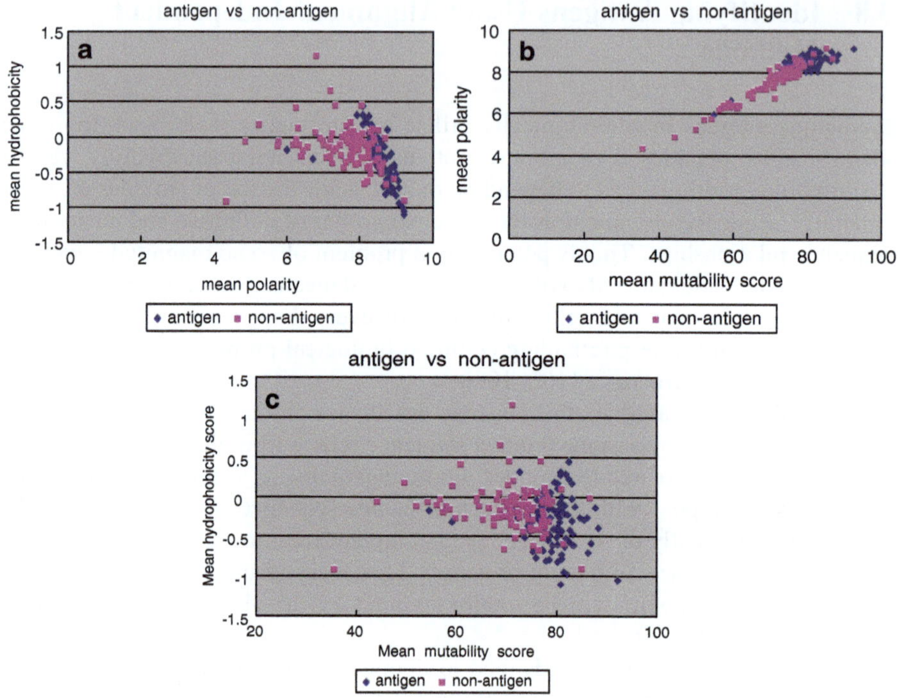

Fig. 3.3 Two scale plots of antigen and non antigen. (**a**) Proteins separated in terms of mean hydrophobicity versus mean polarity. (**b**) Proteins separated by mean polarity versus mean relative mutability. (**c**) Protein separated by mean hydrophobicity versus mean relative mutability score

Our alignment-independent method for antigen identification uses the auto cross covariance (ACC) transformation originally devised by Wold et al. [117, 118] to transform protein sequences into uniform vectors. The ACC transform has found much application in peptide prediction and protein classification [119–126]. In our method, amino acid residues are represented by the well-known and well-used *z* descriptors [127–129], which characterise the hydrophobicity, molecular size, and polarity of residues. Our method also accounts for the absence of complete independence between distinct sequence positions.

We initially applied our approach to groups of known viral, bacterial, and tumour antigens, developing models capable of identifying antigen. Extra models were subsequently added for fungal and parasite antigens. For bacterial, viral, and tumour antigens, models had prediction accuracies in the 70–89 % range [115, 116, 130]. For the parasite and fungal antigens, models had good predictive ability with 78–97 % accuracy. These models were incorporated into a server for protective antigen prediction called VaxiJen [115] (URL: http://www.darrenflower.info/VaxiJen). VaxiJen is an imperfect but encouraging start; future research will yield significantly more insight as well-characterised protective antigens increase significantly in number [70].

3.9 Antigen Selection and Immunogenicity

As we have said, a number of bioinformatics problems are unique to the discipline of immunology: the greatest of these is the accurate quantitative prediction of immunogenicity. This chapter has in its totality been suffused and pervaded by the idea of immunogenicity and the challenge of predicting this property in silico. Such an endeavour is confounding, yet exciting, and, as a key instrument in developing better, safer, more effective vaccines, is also of undisputed practical utility.

Successful immunogenicity prediction is at its simplest made manifest through the identification of B cell or T cell epitopes. Epitope recognition, when seen as a chemical event, may be understood in terms of the relationships between apparent biological function or activity and basic physicochemical properties. Delineating structure-activity or property-activity relationships of this kind is a key concern of immunoinformatics. At the other end of the spectrum, immunogenicity can be viewed is a cohesive, integrated, system property: a property of the entire and complete immune system and not a series of individual and isolated molecular recognition events. Thus, the task of predicting systems-level immunogenicity is in all likelihood manifold more demanding than predicting peptide-binding say.

The clinical manifestation of vaccine immunogenicity arises from the complex amalgam of many contributing extrinsic and intrinsic factors, which includes pathogen-side and host-side properties, as well as those just coming directly from proteins themselves. See Fig. 3.2. Protein-side properties include the aggregation state of candidate vaccines and the possession of PAMPs. Pathogen-side properties are clearly properties intrinsic to the pathogen, including expression levels of the antigen, the time-course of this expression, as well as its subcellular location. So-called host-side properties are innate recognition properties of host immunity, and most obviously include T cell epitopes or B cell epitopes.

A *bona fide* candidate antigen should be available for immune surveillance and thus highly expressed, constitutively or transiently, as well as having several epitopes. A protein without immunogenicity would logically lack all or some of these characteristics. As a prediction problem, this is, to say the least, not uncomplicated; clearly consisting of a great variety of difficult-to-compute stages. In terms of mechanism, many of these stages are poorly understood. Yet, each can be addressed using standard computational and statistical tools. They can all be predicted, however, presupposing, of course, the presence of relevant data in sufficient quantity.

3.10 Expert Systems for Antigen Discovery

One of the strongest messages to emerge from this review is that immunogenicity is a strongly multi-factorial property: some protein antigens are immunogenic for one reason, or set of reasons, and other immunogenic proteins will be so for another possibly tangential reason or set of reasons. Each such causal manifold is itself complex and potentially confusing. Thus, the prediction of immunogenicity is a problem in multi-factorial prediction, and the search for new antigens is a search through a multi-factorial landscape of contingent causes and discombobulating decoys.

Some of the evidence will be highly precise and quantitative. The kind provided by predictive immunoinformatics, for example. This typically yields exact values for, say, the binding affinity of a peptide to a protein component of the immune system, or an unequivocal yes or no answer to the question: is this peptide sequence an epitope? However, for each such exact prediction, we have some notional associated probability concerning how reliable we regard this result. Different methods evince a range of accuracy, which, in practice, equate to probabilities of reliability: we naturally have more confidence and assume a greater reliability for a highly accurate prediction versus one of average predictability, though it can still give wrong predictions and generally inaccurate predictors may work well for a specific subset of the data.

Other types of forms of evidence will have a distinctly more anecdotal flavour. Take, for example, the case of bacterial exotoxins. Together with endotoxins, such as LPS, and so-called superantigens, exotoxins form the principal varieties of toxin secreted by pathogenic bacteria. Exotoxins have evolved to be the most toxic substances known to science: in terms of the median lethal dose, botulinum toxin—the active ingredient of BOTOX and causative agent of botulism, amongst others—is about ten times as lethal as radioactive isotope polonium-210 and a million times more deadly than mainline poisons, such as arsenic or potassium cyanide. Virtually, all such potent bacterial exotoxins comprise two functionally distinct subunits, either separate proteins or distinct domains, usually denoted A and B. The A subunit is habitually an enzyme, such as a protease, which modifies specific protein targets, thus disrupting key cellular processes with host cells. The B subunit is a protein which binds to host cell surface lipids or proteins, enabling the toxin to be internalised efficiently. The high specificity of this dual action lends exotoxins much of their remarkable lethality.

Exotoxins are also extremely immunogenic, inducing the immune systems to produce high-affinity neutralising antibodies against them, and thus make excellent targets for vaccinology. A toxoid—a toxin which has been treated or inactivated, often by formaldehyde—is in essence a form of subunit vaccine and, as such, requires adjuvant to induce adequate immune responses. Vaccines targeting tetanus and diphtheria, which usually need boosting every decade, are based on toxoids, albeit typically combined with pertussis toxin acting as an adjuvant. Poisoning by exotoxins, on the other hand, requires treatment with antitoxin comprising preformed antibodies.

However, and say that we were offered a newly sequenced pathogen genome, is such a classification for AB toxins helpful when trying to identify a potential exotoxins? The answer is neither yes nor is it no, but lies somewhere between these extremes. Assuming we had extant knowledge or a reliable method predicting the presence of structural and functionally distinct domains, this very simple rule-of-thumb would become a useful tool for eliminating large numbers of possible toxin molecules. It would not directly identify an antigen but would enormously reduce the workload inherent in their discovery.

As well as needing more and more reliable predictors, we also need a way of combining the information we gather from any set of reliable predictors to which we have access. Thus, when analysing a pathogen genome, what we seem to need, at least in order to identify immunogenic proteins, is both a set of reliable and robust tools and a cohesive expert system within which to embed them. Such systems, albeit still at a relatively crude and faltering level, do exist. Because there is an implicit hierarchy of one prediction being based on others, there is a need to balance and judge different pieces of probabilistic evidence. An effective expert system should be capable of such a feat.

To a first approximation, an expert system is a computer programme that undertakes tasks that might otherwise be prosecuted by a human expert ostensively by simulating the apparent judgement and behaviour of an individual or organization with expertise and experience within a particular discipline. An Expert System might make financial forecasts, or play chess; it might diagnose human illnesses or schedule the routes of delivery vehicles. To create an expert system, one first needs to analyse human experts and how they make decisions, before translating this into rules that a computer can follow. Such a system leverages both a knowledge base of accumulated expertise and a set of rules for applying such distilled knowledge to particular situations in order to solve problems. Sophisticated expert systems can be updated with new knowledge and rules and can also learn from the success of its prediction, again mirroring the behaviour of properly performing experts.

At the heart then of an Expert System is the need to combine evidence in order to reach decisions. Combining evidence, and reaching a decision based on that combined evidence, is no easier in the laboratory, be that virtual or actual, than it is in the court room. The problem of combining evidence is encountered across the disciplines, and various solutions have arisen in these different areas.

Within bioinformatic prediction, a particular variety of evidence combination, so-called meta-prediction, is a now a well-established strategy [131, 132]. This approach seeks to amalgamate the output of various predictors, typically internet servers, in an intelligent way so that the combined result is more accurate than any of those coming from a single predictor. Indeed, combining results from multiple prediction tools does often increase overall accuracy. A consensus strategy was first proposed by Mallios [133], who combined SYFPEITHI [60, 61, 134], ProPred [135, 136], and the iterative stepwise discriminant analysis meta-algorithm [137–139]. MULTIPRED [140] integrates HMMs and artificial neural networks (ANN). Six MHC class II predictors were combined by Dai and co-workers [141–143] basing its overall prediction on the probability distributions of the different scores. Trost et al. have used a heuristic method to address class I peptide-MHC binding [144]. Wang et al. [145] applied a consensus method to calculate the median rank of the top three predictive methods for each MHC class II protein initially evaluated so as to rank all possible 8-, 9-, and 10-mers from one protein. This rank was used to identify the top 1 % of peptides from each protein.

In probabilistic reasoning, or reasoning with uncertainty, there are many ways to represent espoused beliefs—or, in our domain, predictions—that effectively encode the uncertainty of propositions. These include fuzzy logic and the evidential method, among many others. For quantitative data, information fusion, in its various guises [146], is one robust route to effective combination. Another requires us to enter the world of Bayesian statistics, or, at least, a special thread within it.

Bayes theory, and the ever-expanding strand of statistics devolving from it, is concerned primarily with updating or revising belief in the light of new evidence, while so-called Dempster–Shafer theory [147] is concerned not with the conditional probabilities of Bayesian statistics but with the direct combination of evidence. It extends the Bayesian theory of subjective probability, by replacing Bayesian probabilities with belief functions that describe degrees of belief for one question in terms of probabilities for another and then combines these using Dempster's rule for merging degrees of belief when based on independent lines of evidence. Such belief functions may or may not have the mathematical properties of probabilities but are seemingly able to combine the rigor of probability theory with the flexibility of rule-based approaches.

Several Expert Systems of different flavours and hues have now become available within the vaccinology arena. Sundaresh et al. developed a specialist software package for the analysis of microarray experiments that could easily be classified as an Expert System and used it in the area of reverse vaccinology. This package, which was written in the open-source statistical package R, was used to help analyse a variety of complex microarray experiments on the bacteria *F. tularensis*, a category A bio-defense pathogen [148]. This programme implements a two-stage process for diagnostic analysis: selection of antigens based on significant immune responses coupled with differential expression analysis, followed by classification of measured antigen responses using a combination of k-Means clustering, support vector machines, and k-nearest neighbours.

We have already discussed VaxiJen [115, 116, 130], and the related server EpiJen [149], which combines various methods for identifying epitopes within extant proteins. These two servers can also be classified as vaccine-related Expert Systems. NERVE is another Expert System, which has been developed to help automate aspects of reverse vaccinology [150]. Using NERVE, the prioritisation of potential candidate antigens consists of several stages: prediction of subcellular localisation; is the antigen an adhesion?; identification of membrane-crossing domains; and comparison to pathogen and human proteomes. Candidates are filtered then ranked and putative antigens graded by provenance and its predicted immunogenicity.

The web-based Expert System, DyNAVacS [151], was developed to facilitate the efficient design of DNA vaccines and is available in the URL: http://miracle.igib.res.in/dynavac. It takes a structured approach for vaccine design, leveraging various key design parameters, including the choice of appropriate expression vectors, safeguarding efficient expression through codon optimization, ensuring high levels of translation by adding specific sequence signals, and engineering of CpG motifs as adjuvant mechanisms exacerbating immune responses. It also allows restriction enzyme mapping, the design of primers, and lists vectors in use for known DNA vaccines.

VAXIGN is another Expert System developed to help facilitate vaccine design [152]. VAXIGN undertakes dynamic vaccine target prediction from sequence. Methodologically, it combines protein subcellular location prediction with prediction of transmembrane helices and adhesins, analysis of the conservation to human and/or mouse proteins with sequence exclusion from the genomes of non-pathogenic strains, and prediction of peptide binding to class I and class II MHC. As a test, VAXIGN has been used to predict vaccine candidates against uropathogenic *Escherichia coli*.

However, NERVE and its various and varied siblings are tasked with such a confounding and difficult undertaking that they are obliged to fall somewhat short of what is required. An obvious first step in tackling the greater problem is to address first subcellular location prediction. Then, we can look at antigen presentation, modelling for each component step, before building these into a fully functional model. We can also develop empirical approaches—such as VaxiJen [115, 116, 130]. We must also factor in antibody-mediated issues, properly address PAMPs, post translational danger signals, expression levels, the role of aggregation, and the capacity of molecular adjuvants to enhance the innate immunogenicity to usable levels. See Fig. 3.2.

3.11 Discussion and Conclusions

The value of vaccines is not yet unchallenged. However, most reasonable people would, in all probability, agree that they are a good thing, albeit with a few minor provisos. The idea underlying all vaccines is a strong and robust one: it is in the reification—that is, the realisation, manifestation, and instantiation—of this abstract concept that the trouble lies, if indeed trouble there is. Existing vaccines are by no means perfect; again, most sensible and well-informed people would no doubt acknowledge this also. One might argue that their intrinsic complexity, and the highly empirical nature of their discovery over decades, and the fraught nature of their manufacture, has much to answer in this regard.

Why should this be? In part, it is due to the extreme complexity of immune response to an administered vaccine, which is largely specific to each individual or at least is different in different sub-groups within the totality of the vaccinated population. The immune responses is comprised, at least for whole-pathogen vaccines, of the adaptive immune response to multiple B cell and T cell epitopes as well as the responses made by the innate immune responses to diverse molecular structures, principally PAMPs. When one considers also the degree to which such a repertoire of responses is augmented and modified by the action of additives, be they designed to increase the durability and stability of vaccines or be they adjuvants, which are intended to raise the level of immune reactions. Add in stochastic and coincidental phenomena, such as reversion to pathogenicity, and we can see immediately that navigating our way through the vaccine minefield is no easy task. All such problems engendered by this intrinsic complexity are themselves compounded by our comparatively weak understanding of immunological mechanisms, since, if we understood the mechanism of responses well enough, we could and would have designed our vaccines to circumvent these issues.

Part of the answer to this cacophony of conflicting and confounding quandaries is the newly emergent discipline of vaccinomics. A proper understanding of the relationships between gene variants and vaccine-specific immune responses may help us to design the next generation of personalised vaccines. Vaccinomics addresses this issue directly. It seeks to identify genetic factors mediating or moderating vaccine-induced immune responses, which are known to be extremely variable within population. Much data indicate that host genetic polymorphisms are key determinants of innate and adaptive response to vaccination. HLA genes, non-HLA genes, and genes of the innate immunity all contribute, and do so in many ways, to the variation observed between individuals for immune responses to microbial vaccines. Vaccinomics offers many techniques that can help illuminate these diverse phenomena. Principal amongst these are population-based gene/SNP association studies between allele or SNP variation and specific responses, supplemented by the application of next-generation sequencing technology and microarray approaches.

Yet, and for all this nay-saying and gainsaying, vaccines and vaccination have demonstrated their worth time after time; yet, to justify the continuing faith we invest in them, new and better ways of making safer and more focussed vaccines must be found. Most current vaccines work via antibody-mediated mechanisms; and most target viruses and the diseases they cause. Unfortunately, the stock of such disease targets is dwindling. Low-hanging fruit has long since been cut down. Only fruit that is well out of reach remains. Vaccines based on APCs and peptides are new but unproven strategies; most modern vaccine development relies instead on effective searches for vaccine antigens.

One of the clearest points to emerge from such work is that there are many competing concepts, thoughts, and ideas that may confound or help efficient identification of immune reactive proteins. Certain such ideas we have outlined. Some are indisputably persuasive, even compelling, yet many strategies—and the technical approaches upon which they are based—have singly failed to deliver on their promise.

Long ago, and based on his lifetime's experience of all things immunological, Professor Peter CL Beverley sketched out a paradigm for protein-focussed vaccine development, which we have formalised further, and which schema is summarised in Fig. 3.4. Some of his factors overlap with the factors from Fig. 3.2. He identified many of the factors that potentially contribute to the immunogenicity of proteins, be they of pathogen origin or another source entirely, and also other features which might make proteins particularly suitable for becoming candidate vaccines. Of these, some are as-yet beyond prediction, such as the attractiveness for APCs or the inability to down-regulate immune responses. The status of proteins as evasins is

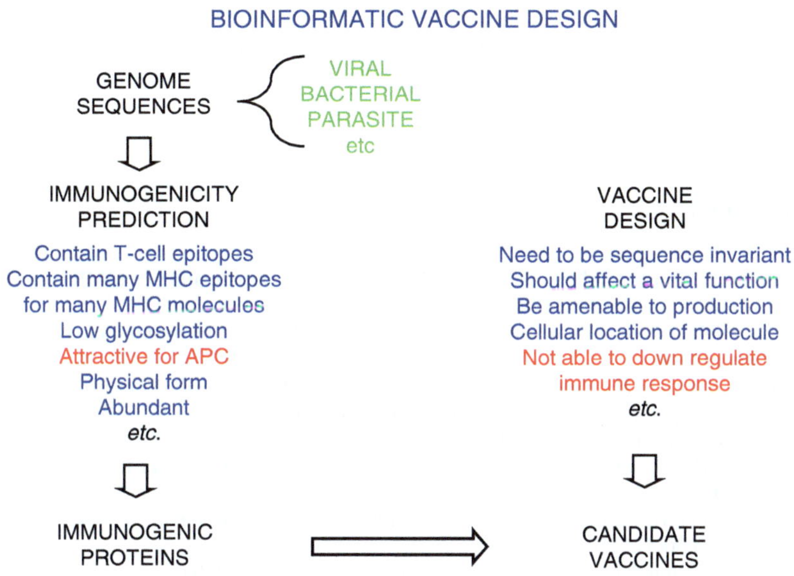

Fig. 3.4 The Beverley paradigm

currently only possibly addressable through sequence similarity-based approaches and likewise for the attractiveness for uptake by APCs is again, though possible there exist motifs, structural or sequence, which could be identified. Currently, the dearth of relevant data precludes prediction of such properties; and, while it is possible to predict some of these properties with some assurance of success, and others are predictable but only incidentally, overall, we are still some way from realising the dream embodied in Fig. 3.4.

Failure occurs for simple reasons: we deal with simplified abstractions and cannot hope to capture all that which is required for prediction by looking superficially at a single factor. Protein immunogenicity comes instead from the dynamic combination of innumerable contributing factors. This is by no means a facile or easily solved informatics conundrum. A vaccine candidate should have epitopes that the host recognises, be available for immune surveillance, and be highly expressed. Factors mediating protein immunogenicity are many; possession of B or T cell epitopes, post-translational danger signals, sub-cellular location, protein expression levels, and aggregation state amongst them. Predicting such diverse, complex, confounding properties is—and remains—a challenge.

Vaccine antigens, once discovered, should, ultimately, and with appropriate manipulation, together with an apt, apposite, and appropriate delivery system and the right choice of adjuvant, become first a candidate for clinical trials, before, hopefully, progressing to regulatory approval. We require an integrative, systems-biology approach to solve this problem. No single approach can be applied universally and with success; what we crave is the full integration of numerous equally partial yet equally valid techniques and strategies which, in turn, draw upon a wealth of relevant, useful data. With an issue of such importance, even an incomplete solution should be sufficient.

References

1. Godlee F, Smith J, Marcovitch H (2011) Wakefield's article linking MMR vaccine and autism was fraudulent. BMJ 342:c7452
2. Flower DR, Davies MN, Ranganathan S: **Bioinformatics for Immunomics**, vol. 3, 1 edn: Springer; 2010.
3. Vivona S, Gardy JL, Ramachandran S, Brinkman FS, Raghava GP, Flower DR, Filippini F (2008) Computer-aided biotechnology: from immuno-informatics to reverse vaccinology. Trends Biotechnol 26(4):190–200
4. Davies MN, Flower DR (2007) Harnessing bioinformatics to discover new vaccines. Drug Discov Today 12(9–10):389–395
5. Lambert PH, Hawkridge T, Hanekom WA (2009) **New vaccines against tuberculosis**. Clin Chest Med 30(4):811–826, x
6. Flower D: **Bioinformatics for Vaccinology**, 1st edn: Wiley; 2008.
7. Plotkin SA (2001) Lessons learned concerning vaccine safety. Vaccine 20(suppl 1):S16–S19, discussion S11
8. Kwok R (2011) Vaccines: the real issues in vaccine safety. Nature 473(7348):436–438
9. Leask J (2011) Target the fence-sitters. Nature 473(7348):443–445
10. Day A (2009) **'An American tragedy'. The Cutter incident and its implications for the Salk polio vaccine in New Zealand 1955–1960**. Health History 11(2):42–61
11. Offit PA (2005) The Cutter incident, 50 years later. N Engl J Med 352(14):1411–1412
12. Nathanson N, Langmuir AD (1995) The Cutter incident. Poliomyelitis following formaldehyde-inactivated poliovirus vaccination in the United States during the Spring of 1955. II. Relationship of poliomyelitis to Cutter vaccine. 1963. Am J Epidemiol 142 (2):109–140, discussion 107–108
13. Flower DR (2008) Bioinformatics for vaccinology. Wiley, Chichester
14. Minor P (2009) Vaccine-derived poliovirus (VDPV): impact on poliomyelitis eradication. Vaccine 27(20):2649–2652
15. Flower DR (2009) Advances in predicting and manipulating the immunogenicity of biotherapeutics and vaccines. BioDrugs 23(4):231–240
16. Bambini S, Rappuoli R (2009) The use of genomics in microbial vaccine development. Drug Discov Today 14(5–6):252–260
17. Serruto D, Rappuoli R (2006) Post-genomic vaccine development. FEBS Lett 580 (12):2985–2992
18. Mora M, Donati C, Medini D, Covacci A, Rappuoli R (2006) Microbial genomes and vaccine design: refinements to the classical reverse vaccinology approach. Curr Opin Microbiol 9 (5):532–536
19. Serruto D, Adu-Bobie J, Capecchi B, Rappuoli R, Pizza M, Masignani V (2004) Biotechnology and vaccines: application of functional genomics to Neisseria meningitidis and other bacterial pathogens. J Biotechnol 113(1–3):15–32
20. Tettelin H, Saunders NJ, Heidelberg J, Jeffries AC, Nelson KE, Eisen JA, Ketchum KA, Hood DW, Peden JF, Dodson RJ et al (2000) Complete genome sequence of Neisseria meningitidis serogroup B strain MC58. Science 287(5459):1809–1815
21. Pizza M, Scarlato V, Masignani V, Giuliani MM, Arico B, Comanducci M, Jennings GT, Baldi L, Bartolini E, Capecchi B et al (2000) Identification of vaccine candidates against serogroup B meningococcus by whole-genome sequencing. Science 287(5459):1816–1820

22. Giuliani MM, Adu-Bobie J, Comanducci M, Arico B, Savino S, Santini L, Brunelli B, Bambini S, Biolchi A, Capecchi B et al (2006) A universal vaccine for serogroup B meningococcus. Proc Natl Acad Sci USA 103(29):10834–10839
23. Ross BC, Czajkowski L, Hocking D, Margetts M, Webb E, Rothel L, Patterson M, Agius C, Camuglia S, Reynolds E et al (2001) Identification of vaccine candidate antigens from a genomic analysis of Porphyromonas gingivalis. Vaccine 19(30):4135–4142
24. Wizemann TM, Heinrichs JH, Adamou JE, Erwin AL, Kunsch C, Choi GH, Barash SC, Rosen CA, Masure HR, Tuomanen E et al (2001) Use of a whole genome approach to identify vaccine molecules affording protection against Streptococcus pneumoniae infection. Infect Immun 69(3):1593–1598
25. Maione D, Margarit I, Rinaudo CD, Masignani V, Mora M, Scarselli M, Tettelin H, Brettoni C, Iacobini ET, Rosini R et al (2005) Identification of a universal Group B streptococcus vaccine by multiple genome screen. Science 309(5731):148–150
26. Weichhart T, Horky M, Sollner J, Gangl S, Henics T, Nagy E, Meinke A, von Gabain A, Fraser CM, Gill SR et al (2003) Functional selection of vaccine candidate peptides from Staphylococcus aureus whole-genome expression libraries in vitro. Infect Immun 71 (8):4633–4641
27. Giefing C, Meinke AL, Hanner M, Henics T, Bui MD, Gelbmann D, Lundberg U, Senn BM, Schunn M, Habel A et al (2008) Discovery of a novel class of highly conserved vaccine antigens using genomic scale antigenic fingerprinting of pneumococcus with human antibodies. J Exp Med 205(1):117–131
28. Eyles JE, Unal B, Hartley MG, Newstead SL, Flick-Smith H, Prior JL, Oyston PC, Randall A, Mu Y, Hirst S et al (2007) Immunodominant Francisella tularensis antigens identified using proteome microarray. Proteomics 7(13):2172–2183
29. Felgner PL, Kayala MA, Vigil A, Burk C, Nakajima-Sasaki R, Pablo J, Molina DM, Hirst S, Chew JS, Wang D et al (2009) A Burkholderia pseudomallei protein microarray reveals serodiagnostic and cross-reactive antigens. Proc Natl Acad Sci USA 106(32):13499–13504
30. Ponomarenko JV, Bourne PE (2007) Antibody-protein interactions: benchmark datasets and prediction tools evaluation. BMC Struct Biol 7:64
31. Blythe MJ, Flower DR (2005) Benchmarking B cell epitope prediction: underperformance of existing methods. Protein Sci 14(1):246–248
32. Lafuente EM, Reche PA (2009) Prediction of MHC-peptide binding: a systematic and comprehensive overview. Curr Pharm Des 15(28):3209–3220
33. Gowthaman U, Agrewala JN (2008) In silico tools for predicting peptides binding to HLA-class II molecules: more confusion than conclusion. J Proteome Res 7(1):154–163
34. El-Manzalawy Y, Dobbs D, Honavar V (2008) On evaluating MHC-II binding peptide prediction methods. PLoS One 3(9):e3268
35. Lin HH, Zhang GL, Tongchusak S, Reinherz EL, Brusic V (2008) **Evaluation of MHC-II peptide binding prediction servers: applications for vaccine research**. BMC Bioinformatics 9(suppl 12):S22
36. Knapp B, Omasits U, Frantal S, Schreiner W (2009) A critical cross-validation of high throughput structural binding prediction methods for pMHC. J Comput Aided Mol Des 23 (5):301–307
37. Zhang H, Wang P, Papangelopoulos N, Xu Y, Sette A, Bourne PE, Lund O, Ponomarenko J, Nielsen M, Peters B (2010) Limitations of Ab initio predictions of peptide binding to MHC class II molecules. PLoS One 5(2):e9272
38. Tynan FE, Burrows SR, Buckle AM, Clements CS, Borg NA, Miles JJ, Beddoe T, Whisstock JC, Wilce MC, Silins SL et al (2005) T cell receptor recognition of a 'super-bulged' major histocompatibility complex class I-bound peptide. Nat Immunol 6(11):1114–1122
39. Tynan FE, Borg NA, Miles JJ, Beddoe T, El-Hassen D, Silins SL, van Zuylen WJ, Purcell AW, Kjer-Nielsen L, McCluskey J et al (2005) High resolution structures of highly bulged viral epitopes bound to major histocompatibility complex class I. Implications for T-cell receptor engagement and T-cell immunodominance. J Biol Chem 280(25):23900–23909

40. Burrows SR, Rossjohn J, McCluskey J (2006) Have we cut ourselves too short in mapping CTL epitopes? Trends Immunol 27(1):11–16
41. Ebert LM, Liu YC, Clements CS, Robson NC, Jackson HM, Markby JL, Dimopoulos N, Tan BS, Luescher IF, Davis ID et al (2009) A long, naturally presented immunodominant epitope from NY-ESO-1 tumor antigen: implications for cancer vaccine design. Cancer Res 69 (3):1046–1054
42. Guy L (2006) Identification and characterization of pathogenicity and other genomic islands using base composition analyses. Future Microbiol 1(3):309–316
43. Ou HY, Chen LL, Lonnen J, Chaudhuri RR, Thani AB, Smith R, Garton NJ, Hinton J, Pallen M, Barer MR et al (2006) A novel strategy for the identification of genomic islands by comparative analysis of the contents and contexts of tRNA sites in closely related bacteria. Nucleic Acids Res 34(1):e3
44. Ou HY, He X, Harrison EM, Kulasekara BR, Thani AB, Kadioglu A, Lory S, Hinton JC, Barer MR, Deng Z et al (2007) MobilomeFINDER: web-based tools for in silico and experimental discovery of bacterial genomic islands. Nucleic Acids Res 35:W97–W104, Web Server issue
45. Hackenberg M, Previti C, Luque-Escamilla PL, Carpena P, Martinez-Aroza J, Oliver JL (2006) CpGcluster: a distance-based algorithm for CpG-island detection. BMC Bioinformatics 7:446
46. Sujuan Y, Asaithambi A, Liu Y (2008) CpGIF: an algorithm for the identification of CpG islands. Bioinformation 2(8):335–338
47. Hutter B, Paulsen M, Helms V (2009) **Identifying CpG islands by different computational techniques**. OMICS 13(2):153–164
48. Su J, Zhang Y, Lv J, Liu H, Tang X, Wang F, Qi Y, Feng Y, Li X (2010) CpG_MI: a novel approach for identifying functional CpG islands in mammalian genomes. Nucleic Acids Res 38(1):e6
49. Langille MG, Hsiao WW, Brinkman FS (2008) Evaluation of genomic island predictors using a comparative genomics approach. BMC Bioinformatics 9:329
50. Hsiao W, Wan I, Jones SJ, Brinkman FS (2003) IslandPath: aiding detection of genomic islands in prokaryotes. Bioinformatics 19(3):418–420
51. Waack S, Keller O, Asper R, Brodag T, Damm C, Fricke WF, Surovcik K, Meinicke P, Merkl R (2006) Score-based prediction of genomic islands in prokaryotic genomes using hidden Markov models. BMC Bioinformatics 7:142
52. Yoon SH, Hur CG, Kang HY, Kim YH, Oh TK, Kim JF (2005) A computational approach for identifying pathogenicity islands in prokaryotic genomes. BMC Bioinformatics 6:184
53. Vernikos GS, Parkhill J (2008) Resolving the structural features of genomic islands: a machine learning approach. Genome Res 18(2):331–342
54. Arvey AJ, Azad RK, Raval A, Lawrence JG (2009) Detection of genomic islands via segmental genome heterogeneity. Nucleic Acids Res 37(16):5255–5266
55. Wang G, Zhou F, Olman V, Li F, Xu Y (2010) Prediction of pathogenicity islands in enterohemorrhagic Escherichia coli O157:H7 using genomic barcodes. FEBS Lett 584 (1):194–198
56. Langille MG, Brinkman FS (2009) IslandViewer: an integrated interface for computational identification and visualization of genomic islands. Bioinformatics 25(5):664–665
57. Yoon SH, Park YK, Lee S, Choi D, Oh TK, Hur CG, Kim JF (2007) Towards pathogenomics: a web-based resource for pathogenicity islands. Nucleic Acids Res 35:D395–D400, Database issue
58. Adamou JE, Heinrichs JH, Erwin AL, Walsh W, Gayle T, Dormitzer M, Dagan R, Brewah YA, Barren P, Lathigra R et al (2001) Identification and characterization of a novel family of pneumococcal proteins that are protective against sepsis. Infect Immun 69(2):949–958
59. Moxon ER, Hood DW, Saunders NJ, Schweda EK, Richards JC (2002) Functional genomics of pathogenic bacteria. Philos Trans R Soc Lond B Biol Sci 357(1417):109–116

60. Schuler MM, Nastke MD, Stevanovikc S (2007) SYFPEITHI: database for searching and T-cell epitope prediction. Methods Mol Biol 409:75–93
61. Rammensee H, Bachmann J, Emmerich NP, Bachor OA, Stevanovic S (1999) SYFPEITHI: database for MHC ligands and peptide motifs. Immunogenetics 50(3–4):213–219
62. Kuiken C, Korber B, Shafer RW (2003) HIV sequence databases. AIDS Rev 5(1):52–61
63. Lata S, Bhasin M, Raghava GP (2009) MHCBN 4.0: a database of MHC/TAP binding peptides and T-cell epitopes. BMC Res Notes 2:61
64. Bhasin M, Singh H, Raghava GP (2003) MHCBN: a comprehensive database of MHC binding and non-binding peptides. Bioinformatics 19(5):665–666
65. Reche PA, Zhang H, Glutting JP, Reinherz EL (2005) EPIMHC: a curated database of MHC-binding peptides for customized computational vaccinology. Bioinformatics 21 (9):2140–2141
66. Toseland CP, Clayton DJ, McSparron H, Hemsley SL, Blythe MJ, Paine K, Doytchinova IA, Guan P, Hattotuwagama CK, Flower DR (2005) AntiJen: a quantitative immunology database integrating functional, thermodynamic, kinetic, biophysical, and cellular data. Immunome Res 1(1):4
67. McSparron H, Blythe MJ, Zygouri C, Doytchinova IA, Flower DR (2003) JenPep: a novel computational information resource for immunobiology and vaccinology. J Chem Inf Comput Sci 43(4):1276–1287
68. Blythe MJ, Doytchinova IA, Flower DR (2002) JenPep: a database of quantitative functional peptide data for immunology. Bioinformatics 18(3):434–439
69. Vita R, Zarebski L, Greenbaum JA, Emami H, Hoof I, Salimi N, Damle R, Sette A, Peters B (2010) The immune epitope database 2.0. Nucleic Acids Res 38:D854–D862, Database issue
70. Ansari HR, Flower DR, Raghava GPS (2010) AntigenDB: an immunoinformatics database of pathogen antigens. Nucleic Acids Res 38:D847–D853
71. Xiang Z, Todd T, Ku KP, Kovacic BL, Larson CB, Chen F, Hodges AP, Tian Y, Olenzek EA, Zhao B et al (2008) VIOLIN: vaccine investigation and online information network. Nucleic Acids Res 36:D923–D928, Database issue
72. Kanduc D (2009) Epitopic peptides with low similarity to the host proteome: towards biological therapies without side effects. Expert Opin Biol Ther 9(1):45–53
73. Kanduc D (2005) Peptimmunology: immunogenic peptides and sequence redundancy. Curr Drug Discov Technol 2(4):239–244
74. Singh NJ, Schwartz RH (2006) Primer: mechanisms of immunologic tolerance. Nat Clin Pract Rheumatol 2(1):44–52
75. Miao CH (2007) Recent advances in immune modulation. Curr Gene Ther 7(5):391–402
76. Barron L, Knoechel B, Lohr J, Abbas AK (2008) Cutting edge: contributions of apoptosis and anergy to systemic T cell tolerance. J Immunol 180(5):2762–2766
77. Ramakrishnan K, Flower DR (2010) Discriminating antigen and non-antigen using proteome dissimilarity III: tumour and parasite antigens. Bioinformation 5(1):39–42
78. Ramakrishnan K, Flower DR (2010) Discriminating antigen and non-antigen using proteome dissimilarity II: viral and fungal antigens. Bioinformation 5(1):35–38
79. Ramakrishnan K, Flower DR (2010) Discriminating antigen and non-antigen using proteome dissimilarity: bacterial antigens. Bioinformation 4(10):445–447
80. Altschul SF, Madden TL, Schaffer AA, Zhang J, Zhang Z, Miller W, Lipman DJ (1997) Gapped BLAST and PSI-BLAST: a new generation of protein database search programs. Nucleic Acids Res 25(17):3389–3402
81. Radisky DC, Stallings-Mann M, Hirai Y, Bissell MJ (2009) Single proteins might have dual but related functions in intracellular and extracellular microenvironments. Nat Rev Mol Cell Biol 10(3):228–234
82. Emanuelsson O, Brunak S, von Heijne G, Nielsen H (2007) Locating proteins in the cell using TargetP, SignalP and related tools. Nat Protoc 2(4):953–971
83. Bendtsen JD, Nielsen H, von Heijne G, Brunak S (2004) Improved prediction of signal peptides: SignalP 3.0. J Mol Biol 340(4):783–795

84. Choo KH, Tan TW, Ranganathan S (2009) **A comprehensive assessment of N-terminal signal peptides prediction methods**. BMC Bioinformatics 10(suppl 15):S2
85. Horton P, Park KJ, Obayashi T, Fujita N, Harada H, Adams-Collier CJ, Nakai K (2007) WoLF PSORT: protein localization predictor. Nucleic Acids Res 35:W585–W587, Web Server issue
86. Chen Y, Yu P, Luo J, Jiang Y (2003) Secreted protein prediction system combining CJ-SPHMM, TMHMM, and PSORT. Mamm Genome 14(12):859–865
87. Gardy JL, Spencer C, Wang K, Ester M, Tusnady GE, Simon I, Hua S, deFays K, Lambert C, Nakai K et al (2003) **PSORT-B: improving protein subcellular localization prediction for Gram-negative bacteria**. Nucleic Acids Res 31(13):3613–3617
88. Nakai K, Horton P (1999) PSORT: a program for detecting sorting signals in proteins and predicting their subcellular localization. Trends Biochem Sci 24(1):34–36
89. Bulashevska A, Eils R (2006) Predicting protein subcellular locations using hierarchical ensemble of Bayesian classifiers based on Markov chains. BMC Bioinformatics 7:298
90. Chen H, Huang N, Sun Z (2006) SubLoc: a server/client suite for protein subcellular location based on SOAP. Bioinformatics 22(3):376–377
91. Shen HB, Chou KC (2007) Gpos-PLoc: an ensemble classifier for predicting subcellular localization of Gram-positive bacterial proteins. Protein Eng Des Sel 20(1):39–46
92. Kall L, Krogh A, Sonnhammer EL (2007) Advantages of combined transmembrane topology and signal peptide prediction–the Phobius web server. Nucleic Acids Res 35:W429–W432, Web Server issue
93. Juncker AS, Willenbrock H, Von Heijne G, Brunak S, Nielsen H, Krogh A (2003) Prediction of lipoprotein signal peptides in Gram-negative bacteria. Protein Sci 12(8):1652–1662
94. Bendtsen JD, Nielsen H, Widdick D, Palmer T, Brunak S (2005) Prediction of twin-arginine signal peptides. BMC Bioinformatics 6:167
95. Restrepo-Montoya D, Vizcaino C, Nino LF, Ocampo M, Patarroyo ME, Patarroyo MA (2009) Validating subcellular localization prediction tools with mycobacterial proteins. BMC Bioinformatics 10:134
96. Taylor PD, Attwood TK, Flower DR (2006) Toward bacterial protein sub-cellular location prediction: single-class discrimminant models for all gram- and gram+ compartments. Bioinformation 1(8):276–280
97. Taylor PD, Attwood TK, Flower DR (2006) Multi-class subcellular location prediction for bacterial proteins. Bioinformation 1(7):260–264
98. Taylor PD, Toseland CP, Attwood TK, Flower DR (2006) Alpha helical trans-membrane proteins: enhanced prediction using a Bayesian approach. Bioinformation 1(6):234–236
99. Taylor PD, Toseland CP, Attwood TK, Flower DR (2006) Beta barrel trans-membrane proteins: enhanced prediction using a Bayesian approach. Bioinformation 1(6):231–233
100. Taylor PD, Toseland CP, Attwood TK, Flower DR (2006) A predictor of membrane class: discriminating alpha-helical and beta-barrel membrane proteins from non-membranous proteins. Bioinformation 1(6):208–213
101. Taylor PD, Toseland CP, Attwood TK, Flower DR (2006) TATPred: a Bayesian method for the identification of twin arginine translocation pathway signal sequences. Bioinformation 1 (5):184–187
102. Taylor PD, Toseland CP, Attwood TK, Flower DR (2006) LIPPRED: a web server for accurate prediction of lipoprotein signal sequences and cleavage sites. Bioinformation 1 (5):176–179
103. Taylor PD, Attwood TK, Flower DR (2006) Combining algorithms to predict bacterial protein sub-cellular location: parallel versus concurrent implementations. Bioinformation 1 (8):285–289
104. Scott MS, Oomen R, Thomas DY, Hallett MT (2006) Predicting the subcellular localization of viral proteins within a mammalian host cell. Virol J 3:24
105. Shen HB, Chou KC (2007) Virus-PLoc: a fusion classifier for predicting the subcellular localization of viral proteins within host and virus-infected cells. Biopolymers 85(3):233–240

106. Flower DR, North AC, Attwood TK (1993) Structure and sequence relationships in the lipocalins and related proteins. Protein Sci 2(5):753–761
107. Flower DR (1993) Structural Relationship of Streptavidin to the Calycin Protein Superfamily. FEBS Lett 333(1–2):99–102
108. Mayers C, Duffield M, Rowe S, Miller J, Lingard B, Hayward S, Titball RW (2003) Analysis of known bacterial protein vaccine antigens reveals biased physical properties and amino acid composition. Comp Funct Genomics 4(5):468–478
109. Andrade MA, O'Donoghue SI, Rost B (1998) Adaptation of protein surfaces to subcellular location. J Mol Biol 276(2):517–525
110. Secker A, Davies MN, Freitas AA, Clark EB, Timmis J, Flower DR (2010) Hierarchical classification of G-protein-coupled receptors with data-driven selection of attributes and classifiers. Int J Data Min Bioinform 4(2):191–210
111. Davies MN, Secker A, Halling-Brown M, Moss DS, Freitas AA, Timmis J, Clark E, Flower DR (2008) GPCRTree: online hierarchical classification of GPCR function. BMC Res Notes 1:67
112. Davies MN, Secker A, Freitas AA, Clark E, Timmis J, Flower DR (2008) Optimizing amino acid groupings for GPCR classification. Bioinformatics 24(18):1980–1986
113. Davies MN, Secker A, Freitas AA, Mendao M, Timmis J, Flower DR (2007) On the hierarchical classification of G protein-coupled receptors. Bioinformatics 23(23):3113–3118
114. Davies MN, Gloriam DE, Secker A, Freitas AA, Mendao M, Timmis J, Flower DR (2007) Proteomic applications of automated GPCR classification. Proteomics 7(16):2800–2814
115. Doytchinova IA, Flower DR (2007) **VaxiJen: a server for prediction of protective antigens, tumour antigens and subunit vaccines**. BMC Bioinformatics 8:4
116. Doytchinova IA, Flower DR (2007) Identifying candidate subunit vaccines using an alignment-independent method based on principal amino acid properties. Vaccine 25 (5):856–866
117. Wold S, Jonsson J, Sjostrom M, Sandberg M, Rannar S (1993) DNA and peptide sequences and chemical processes multivariately modeled by principal component analysis and partial least-squares projections to latent structures. Anal Chim Acta 277(2):239–253
118. Wold S, Eriksson L, Hellberg S, Jonsson J, Sjostrom M, Skagerberg B, Wikstrom C (1987) Principal property-values for 6 nonnatural amino-acids and their application to a structure activity relationship for oxytocin peptide analogs. Can J Chem 65(8):1814–1820
119. Dimitrov I, Garnev P, Flower DR, Doytchinova I (2010) Peptide binding to the HLA-DRB1 supertype: a proteochemometrics analysis. Eur J Med Chem 45(1):236–243
120. Kontijevskis A, Petrovska R, Yahorava S, Komorowski J, Wikberg JE (2009) Proteochemometrics mapping of the interaction space for retroviral proteases and their substrates. Bioorg Med Chem 17(14):5229–5237
121. Prusis P, Lapins M, Yahorava S, Petrovska R, Niyomrattanakit P, Katzenmeier G, Wikberg JE (2008) Proteochemometrics analysis of substrate interactions with dengue virus NS3 proteases. Bioorg Med Chem 16(20):9369–9377
122. Strombergsson H, Kryshtafovych A, Prusis P, Fidelis K, Wikberg JE, Komorowski J, Hvidsten TR (2006) Generalized modeling of enzyme-ligand interactions using proteochemometrics and local protein substructures. Proteins 65(3):568–579
123. Strombergsson H, Prusis P, Midelfart H, Lapinsh M, Wikberg JE, Komorowski J (2006) Rough set-based proteochemometrics modeling of G-protein-coupled receptor-ligand interactions. Proteins 63(1):24–34
124. Lapinsh M, Prusis P, Uhlen S, Wikberg JE (2005) Improved approach for proteochemometrics modeling: application to organic compound–amine G protein-coupled receptor interactions. Bioinformatics 21(23):4289–4296
125. Wikberg JE, Mutulis F, Mutule I, Veiksina S, Lapinsh M, Petrovska R, Prusis P (2003) Melanocortin receptors: ligands and proteochemometrics modeling. Ann N Y Acad Sci 994:21–26

126. Lapinsh M, Prusis P, Lundstedt T, Wikberg JE (2002) Proteochemometrics modeling of the interaction of amine G-protein coupled receptors with a diverse set of ligands. Mol Pharmacol 61(6):1465–1475
127. Hellberg S, Sjostrom M, Skagerberg B, Wold S (1987) Peptide quantitative structure-activity-relationships, a multivariate approach. J Med Chem 30(7):1126–1135
128. Jonsson J, Eriksson L, Hellberg S, Sjostrom M, Wold S (1989) Multivariate parametrization of 55 coded and non-coded amino-acids. Quant Struct Act Rel 8(3):204–209
129. Sandberg M, Eriksson L, Jonsson J, Sjostrom M, Wold S (1998) New chemical descriptors relevant for the design of biologically active peptides. A multivariate characterization of 87 amino acids. J Med Chem 41(14):2481–2491
130. Doytchinova IA, Flower DR (2008) Bioinformatic approach for identifying parasite and fungal candidate subunit vaccines. Open Vaccine J 1(1):4
131. Friedberg I, Harder T, Godzik A (2006) JAFA: a protein function annotation meta-server. Nucleic Acids Res 34:W379–W381, Web Server issue
132. Pawlowski M, Gajda MJ, Matlak R, Bujnicki JM (2008) MetaMQAP: a meta-server for the quality assessment of protein models. BMC Bioinformatics 9:403
133. Mallios RR (2003) A consensus strategy for combining HLA-DR binding algorithms. Hum Immunol 64(9):852–856
134. Dong HL, Sui YF (2005) Prediction of HLA-A2-restricted CTL epitope specific to HCC by SYFPEITHI combined with polynomial method. World J Gastroenterol 11(2):208–211
135. Mustafa AS, Shaban FA (2006) ProPred analysis and experimental evaluation of promiscuous T-cell epitopes of three major secreted antigens of Mycobacterium tuberculosis. Tuberculosis (Edinb) 86(2):115–124
136. Singh H, Raghava GP (2001) ProPred: prediction of HLA-DR binding sites. Bioinformatics 17(12):1236–1237
137. Mallios RR (2001) Predicting class II MHC/peptide multi-level binding with an iterative stepwise discriminant analysis meta-algorithm. Bioinformatics 17(10):942–948
138. Mallios RR (1999) Class II MHC quantitative binding motifs derived from a large molecular database with a versatile iterative stepwise discriminant analysis meta-algorithm. Bioinformatics 15(6):432–439
139. Mallios RR (1998) Iterative stepwise discriminant analysis: a meta-algorithm for detecting quantitative sequence motifs. J Comput Biol 5(4):703–711
140. Zhang GL, Khan AM, Srinivasan KN, August JT, Brusic V (2005) Neural models for predicting viral vaccine targets. J Bioinform Comput Biol 3(5):1207–1225
141. Huang L, Karpenko O, Murugan N, Dai Y (2007) Building a meta-predictor for MHC class II-binding peptides. Methods Mol Biol 409:355–364
142. Karpenko O, Huang L, Dai Y (2008) A probabilistic meta-predictor for the MHC class II binding peptides. Immunogenetics 60(1):25–36
143. Huang L, Karpenko O, Murugan N, Dai Y (2006) A meta-predictor for MHC class II binding peptides based on Naive Bayesian approach. Conf Proc IEEE Eng Med Biol Soc 1:5322–5325
144. Trost B, Bickis M, Kusalik A (2007) Strength in numbers: achieving greater accuracy in MHC-I binding prediction by combining the results from multiple prediction tools. Immunome Res 3:5
145. Wang P, Sidney J, Dow C, Mothe B, Sette A, Peters B (2008) A systematic assessment of MHC class II peptide binding predictions and evaluation of a consensus approach. PLoS Comput Biol 4(4):e1000048
146. Salim N, Holliday J, Willett P (2003) Combination of fingerprint-based similarity coefficients using data fusion. J Chem Inf Comput Sci 43(2):435–442
147. Basir O, Karray F, Zhu H (2005) Connectionist-based Dempster-Shafer evidential reasoning for data fusion. IEEE Trans Neural Netw 16(6):1513–1530

148. Sundaresh S, Randall A, Unal B, Petersen JM, Belisle JT, Hartley MG, Duffield M, Titball RW, Davies DH, Felgner PL et al (2007) From protein microarrays to diagnostic antigen discovery: a study of the pathogen Francisella tularensis. Bioinformatics 23(13):i508–i518
149. Doytchinova IA, Guan P, Flower DR (2006) EpiJen: a server for multistep T cell epitope prediction. BMC Bioinformatics 7:131
150. Vivona S, Bernante F, Filippini F (2006) NERVE: new enhanced reverse vaccinology environment. BMC Biotechnol 6:35
151. Harish N, Gupta R, Agarwal P, Scaria V, Pillai B (2006) DyNAVacS: an integrative tool for optimized DNA vaccine design. Nucleic Acids Res 34:W264–W266, Web Server issue
152. He Y, Xiang Z, Mobley HL (2010) Vaxign: the first web-based vaccine design program for reverse vaccinology and applications for vaccine development. J Biomed Biotechnol 2010:297505
153. Fell DA (2005) Enzymes, metabolites and fluxes. J Exp Bot 56(410):267–272

[illegible]

Chapter 4
Post-genomic Antigen Discovery: Bioinformatical Approaches to Reveal Novel T Cell Antigens of *Mycobacterium bovis*

Martin Vordermeier, Gareth J. Jones, Samantha Sampson, and Stephen V. Gordon

Abstract The elucidation of the genomes of pathogenic mycobacteria and the application of bioinformatic tools has greatly assisted the process of defining antigenic proteins for diagnosis of, and subunit vaccination against, bovine tuberculosis. By applying in silico genome comparisons or transcriptome comparisons, it was possible to prioritise potentially specific and immunogenic proteins for testing in infected or vaccinated cattle. These approaches led to the identification of antigens supporting discrimination of infected from vaccinated animals (DIVA diagnosis) or subunit vaccine candidates. Some progress has also been made to develop algorithms predicting peptides binding to bovine major histocompatibility complex class II molecules. The following chapter will review these advances and consider them in the context of bovine TB vaccine development programmes.

4.1 Novel Cattle Tuberculosis Vaccines

Bovine TB in cattle, caused mainly by *Mycobacterium bovis* (*M. bovis*), remains a major global animal health problem [1, 2] In England and Wales. The disease incidence has risen steadily since the mid-1980s and still remains high. Vaccination of cattle against *M. bovis* infection is being considered as one of the long-term policy options for reducing the risk and incidence of bovine TB in England, and progress in developing TB vaccines for cattle has been reviewed in a number of recent articles [3–6]. The most-promising and effective vaccination strategies against bovine TB in cattle are based on priming the immune system with BCG followed by boosting with subunit vaccines (*heterologous prime-boost strategy*), based on DNA [7, 8], protein [9], or viral subunit vaccines [10–12]. As these immunisation strategies result in

M. Vordermeier (✉)
Animal Health & Veterinary Laboratories Agency—Weybridge, Department for Bovine Tuberculosis, New Haw, Addlestone, Surrey, UK
e-mail: martin.vordermeier@ahvla.gsi.gov.uk

D.R. Flower and Y. Perrie (eds.), *Immunomic Discovery of Adjuvants and Candidate Subunit Vaccines*, Immunomics Reviews: 5, DOI 10.1007/978-1-4614-5070-2_4,

animals becoming tuberculin-test positive, complementary diagnostic reagents allowing the discrimination of infected from vaccinated animals (DIVA) are an essential requirement to continue with test and slaughter TB control strategies alongside vaccination. Bioinformatic approaches have been successfully applied over the last decade both in the search for DIVA targets and subunit vaccine candidates, and this review will present some of these findings.

Immune responses to TB in cattle are characterised by early and sustained cell-mediated immune responses post-infection with detectable serum responses emerging later in the infection cycle [13–15]. Consequently, the most widely used diagnostic assays, such as tuberculin skin testing or in vitro cytokine detection assays (e.g. the Bovigam interferon-gamma (IFN-γ) assay) are targeted at measuring cell-mediated immune responses.

In its original form, the Bovigam assay measures IFN-γ after stimulation of whole blood with avian or bovine tuberculin purified protein derivative (PPD) produced from *M. avium* or *M. bovis*, respectively [16, 17]. However, as PPD comprises a mix of hundreds of mycobacterial antigens, the specificity of the Bovigam assay in this form is compromised by BCG vaccination [18, 19]. Fortunately, the Bovigam test can be readily modified to accommodate specific antigens more suitable as DIVA antigens, allowing discrimination between infected and vaccinated animals.

4.2 DIVA: Proof of Principle Antigens

Two major antigenic DIVA targets recognised by T cells from infected cattle or humans are ESAT-6 and CFP-10 [20, 21], encoded by genes in the RD1 region of the *M. bovis* genome, a locus that is deleted from all BCG strains [22–25]. When used as a diagnostic antigen, ESAT-6 discriminated between infected and BCG-vaccinated cattle [18, 19, 26]. Peptides derived from ESAT-6 and CFP-10 induced equivalent responses to recombinant proteins in *M. bovis*-infected cattle, but did not elicit responses in BCG-vaccinated cattle. In contrast, bovine PPD-biased responses were detected in more than 70 % of BCG-vaccinated animals [26]. Unfortunately, the sensitivity ESAT-6 and CFP-10 was still below that of tuberculin, necessitating the identification of further antigens to increase overall test sensitivity.

4.3 Elucidation of Sequences of Mycobacterial Species

Since the first mycobacterial genome (*M. tuberculosis* [27]) was completed in 1998, the genomes of many pathogenic and non-pathogenic mycobacterial species have been elucidated including *M. bovis* [23, 28], *M. bovis* BCG Pasteur [29], *M. avium* subsp. *paratuberculosis* [30], and *M. avium* subsp. *avium*. A comprehensive mycobacterial genome resource, therefore, exists which allows the systematic search for additional differential diagnostic candidates (Table 4.1). In addition, micro-array

Table 4.1 Characteristics of mycobacterial genomes

Species	Size (Mb)	CDS[a]	% GC	Accession
M. tuberculosis H37Rv	4.4	4,012	65.9	NC_000962
M. bovis 2122/97	4.3	3,952	65.6	NC_002945
M. bovis BCG Pasteur	4.4	3,954	65.6	NC_008769
M. leprae TN	3.3	1,604	57.8	NC_002677
M. avium 104	5.5	5,120	69.2	NC_008595
M. avium subsp. paratuberculosis K10	4.8	4,350	69.3	NC_002944
M. smegmatis mc^{2}155	6.9	6,716	67.4	NC_008596

[a]based on most recent version of annotation

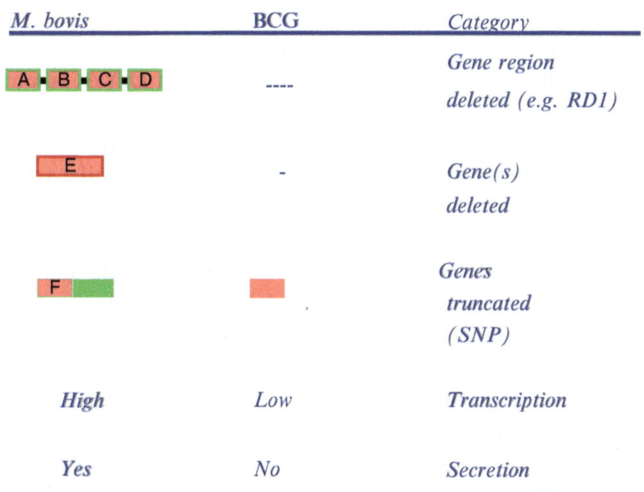

Fig. 4.1 Antigen mining strategies applied to define antigens for DIVA diagnosis

technology has made the systematic evaluation of mycobacterial gene expression possible. Based on these technologies, a number of approaches have been applied for rational antigen mining. These include: comparative genome analysis to identify antigen-encoding regions or individual genes deleted from BCG; comparative transcriptome analysis with the aim of defining genes that are highly expressed in *M. bovis* but lowly or not expressed in BCG; or identification of secreted or potentially secreted antigens (see Fig. 4.1). We will briefly describe some of the results obtained with these approaches in the next section.

4.4 Mining Genome Information

4.4.1 Antigens Encoded by Genome Regions Deleted from BCG

Twenty-eight potential DIVA antigens are encoded by the RD1, RD2, and RD14 gene regions that are deleted from the genome of BCG Pasteur [23, 29]. Cockle et al. determined their immunogenicity and specificity in *M. bovis*-infected or BCG-vaccinated cattle. For this and all the other studies described below from our laboratories, we have applied a high-throughput, cost-effective biological screening system which utilises overlapping pools of synthetic peptides spanning the complete sequences of the target proteins combined with a whole blood IFN-γ secretion assay. This screening system revealed that seven of these RD-encoded proteins were recognised at high frequencies (41–86 %) in infected cattle. However, despite all seven genes being deleted from the BCG genome, only three proteins (Rv1986, Rv3872, and Rv3878) were not recognised by T cells from BCG-vaccinated cattle [31]. The most frequently recognised peptides from Rv1986, Rv3872, and Rv3878, as well as similar peptides from Rv3873, Rv3879c, Rv0288, and Rv3019c were identified and formulated together with peptides from ESAT-6 and CFP-10 into a larger peptide cocktail [32]. Some of these antigens were also described as specific for *M. bovis* in other studies [33, 34], although their DIVA potential was not assessed in these studies.

This peptide cocktail was significantly better than tuberculin for identifying skin test-negative animals with confirmed bovine tuberculosis, whilst still maintaining its DIVA potential. This result indicated that the identification of potentially discriminatory peptides is not necessarily restricted to antigens that in their entirety are not recognised by T cells from BCG-vaccinated cattle (such as Rv1986, Rv3872, and Rv3878); it is also possible to define empirically by epitope surgery DIVA peptides within the sequences of apparently non-specific antigens that as complete proteins are recognised in BCG-vaccinated cattle [32]. Additional studies with this peptide cocktail, however, suggested that its sensitivity advantage could largely be realised only in freshly sampled blood, but not in blood stored overnight before the blood cultures were initiated (Vordermeier, unpublished data). As the Bovigam test in GB is routinely performed on blood stored overnight [35], additional antigens had to be found to improve ESAT-6 and CFP-10 sensitivity in this testing strategy.

It should be noted here that antigens that prove unsuitable for DIVA diagnosis can still be useful for other applications, for example, as subunit vaccine candidates particularly when used in heterologous prime-boost scenarios in combination with BCG. Indeed, for this application, recognition after BCG vaccination is a requirement for antigens to be able to function as a booster vaccine. An example of such an antigen is the ESAT-6 family member TB10.4 (Rv0288) that is strongly recognised by humans and cattle infected with *M. bovis* or *M. tuberculosis*. It is now being assessed as a vaccine candidate for human [36] and bovine tuberculosis (Hogarth, Vordermeier et al., unpublished data).

4.4.2 T Cell Cross-Reactivity

To explore why four of the seven antigens discussed in the previous paragraph were not specific despite being deleted from the BCG Pasteur genome, we identified the

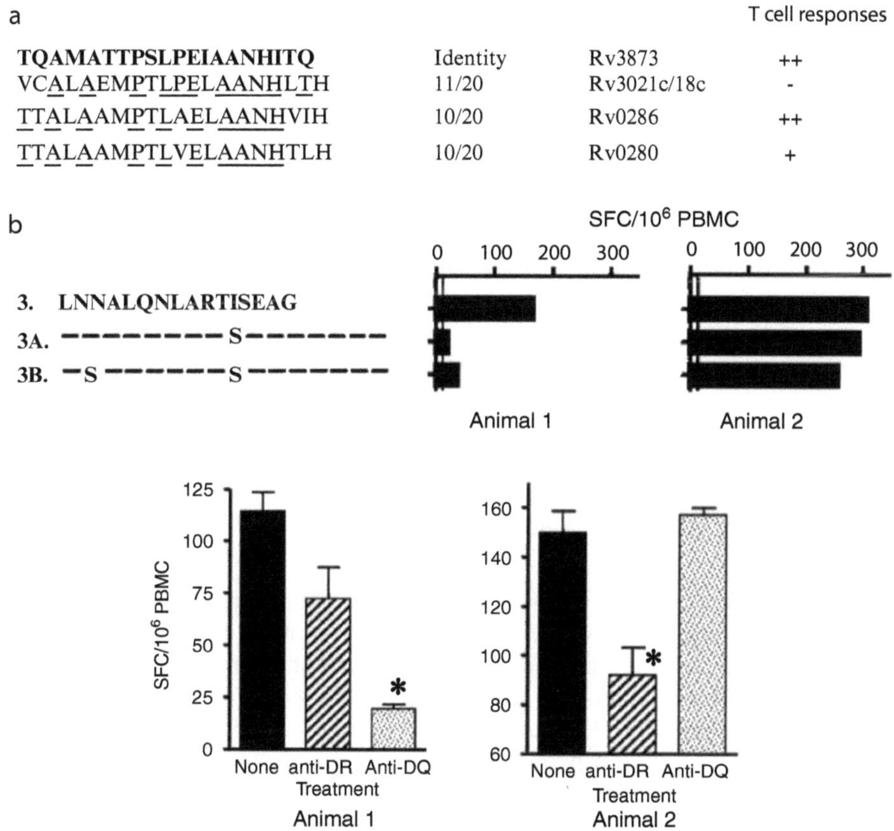

Fig. 4.2 The challenge of predicting T cell cross-reactivity between proteins. A. Recognition of closely related peptide sequences derived from otherwise unrelated proteins. B. Recognition of closely related ESAT-6-derived peptide homologues from *M. bovis* (peptide 3) and two *M. kansasii* isolates (3A and 3B). Read-out system: IFN-γ ELIPSOT assays. Recognition of peptide 3 was BoLA-DQ-restriced in animal 1, and BoLA-DR restricted in animal 2 (bottom left and bottom right panels, respectively). Modified from [38]

epitope-carrying peptides within their sequences by testing individual peptides rather than peptide pools. We then performed BLAST searches using these 20-mer peptide sequences, instead of the whole protein sequences, to search for sequence identity between them and proteins encoded outside the RD regions. We found small regions with high degrees of amino acid sequence identity in otherwise unrelated proteins [37]. When we synthesised the encoded peptides and used them in IFN-γ assays, we could demonstrate that they were cross-reactive; this, therefore, explains the lack of DIVA specificity of these antigens (Figure 4.2a shows an epitope from Rv3873 and its sequence match across Rv0280, Rv0286 and Rv3018c/3021c, Rv0286). Interestingly, the degree of sequence identity or similarity alone did not necessarily predict cross-reactivity (Fig. 4.2a). This makes it difficult to predict T cell cross-reactivity based solely on the primary epitope sequence. The complexity of T cell cross-reactivity was further illustrated in a study evaluating the epitope specificity between *M. bovis* ESAT-6 and its *M. kansasii* homologues that exhibit >95 % sequence identity overall. To our surprise, we could demonstrate that *M. kansasii*-derived peptides that shared 14/16 and 15/16 amino acids with the corresponding epitopic *M. bovis* peptide were not recognised by T cells from a proportion of *M. bovis*-infected cows, whilst other *M. bovis*-infected cattle reacted to all three peptides, i.e. displayed complete cross-reactivity (Fig. 4.2b) [38]. On closer analysis, we demonstrated that these peptides were recognised in the context of different major histocompatibility complex (MHC) class II restriction elements: the 'specific' epitope within this peptide was recognised in the context of BoLA-DQ, whilst the 'cross-reactive' epitope was recognised in the context of BoLA-DR (Fig. 4.2b) [38].

4.4.3 Antigens Deleted from the BCG Genome, or with Truncated or Frame-Shifted Amino Acid Portions

Iterative bioinformatic analysis was performed to identify potential antigens for which the encoding genes were deleted from BCG compared to *M. bovis*, or that harboured mutations that truncated coding sequences, or that altered the amino acid sequence of the encoded protein. The file of 3,592 *M. bovis* genes was then used to perform stand-alone BLASTP and TBLASTN searches against the *M. avium* subsp. *avium* and *M. avium* subsp. *paratuberculosis* genome sequences to identify *M. bovis* proteins with low score and E values (*M. bovis* unique proteins). In total, 40 such genes were selected for immunological analysis. However, none of them were recognised well in *M. bovis*-infected cattle (responder frequencies <25 %), nor did any of them complement ESAT-6/CFP-10 by increasing overall test sensitivity (Vordermeier, Ewer, Gordon, unpublished results).

4.4.4 Analysis of Proteins Predicted to Be Secreted (Secretome Antigens)

A longstanding hypothesis in tuberculosis research is that active secretion of antigenic proteins by mycobacteria induces strong cellular immune responses in the host. Thus, we prepared a list of all predicted potentially secreted *M. bovis* antigens (secretome) by the in silico analysis of the *M. tuberculosis* H37Rv genome. Selection criteria were (i) the presence of signal sequences (e.g. Rv0192A, Rv0559c, etc.), (ii) linkage to ESX loci (e.g. Rv3449, Rv3883c, etc.), (iii) members of the ESX family (e.g. Rv1197, Rv1198, etc.), or (iv) prior evidence for secretion from the literature. Pools of overlapping peptides spanning 119 *M. bovis* secretome proteins were screened for their ability to stimulate an IFN-γ

response using blood from either TB-reactor or BCG-vaccinated cattle. A hierarchy of immunogenicity of the secretome antigens was observed in TB-reactor animals, with members of the ESAT-6 protein family being amongst the most immunodominant proteins thus identified [39]. In order to identify potential DIVA reagents, the full complement of secretome antigens were also screened in BCG-vaccinated cattle [39]. Of the eight most frequently recognised peptide pools (i.e. those that induced an IFN-γ response in over half of *M. bovis*-infected animals studied), pools corresponding to Rv3020c and Rv2346c were not recognised by any of the BCG-vaccinated animals, suggesting that they may contain peptides with potential application as DIVA reagents. Although the other six peptide pools induced IFN-γ responses in some BCG-vaccinated animals, elucidation of the individual peptide recognised by T cells from infected cattle revealed individual peptides that were specific and induced IFN-γ responses in TB-reactor animals only [40]. These results informed the formulation of a cocktail of nine peptides representing multiple antigen targets. This cocktail was recognised by 54 % of TB-reactor animals but did not induce responses in any BCG-vaccinated animal studied, although our study using a relatively small number of animals did not demonstrate that these reagents increased overall sensitivity compared to ESAT-6/CFP-10 alone. Thus, larger field trials are required to demonstrate the potential of these antigens to increase ESAT-6-/CFP-10-dependent diagnostic sensitivity without compromising specificity in BCG-vaccinated animals.

4.5 Transcriptome Analysis

4.5.1 Comparative Transcriptome Analysis

The transcriptome represents the complete gene expression profile of an organism under defined conditions. By DNA microarray technology, we compared the transcriptomes of BCG and *M. bovis* after infection of bovine macrophages (*comparative transcriptomics*), in the hope of identifying antigen-encoding genes induced by *M. bovis*, but not BCG, in vivo. Genes strongly expressed across different in vitro growth conditions (the invarisome, [41]) were also assessed. The feasibility of the transcriptome approach, for example, was supported by the study of the serodominant antigens MPB70 and MPB83 that are weakly expressed in some BCG strains compared to *M. bovis* [42, 43]. Overall, our studies did not establish a strong correlation between the level of a gene's expression and immunogenicity [44]. This approach may need to be revisited, however, as a recent study using humans infected with *M. tuberculosis* indicated that expression data combined with epitope prediction targeted at HLA-DR alleles dominant in given target populations might be able to predict antigenicity (Wilkinson et al., unpublished observation).

Only the novel antigen Rv3615c was recognised by blood cells isolated from *M. bovis*-infected animals [44], but not by blood cells from uninfected or BCG-vaccinated cattle [44]. Further, Rv3615c was recognised strongly in a subset of infected cattle that escaped detection by ESAT-6/CFP-10. The application of this protein in combination with ESAT-6 and CFP-10, therefore, increased the overall DIVA performance [44], and studies are underway to extend these data in international field studies in different cattle populations. Recently, our findings have been confirmed by a study of human tuberculosis patients [45]. Interestingly, Rv3615c is expressed in BCG and it is therefore not immediately obvious why it is not recognised after BCG vaccination. Our hypothesis was that unlike in *M. bovis*, Rv3615c would not be secreted by BCG because its secretion is dependent on the presence of the intact esx-1 locus, encoded by the RD1 region which is deleted in BCG (reviewed in [46]). ESX-1-dependent secretion of Rv3615c was originally demonstrated using defined *M. tuberculosis* mutants (REF), and has subsequently been verified for BCG [45].

4.5.2 Stage-Specific Antigens

Long latency periods are a hallmark of *M. tuberculosis* infection of humans and efforts are underway to define antigens that are specific for this stage of disease. Thus, several stage-specific 'latency antigens' of the DosR regulon [47] genes are more strongly recognised in latently infected humans compared to patients with active tuberculosis [48–51]. Another class of potential stage-specific antigens could derive from genes of the enduring hypoxia response (EHR) [52]. The EHR defines a group of *M. tuberculosis* genes that are specifically induced when the bacilli are exposed in vitro to low oxygen conditions, which is thought to mimic the environment encountered by mycobacteria during latent infection. Although well described in humans, latent mycobacterial infection in cattle remains poorly understood. We have tested a selection of DosR regulon and EHR gene products for their antigenicity in infected and vaccinated cattle, with the aim of identifying antigens that may potentially disclose cattle with latent *M. bovis* infection. As all of the DosR regulon proteins screened were poorly recognised by *M. bovis*-infected animals [53], we focused our attention on the panel of EHR antigens. Thus, 29 EHR antigens were screened for their ability to stimulate an immune response in TB-reactor cattle. The data demonstrated a hierarchy of responder frequencies, with some proteins recognised by about half of the infected animals tested with responses largely IFN-γ biased [53]. The EHR antigen Rv0188 was recognised predominantly in animals presenting with limited visible pathology, whereas responses to ESAT-6/CFP-10 or the other EHR antigens were prevalent across the pathology spectrum [53]. This could support the concept for their role in latency. However, when we determined the production of additional bovine PPD-induced biomarkers significantly greater production of the pro-inflammatory cytokine IL-1β was found in animals recognising Rv0188 (i.e. those with limited pathology) [53]. These results, therefore, supported the idea that animals recognising the EHR antigen Rv0188 are at early stages of infection rather than in a state of latency. Studies to determine if Rv0188 can be used as a DIVA antigen are underway. Alternatively, responses to Rv0188 may identify a subset of animals that is capable of limiting infection.

4.5.3 Potential Antigen Mining Based on Small Antisense RNA

Small RNAs (sRNA) are short RNA molecules of 50–500 nucleotides in length that were first identified in bacterial plasmids. The advent of next-generation sequencing technologies and oligonuceotide tiling arrays has allowed the discovery of sRNA molecules in many bacteria, including *Escherichia coli* and *Salmonella enterica* Typhimurium. Arnvig and Young first described nine sRNAs in *M. tuberculosis,* while McDonough and colleagues reported 34 novel sRNAs in *M. bovis* BCG [54, 55]. The role of these sRNA molecules is generally in gene regulation, with the majority acting to silence or enhance gene transcription or translation [56]. While sometimes referred to as 'non-coding' RNAs, this nomenclature is incorrect, as it is known that some sRNA molecules encode peptides. Recent work has identified peptides encoded by sRNAs in *Bacillus subtilis* [57], *Staphylococcus aureus* [58], and *E. coli* [59]. Hence it appears that sRNAs are a previously unappreciated source of short peptides produced by the bacterial cell. In our initial work with *M. bovis,* we have analysed the sRNAs produced by four molecular types of *M. bovis* that encompass the genetic diversity of GB *M. bovis* strains. These data revealed a set of differentially expressed sRNA molecules across the *M. bovis* strains associated and frequently linked to single nucleotide mutations (SNPs) in their genomes. The genome sequences of *M. bovis* and BCG have revealed more than 700 point mutations across the two strains; hence it is probable that some of this SNP variation leads to differential expression of sRNAs across *M. bovis* and BCG. As some sRNAs encode peptides which may be antigenic, screening of sRNAs across *M. bovis* and BCG could lead the identification of novel antigens to be used in differential diagnostics. We are currently testing this hypothesis in our laboratories.

4.6 Predicting Epitopes Recognised by Bovine MHC-Class II Restricted CD4$^+$ T Cells

BoLA class II complex consists of one DR gene pair and up to two DQ gene pairs per haplotype, and is highly polymorphic [60, 61]. Pathogen-derived epitopes can be recognised both in the context of BoLA-DR and BoLA-DQ [62]. Moreover, identical peptides from mycobacterial antigens can be recognised in cattle both in the context of BoLA-DR and BoLA-DQ molecules [38]. Knowledge of MHC restriction and anchor residues of epitopes recognised by bovine T cells is limited, with binding motifs defined only for a small number of BoLA class I molecules [63, 64] and even more tentative data available for motifs predicting binding to BoLA class II molecules [64, 65]. In contrast to other species (e.g. humans and mice), experimental peptide-binding data for BoLA class II-restricted peptides are therefore limited and no dedicated computational prediction tools are currently available to predict BoLA class II-restricted peptides, although a programme predicting peptides binding to the BoLA class I allele A11 has been described [66].

Previously, we achieved some success using ProPred software (which calculates the likelihood of peptides binding to human HLA-DR alleles (http://www.imtech.res.in/raghava/ProPred [67])) to predict peptides recognised by bovine T cells [68]. In a recent study [69], a novel structure-based prediction method (Hepitom) was developed based upon evaluating the binding free energies between BoLA DRB3 and a panel of peptides derived from the sequences of 13 *M. bovis* antigens (Fig. 4.3a). Using immunogenicity data derived from responses of *M. bovis*-infected cattle after stimulation with 105 individual overlapping peptides, we have compared the sensitivity and specificity of both the Hepitom and the ProPred models to predict peptides that are recognised by bovine T cells [69]. A range of immunogenicity cut-offs were evaluated, the most stringent being the prediction of the most promiscuous epitopic peptides recognised by more than 40 % of infected animals (responder frequencies >40 %). With this most stringent cut-off, Hepitom and ProPred models predicted 62 % and 77 % of the empirically defined immunogenic peptides (sensitivity). In contrast, 66 % and 34 % of the non-immunogenic peptides were predicted to be non-binder (specificity). Thus, the Hepitom model was able to identify a larger proportion peptides correctly than ProPred (diagnostic accuracy = 0.9 and 0.74, respectively, Fig. 4.3b) [69].

The advantages of applying predictive algorithms to pre-select peptides include the use of fewer peptides in antigen screening assays, saving time and costs. However, one requirement of this approach would be that the use of selected peptides only does not compromise the ability to detect a similar number of immunogenic antigens when compared to using the full complement of overlapping peptides. To validate the different approaches, we compared the IFN-γ responses of TB-reactor animals to 11 secreted proteins using either the full complement of overlapping peptides ($n = 85$), or those peptides predicted by either the Hepitom model ($n = 31$) or ProPred ($n = 59$) to contain binding motifs. Using the most stringent cut-off level for immunogenicity, 7 out of the 11 proteins were identified using the full complement of overlapping peptides. Encouragingly, all but one of these seven antigens were also identified as immunogenic when just the 31 peptides predicted by the Hepitom model were used. In contrast, when using the ProPred-predicted peptides, only four of the seven antigens gave responder frequencies comparable to the unbiased complete set of peptides [69]. Thus, whilst having only medium sensitivity and specificity to correctly predict peptides recognised by bovine CD4+ T cells, the Hepitom model can be used to reduce the number of peptides required and thus their purchase costs, without loss of the sensitivity to identify strong antigens correctly.

4.7 All Proteins Are Equal but Some Are more Equal than Others

Over the last decade, we have assessed the immunogenicity in infected cattle of more than 500 proteins. The observed hierarchy of responses is shown in Fig. 4.4 and ranges from proteins not recognised at all (0 % responder frequencies) to antigens being recognised by more than 90 % of animals tested. Although the selection of proteins tested was not unbiased, with secreted antigens, for example, being over-represented, it is still possible to determine if some classes of proteins are better recognised than others. We grouped the proteins in two categories based on their responder frequencies; those that were recognised by at least 30 % of infected cattle (high responders) and those that were recognised below 30 % (medium to low responders). This split the dataset into 80 proteins that were highly recognised and 425 in the low/medium recognition group. Although antigens predicted to be secreted (secretome) were distributed across both groups, they were significantly more highly represented in the high-responder group (Fig. 4.4, insert, $P < 0.0001$). Interestingly, just being secreted did not necessarily mean that proteins are highly recognised (Fig. 4.3, insert), because this predominance of secreted proteins in the high response group was largely due to the strong recognition of proteins of the ESAT-6 family of proteins: all of the ESAT-6 family members tested clustered in the high-responder group and indeed constituted more than 50 % of the highly recognised secretome proteins (21/41, Fig. 4.4 insert). In addition, proteins of the PE and PPE protein families were also significantly overrepresented in the high-responder group (Fig. 4.4, insert, $P = 0.001$). These families of around 200 genes are characterised by conserved proline-glutamic acid (PE) or proline-proline-glutamic acid (PPE) motifs near their N-termini [27].

What could be the reason for the immunodominance of ESAT-6 family members and PE and PPE family proteins? The genes encoding ten of these ESAT-6 family proteins studied are located within the ESX1-5 loci, which encode novel type VII secretion systems responsible for the export of ESAT-6 family proteins, as well as other proteins [46]. The remainder are encoded by genes located outside of these intact loci [70], raising questions as to how, or if, these proteins are secreted. Given the high degree of amino acid similarity and the fact that immunogenicity was not dependent on the inclusion of the proteins in distinct ESX secretory systems, we speculated that the immune response to these antigens was, in part, driven by the recognition of antigenic epitopes located in conserved regions shared among numerous proteins, effectively increasing the antigenic load. Indeed, peptide-mapping experiments revealed that a proportion of (but not all) antigenic epitopes were located in the highly conserved regions shared between numerous ESAT-6

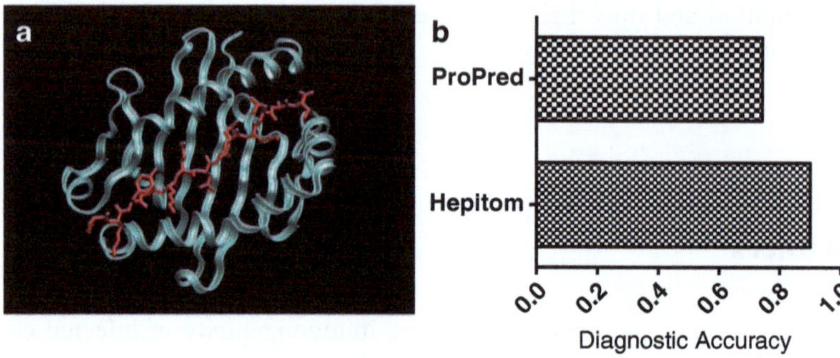

Fig. 4.3 Predicting peptides recognised by bovine T cells. (**a**) Predicted structure of the BoLA DRB3/peptide complex restricted to the peptide binding groove only. The BoLA DRB3 molecule is shown in blue while an influenza reference peptide PKYVKQNTLKLAT is shown in red. (**b**). Proportion of peptides correctly assigned (Diagnostic accuracy) by ProPred or Hepitom models. Based on 13/105 assessed peptides to be recognised by more than 40 % of infected cattle (prevalence = 0.12). Diagnostic accuracy = Prevalence × sensitivity + (1−Prevalence/specificity)

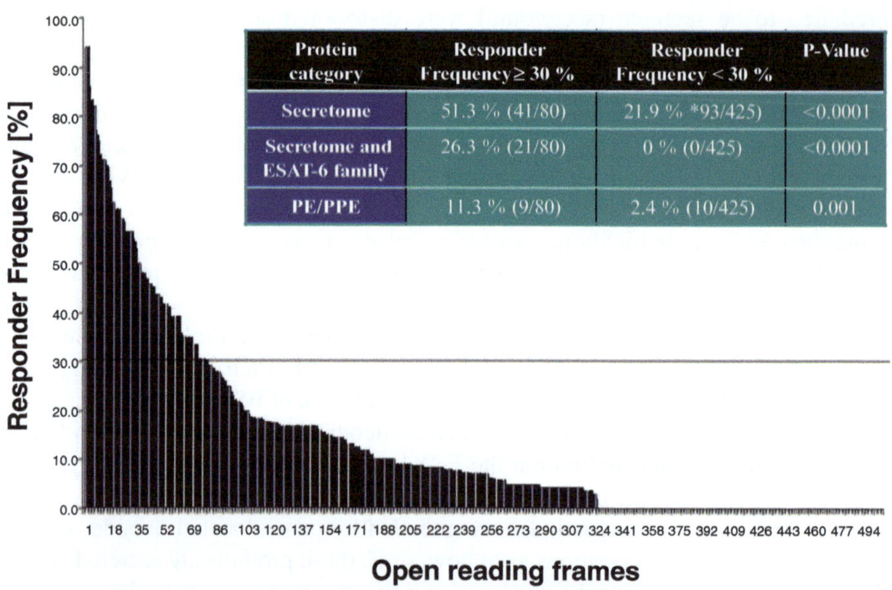

Protein category	Responder Frequency ≥ 30 %	Responder Frequency < 30 %	P-Value
Secretome	51.3 % (41/80)	21.9 % *93/425)	<0.0001
Secretome and ESAT-6 family	26.3 % (21/80)	0 % (0/425)	<0.0001
PE/PPE	11.3 % (9/80)	2.4 % (10/425)	0.001

Fig. 4.4 Response hierarchy of a set of *M. bovis*/*M. tuberculosis* antigens tested in infected cattle. Data for 505 proteins screened as peptide cocktails using IFN-γ secretion as read-out system. Results are expressed as the proportion of animals recognising a given protein (responder frequency in %). Horizontal line segregates proteins recognised by at least 30 % of animals (high responders) from those recognised by less than 30 % (medium to non-responders). Insert: Distribution of secreted (secretome), ESAT-6 or PE/PPE family members in the high and medium to non-responder subsets. P-values were determined using the Fisher's exact test

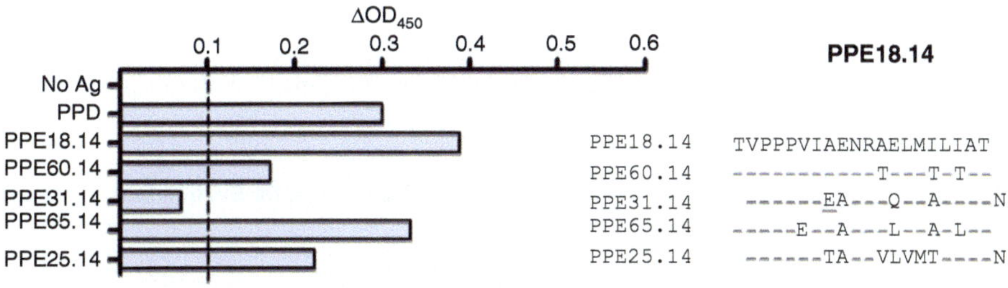

Fig. 4.5 IFN-γ responses of short-term T cell lines to potentially cross-reactive PPE peptides. Short-term T cell lines were raised by primary stimulation of bovine PBMC with individual peptides. Cells were restimulated with selected peptides, predicted to be immunologically cross-reactive. The amino acid sequence of the initial stimulation peptide is shown in alignment with restimulation peptides. Responses are shown as ΔOD450 values, and the dashed line indicates the positivity cut-off value of 0.1

proteins [39]. Recently, a comprehensive analysis of the immunogenicity of 36 PE/PPE proteins in cattle infected with *M. bovis* was performed, leading to the identification of immunogenic PE/PPE-derived peptides. Sequence analysis of these immunogenic peptides also revealed wide-spread antigenic cross-reactivity associated with their recognition. An example for one such peptide is presented in Fig. 4.5, where a T cell line raised against peptide PPE18.14 produced IFN-γ in response to stimulation with a number of closely related peptides derived from other PPE proteins [71]. Thus, these observations studying two independent protein families support the hypothesis raised above that their immunogenicity is in part related to the immunodominance of epitopes that are shared across family members. In addition, these observations are not congruent with the hypothesis that these proteins (ESAT-6 family, PE/PPE) contribute to antigenic variation in tuberculosis.

4.8 Conclusions

The elucidation of the genomes of pathogenic mycobacteria has revolutionised the art of defining antigenic proteins for diagnosis and subunit vaccination. However, our data also highlighted the limitations of these approaches, namely that approaches based exclusively on bioinformatics can neither reliably predict the immunogenicity/antigenicity of a mycobacterial protein, nor its specificity. Therefore, once potential antigens have been predicted by either in silico comparisons or expression profiling, they still need to be empirically and individually screened by testing infected or vaccinated cattle. Nonetheless, the use of bioinformatical analysis approaches discussed herein has led to the identification of antigens supporting DIVA diagnosis such as Rv3615c, or vaccine candidates such as Rv0288. These antigens are now being validated in larger trials (DIVA antigens) or tested in vaccination/experimental *M. bovis* challenge models (subunit candidates).

Application of DIVA antigens as skin test reagents is also being actively pursued [72]. Thus, we believe that bioinformatic approaches represent valuable tools to help prioritise potential antigens for empirical immunological evaluation for maximum benefit where resources are limited.

Acknowledgments These studies were supported by the Department for Environment, Food and Rural Affairs UK and the Wellcome Trust.

References

1. LoBue PA, Enarson DA, Thoen CO (2010) Tuberculosis in humans and animals: an overview. Int J Tuberc Lung Dis 14(9):1075–1078
2. Thoen CO, Lobue PA, Enarson DA, Kaneene JB, de Kantor IN (2009) Tuberculosis: a re-emerging disease in animals and humans. Vet Ital 45(1):135–181
3. Buddle BM, Wedlock DN, Denis M (2006) Progress in the development of tuberculosis vaccines for cattle and wildlife. Vet Microbiol 112(2–4):191–200
4. Buddle BM, Wedlock DN, Denis M, Vordermeier HM, Hewinson RG (2011) Update on vaccination of cattle and wildlife populations against tuberculosis. Vet Microbiol 151 (1–2):14–22. doi:S0378-1135(11)00102-7 [pii] 10.1016/j.vetmic.2011.02.021
5. Hogarth PJ, Hewinson RG, Vordermeier HM (2006) Development of vaccines against bovine tuberculosis. J Pharm Pharmacol 58(6):749–757
6. Vordermeier HM, Chambers MA, Buddle BM, Pollock JM, Hewinson RG (2006) Progress in the development of vaccines and diagnostic reagents to control tuberculosis in cattle. Vet J 171 (2):229–244
7. Skinner MA, Buddle BM, Wedlock DN, Keen D, de Lisle GW, Tascon RE, Ferraz JC, Lowrie DB, Cockle PJ, Vordermeier HM, Hewinson RG (2003) A DNA prime-Mycobacterium bovis BCG boost vaccination strategy for cattle induces protection against bovine tuberculosis. Infect Immun 71(9):4901–4907
8. Skinner MA, Wedlock DN, de Lisle GW, Cooke MM, Tascon RE, Ferraz JC, Lowrie DB, Vordermeier HM, Hewinson RG, Buddle BM (2005) The order of prime-boost vaccination of neonatal calves with Mycobacterium bovis BCG and a DNA vaccine encoding mycobacterial proteins Hsp65, Hsp70, and Apa is not critical for enhancing protection against bovine tuberculosis. Infect Immun 73(7):4441–4444
9. Wedlock DN, Skinner MA, de Lisle GW, Vordermeier HM, Hewinson RG, Hecker R, van Drunen Littel-van den Hurk S, Babiuk LA, Buddle BM (2005) Vaccination of cattle with Mycobacterium bovis culture filtrate proteins and CpG oligodeoxynucleotides induces protection against bovine tuberculosis. Vet Immunol Immunopathol 106(1–2):53–63
10. Vordermeier HM, Huygen K, Singh M, Hewinson RG, Xing Z (2006) Immune responses induced in cattle by vaccination with a recombinant adenovirus expressing Mycobacterial antigen 85A and Mycobacterium bovis BCG. Infect Immun 74(2):1416–1418
11. Vordermeier HM, Rhodes SG, Dean G, Goonetilleke N, Huygen K, Hill AV, Hewinson RG, Gilbert SC (2004) Cellular immune responses induced in cattle by heterologous prime-boost vaccination using recombinant viruses and bacille Calmette-Guerin. Immunology 112 (3):461–470
12. Vordermeier HM, Villarreal-Ramos B, Cockle PJ, McAulay M, Rhodes SG, Thacker T, Gilbert SC, McShane H, Hill AV, Xing Z, Hewinson RG (2009) Viral booster vaccines improve Mycobacterium bovis BCG-induced protection against bovine tuberculosis. Infect Immun 77(8):3364–3373. doi:IAI.00287-09 [pii] 10.1128/IAI.00287-09

13. Neill SD, Bryson DG, Pollock JM (2001) Pathogenesis of tuberculosis in cattle. Tuberculosis (Edinb) 81(1–2):79–86
14. Pollock JM, McNair J, Welsh MD, Girvin RM, Kennedy HE, Mackie DP, Neill SD (2001) Immune responses in bovine tuberculosis. Tuberculosis (Edinb) 81(1–2):103–107
15. Ritacco V, Lopez B, De Kantor IN, Barrera L, Errico F, Nader A (1991) Reciprocal cellular and humoral immune responses in bovine tuberculosis. Res Vet Sci 50(3):365–367
16. Rothel JS, Jones SL, Corner LA, Cox JC, Wood PR (1990) A sandwich enzyme immunoassay for bovine interferon-gamma and its use for the detection of tuberculosis in cattle. Aust Vet J 67(4):134–137
17. Rothel JS, Jones SL, Corner LA, Cox JC, Wood PR (1992) The gamma-interferon assay for diagnosis of bovine tuberculosis in cattle: conditions affecting the production of gamma-interferon in whole blood culture. Aust Vet J 69(1):1–4
18. Buddle BM, Parlane NA, Keen DL, Aldwell FE, Pollock JM, Lightbody K, Andersen P (1999) Differentiation between Mycobacterium bovis BCG-vaccinated and M. bovis-infected cattle by using recombinant mycobacterial antigens. Clin Diagn Lab Immunol 6(1):1–5
19. Vordermeier HM, Cockle PC, Whelan A, Rhodes S, Palmer N, Bakker D, Hewinson RG (1999) Development of diagnostic reagents to differentiate between Mycobacterium bovis BCG vaccination and M. bovis infection in cattle. Clin Diagn Lab Immunol 6(5):675–682
20. Pollock JM, Andersen P (1997) Predominant recognition of the ESAT-6 protein in the first phase of interferon with Mycobacterium bovis in cattle. Infect Immun 65(7):2587–2592
21. Pollock JM, Andersen P (1997) The potential of the ESAT-6 antigen secreted by virulent mycobacteria for specific diagnosis of tuberculosis. J Infect Dis 175(5):1251–1254
22. Behr MA, Wilson MA, Gill WP, Salamon H, Schoolnik GK, Rane S, Small PM (1999) Comparative genomics of BCG vaccines by whole-genome DNA microarray. Science 284 (5419):1520–1523
23. Garnier T, Eiglmeier K, Camus JC, Medina N, Mansoor H, Pryor M, Duthoy S, Grondin S, Lacroix C, Monsempe C, Simon S, Harris B, Atkin R, Doggett J, Mayes R, Keating L, Wheeler PR, Parkhill J, Barrell BG, Cole ST, Gordon SV, Hewinson RG (2003) The complete genome sequence of Mycobacterium bovis. Proc Natl Acad Sci USA 100(13):7877–7882
24. Gordon SV, Brosch R, Billault A, Garnier T, Eiglmeier K, Cole ST (1999) Identification of variable regions in the genomes of tubercle bacilli using bacterial artificial chromosome arrays. Mol Microbiol 32(3):643–655
25. Mahairas GG, Sabo PJ, Hickey MJ, Singh DC, Stover CK (1996) Molecular analysis of genetic differences between Mycobacterium bovis BCG and virulent M. bovis. J Bacteriol 178 (5):1274–1282
26. Vordermeier HM, Whelan A, Cockle PJ, Farrant L, Palmer N, Hewinson RG (2001) Use of synthetic peptides derived from the antigens ESAT-6 and CFP-10 for differential diagnosis of bovine tuberculosis in cattle. Clin Diagn Lab Immunol 8(3):571–578
27. Cole ST, Brosch R, Parkhill J, Garnier T, Churcher C, Harris D, Gordon SV, Eiglmeier K, Gas S, Barry CE, Tekaia F, Badcock K, Basham D, Brown D, Chillingworth T, Connor R, Davies R, Devlin K, Feltwell T, Gentles S, Hamlin N, Holroyd S, Hornsby T, Jagels K, Krogh A, McLean J, Moule S, Murphy L, Oliver K, Osborne J, Quail MA, Rajandream MA, Rogers J, Rutter S, Seeger K, Skelton J, Squares R, Squares S, Sulston JE, Taylor K, Whitehead S, Barrell BG (1998) Deciphering the biology of Mycobacterium tuberculosis from the complete genome sequence. Nature 393(6685):537–544
28. Waters WR, Palmer MV, Nonnecke BJ, Thacker TC, Scherer CF, Estes DM, Hewinson RG, Vordermeier HM, Barnes SW, Federe GC, Walker JR, Glynne RJ, Hsu T, Weinrick B, Biermann K, Larsen MH, Jacobs WR Jr (2009) Efficacy and immunogenicity of Mycobacterium bovis DeltaRD1 against aerosol M. bovis infection in neonatal calves. Vaccine 27 (8):1201–1209. doi:S0264-410X(08)01752-0 [pii] 10.1016/j.vaccine.2008.12.018
29. Brosch R, Gordon SV, Garnier T, Eiglmeier K, Frigui W, Valenti P, Dos Santos S, Duthoy S, Lacroix C, Garcia-Pelayo C, Inwald JK, Golby P, Garcia JN, Hewinson RG, Behr MA, Quail

MA, Churcher C, Barrell BG, Parkhill J, Cole ST (2007) Genome plasticity of BCG and impact on vaccine efficacy. Proc Natl Acad Sci USA 104(13):5596–5601
30. Li L, Bannantine JP, Zhang Q, Amonsin A, May BJ, Alt D, Banerji N, Kanjilal S, Kapur V (2005) The complete genome sequence of Mycobacterium avium subspecies paratuberculosis. Proc Natl Acad Sci USA 102(35):12344–12349
31. Cockle PJ, Gordon SV, Lalvani A, Buddle BM, Hewinson RG, Vordermeier HM (2002) Identification of novel Mycobacterium tuberculosis antigens with potential as diagnostic reagents or subunit vaccine candidates by comparative genomics. Infect Immun 70 (12):6996–7003
32. Cockle PJ, Gordon SV, Hewinson RG, Vordermeier HM (2006) Field evaluation of a novel differential diagnostic reagent for detection of Mycobacterium bovis in cattle. Clin Vaccine Immunol 13(10):1119–1124
33. Aagaard C, Govaerts M, Meikle V, Vallecillo AJ, Gutierrez-Pabello JA, Suarez-Guemes F, McNair J, Cataldi A, Espitia C, Andersen P, Pollock JM (2006) Optimizing antigen cocktails for detection of Mycobacterium bovis in herds with different prevalences of bovine tuberculosis: ESAT6-CFP10 mixture shows optimal sensitivity and specificity. J Clin Microbiol 44 (12):4326–4335. doi:JCM.01184-06 [pii] 10.1128/JCM.01184-06
34. Aagaard C, Govaerts M, Meng Okkels L, Andersen P, Pollock JM (2003) Genomic approach to identification of Mycobacterium bovis diagnostic antigens in cattle. J Clin Microbiol 41 (8):3719–3728
35. Vordermeier M, Goodchild A, Clifton-Hadley R, de la Rua R (2004) The interferon-gamma field trial: background, principles and progress. Vet Rec 155(2):37–38
36. Aagaard C, Hoang TT, Izzo A, Billeskov R, Troudt J, Arnett K, Keyser A, Elvang T, Andersen P, Dietrich J (2009) Protection and polyfunctional T cells induced by Ag85B-TB10.4/IC31 against Mycobacterium tuberculosis is highly dependent on the antigen dose. PLoS One 4(6): e5930. doi:10.1371/journal.pone.0005930
37. Hewinson RG, Vordermeier HM, Smith NH, Gordon SV (2006) Recent advances in our knowledge of Mycobacterium bovis: a feeling for the organism. Vet Microbiol 112 (2–4):127–139
38. Vordermeier HM, Brown J, Cockle PJ, Franken WP, Drijfhout JW, Arend SM, Ottenhoff TH, Jahans K, Hewinson RG (2007) Assessment of cross-reactivity between Mycobacterium bovis and M. kansasii ESAT-6 and CFP-10 at the T-cell epitope level. Clin Vaccine Immunol 14 (9):1203–1209. doi:CVI.00116-07 [pii] 10.1128/CVI.00116-07
39. Jones GJ, Gordon SV, Hewinson RG, Vordermeier HM (2010) Screening of predicted secreted antigens from Mycobacterium bovis reveals the immunodominance of the ESAT-6 protein family. Infect Immun 78(3):1326–1332. doi:IAI.01246-09 [pii] 10.1128/IAI.01246-09
40. Jones GJ, Hewinson RG, Vordermeier HM (2010) Screening of predicted secreted antigens from Mycobacterium bovis identifies potential novel differential diagnostic reagents. Clin Vaccine Immunol 17(9):1344–1348. doi:CVI.00261-10 [pii] 10.1128/CVI.00261-10
41. Sidders B, Withers M, Kendall SL, Bacon J, Waddell SJ, Hinds J, Golby P, Movahedzadeh F, Cox RA, Frita R, Ten Bokum AM, Wernisch L, Stoker NG (2007) Quantification of global transcription patterns in prokaryotes using spotted microarrays. Genome Biol 8(12):R265. doi: gb-2007-8-12-r265 [pii] 10.1186/gb-2007-8-12-r265
42. Charlet D, Mostowy S, Alexander D, Sit L, Wiker HG, Behr MA (2005) Reduced expression of antigenic proteins MPB70 and MPB83 in Mycobacterium bovis BCG strains due to a start codon mutation in sigK. Mol Microbiol 56(5):1302–1313. doi:MMI4618 [pii] 10.1111/j.1365-2958.2005.04618.x
43. Wiker HG (2009) MPB70 and MPB83–major antigens of Mycobacterium bovis. Scand J Immunol 69(6):492–499. doi:SJI2256 [pii] 10.1111/j.1365-3083.2009.02256.x
44. Sidders B, Pirson C, Hogarth PJ, Hewinson RG, Stoker NG, Vordermeier HM, Ewer K (2008) Screening of highly expressed mycobacterial genes identifies Rv3615c as a useful differential diagnostic antigen for the Mycobacterium tuberculosis complex. Infect Immun 76 (9):3932–3939. doi:IAI.00150-08 [pii] 10.1128/IAI.00150-08

45. Millington KA, Fortune SM, Low J, Garces A, Hingley-Wilson SM, Wickremasinghe M, Kon OM, Lalvani A (2011) Rv3615c is a highly immunodominant RD1 (Region of Difference 1)-dependent secreted antigen specific for Mycobacterium tuberculosis infection. Proc Natl Acad Sci USA 108(14):5730–5735. doi:1015153108 [pii] 10.1073/pnas.1015153108
46. DiGuiseppe Champion PA, Cox JS (2007) Protein secretions systems in Mycobacteria. Cell Microbiol 9:1376–1384
47. Schnappinger D, Ehrt S, Voskuil MI, Liu Y, Mangan JA, Monahan IM, Dolganov G, Efron B, Butcher PD, Nathan C, Schoolnik GK (2003) Transcriptional Adaptation of Mycobacterium tuberculosis within Macrophages: insights into the Phagosomal Environment. J Exp Med 198 (5):693–704
48. Demissie A, Leyten EM, Abebe M, Wassie L, Aseffa A, Abate G, Fletcher H, Owiafe P, Hill PC, Brookes R, Rook G, Zumla A, Arend SM, Klein M, Ottenhoff TH, Andersen P, Doherty TM (2006) Recognition of stage-specific mycobacterial antigens differentiates between acute and latent infections with Mycobacterium tuberculosis. Clin Vaccine Immunol 13(2):179–186
49. Geluk A, Lin MY, van Meijgaarden KE, Leyten EM, Franken KL, Ottenhoff TH, Klein MR (2007) T-cell recognition of the HspX protein of Mycobacterium tuberculosis correlates with latent M. tuberculosis infection but not with M. bovis BCG vaccination. Infect Immun 75 (6):2914–2921
50. Leyten EM, Lin MY, Franken KL, Friggen AH, Prins C, van Meijgaarden KE, Voskuil MI, Weldingh K, Andersen P, Schoolnik GK, Arend SM, Ottenhoff TH, Klein MR (2006) Human T-cell responses to 25 novel antigens encoded by genes of the dormancy regulon of Mycobacterium tuberculosis. Microbes Infect 8(8):2052–2060
51. Lin MY, Geluk A, Smith SG, Stewart AL, Friggen AH, Franken KL, Verduyn MJ, van Meijgaarden KE, Voskuil MI, Dockrell HM, Huygen K, Ottenhoff TH, Klein MR (2007) Lack of Immune Responses to Mycobacterium tuberculosis DosR Regulon Proteins following Mycobacterium bovis BCG Vaccination. Infect Immun 75(7):3523–3530
52. Rustad TR, Harrell MI, Liao R, Sherman DR (2008) The enduring hypoxic response of Mycobacterium tuberculosis. PLoS One 3(1):e1502
53. Jones GJ, Pirson C, Gideon HP, Wilkinson KA, Sherman DR, Wilkinson RJ, Hewinson RG, Vordermeier HM (2011) Immune responses to the Enduring Hypoxia Response antigen Rv0188 are preferentially detected in *Mycobacterium bovis infected cattle with low pathology*. PLoS One 6(6):e21371
54. Arnvig KB, Young DB (2009) Identification of small RNAs in Mycobacterium tuberculosis. Mol Microbiol 73(3):397–408. doi:MMI6777 [pii] 10.1111/j.1365-2958.2009.06777.x
55. DiChiara JM, Contreras-Martinez LM, Livny J, Smith D, McDonough KA, Belfort M (2010) Multiple small RNAs identified in Mycobacterium bovis BCG are also expressed in Mycobacterium tuberculosis and Mycobacterium smegmatis. Nucleic Acids Res 38(12):4067–4078. doi:gkq101 [pii] 10.1093/nar/gkq101
56. Liu Q, Paroo Z (2010) Biochemical principles of small RNA pathways. Annu Rev Biochem 79:295–319. doi:10.1146/annurev.biochem.052208.151733
57. Gimpel M, Heidrich N, Mader U, Krugel H, Brantl S (2010) A dual-function sRNA from B. subtilis: SR1 acts as a peptide encoding mRNA on the gapA operon. Mol Microbiol 76 (4):990–1009. doi:MMI7158 [pii] 10.1111/j.1365-2958.2010.07158.x
58. Boisset S, Geissmann T, Huntzinger E, Fechter P, Bendridi N, Possedko M, Chevalier C, Helfer AC, Benito Y, Jacquier A, Gaspin C, Vandenesch F, Romby P (2007) Staphylococcus aureus RNAIII coordinately represses the synthesis of virulence factors and the transcription regulator Rot by an antisense mechanism. Genes Dev 21(11):1353–1366. doi:21/11/1353 [pii] 10.1101/gad.423507
59. Wadler CS, Vanderpool CK (2007) A dual function for a bacterial small RNA: SgrS performs base pairing-dependent regulation and encodes a functional polypeptide. Proc Natl Acad Sci USA 104(51):20454–20459. doi:0708102104 [pii] 10.1073/pnas.0708102104
60. Amills M, Ramiya V, Norimine J, Lewin HA (1998) The major histocompatibility complex of ruminants. Rev Sci Tech 17(1):108–120

61. Lewin HA, Russell GC, Glass EJ (1999) Comparative organization and function of the major histocompatibility complex of domesticated cattle. Immunol Rev 167:145–158
62. Glass EJ (2004) Genetic variation and responses to vaccines. Anim Health Res Rev 5:197–208
63. Bamford AI, Douglas A, Friede T, Stevanovic S, Rammensee HG, Adair BM (1995) Peptide motif of a cattle MHC class I molecule. Immunol Lett 45(1–2):129–136
64. Hegde NR, Deshpande MS, Godson DL, Babiuk LA, Srikumaran S (1999) Bovine lymphocyte antigen-A11–specific peptide motif as a means to identify cytotoxic T-lymphocyte epitopes of bovine herpesvirus 1. Viral Immunol 12(2):149–161
65. Gerner W, Hammer SE, Wiesmuller KH, Saalmuller A (2009) Identification of major histocompatibility complex restriction and anchor residues of foot-and-mouth disease virus-derived bovine T-cell epitopes. J Virol 83(9):4039–4050. doi:JVI.01534-08 [pii] 10.1128/JVI.01534-08
66. De Groot AS, Nene V, Hegde NR, Srikumaran S, Rayner J, Martin W (2003) T cell epitope identification for bovine vaccines: an epitope mapping method for BoLA A-11. Int J Parasitol 33(5–6):641–653. doi:S0020751903000511 [pii]
67. Singh H, Raghava GP (2001) ProPred: prediction of HLA-DR binding sites. Bioinformatics 17 (12):1236–1237
68. Vordermeier M, Whelan AO, Hewinson RG (2003) Recognition of mycobacterial epitopes by T cells across mammalian species and use of a program that predicts human HLA-DR binding peptides to predict bovine epitopes. Infect Immun 71(4):1980–1987
69. Jones GJ, Bagaini F, Hewinson RG, Vordermeier HM (2011) The use of binding-prediction models to identify M. bovis-specific antigenic peptides for screening assays in bovine tuberculosis. Vet Immunol Immunopathol 141(3–4):239–245. doi:S0165-2427(11)00089-4 [pii] 10.1016/j.vetimm.2011.03.006
70. Gey Van Pittius NC, Gamieldien J, Hide W, Brown GD, Siezen RJ, Beyers AD (2001) The ESAT-6 gene cluster of Mycobacterium tuberculosis and other high G+C Gram-positive bacteria. Genome Biol 2(10), RESEARCH0044
71. Vordermeier HM, Hewinson RG, Wilkinson RJ, Wilkinson KA, Gideon HP, Young DB, Sampson SL (2012) Conserved Immune Recognition Hierarchy of Mycobacterial PE/PPE Proteins during Infection in Natural Hosts. PLoS One. 7:e40890
72. Whelan AO, Clifford D, Upadhyay B, Breadon EL, McNair J, Hewinson GR, Vordermeier MH (2010) Development of a skin test for bovine tuberculosis for differentiating infected from vaccinated animals. J Clin Microbiol 48(9):3176–3181. doi:JCM.00420-10 [pii] 10.1128/JCM.00420-10

Chapter 5
Genome-Based Computational Vaccine Discovery by Reverse Vaccinology

Yongqun He

Abstract Reverse vaccinology starts with bioinformatics analysis of genome sequences to predict best vaccine candidates. With more and more genomes sequenced for any given microbial pathogens, reverse vaccinology becomes an emerging and important vaccine development strategy. Different criteria have been designed for reverse vaccinology prediction, ranging from the prediction of protein subcellular localization, transmembrane helices, adhesin probability, to pangenome sequence conservation prediction. The prediction of MHC class I and class II binding epitopes is also a critical feature for ranking protein antigenicity. Vaxign is the first web-based software program that targets for vaccine design using the genome-wide reverse vaccinology strategy and epitope prediction. As a use case study, Vaxign was used to predict protein targets for vaccine development against infections with virulent *Francisella tularensis*. In total 12 outer membrane proteins from *F. tularensis* strain SCHU S4 were predicted to be adhesins and conserved within seven other strains of *F. tularensis* subspecies *tularensis*, *holarctica*, *mediasiatica*, and *novicida*. Among them, an extracellular lipoprotein FTT0482c is absent from *F. philomiragia*. MHC class I epitopes predicted by the Vaxign/Vaxitop program overlaps with the results predicted by the IEDB consensus prediction method. Compared to the IEDB method, a smaller number of epitope hits are typically predicted by Vaxign/Vaxitop (P-value < 0.05).

Y. He (✉)
Unit for Laboratory Animal Medicine, Department of Microbiology and Immunology, Center for Computational Medicine and Bioinformatics, University of Michigan Medical School, Ann Arbor, MI, USA
e-mail: yongqunh@med.umich.edu

D.R. Flower and Y. Perrie (eds.), *Immunomic Discovery of Adjuvants and Candidate Subunit Vaccines*, Immunomics Reviews: 5, DOI 10.1007/978-1-4614-5070-2_5,

5.1 Introduction

Since the publication of the first complete genome sequence of *Haemophilus influenza* Rd in 1995 [1], over 1,700 microbial genomes have been sequenced (http://www.ncbi.nlm.nih.gov/genomes/MICROBES/microbial_growth.html). With the increasing number of sequenced bacterial genomes, it becomes possible to rely on genome sequence analysis and multiple genome comparison for vaccine discovery.

The idea of predicting vaccine targets based on genome sequences is the basis of the reverse vaccinology, an emerging and novel vaccine design strategy. With the large protein sequence data, it is also possible to predict MHC class I and II epitopes for individual proteins in an entire genome and rank their antigenicity based on the epitope prediction. Different tools have been developed to support genome-wide vaccine discovery. The Vaxign vaccine design software is the first web-based program that targets for vaccine design using the genome-wide reverse vaccinology strategy and epitope prediction.

In this chapter, I will first introduce the concepts and criteria of reverse vaccinology vaccine design and its use in genome-wide vaccine prediction. The Vaxign reverse vaccinology method will then be introduced, followed by description of a specific use case study, that is, applying Vaxign to predict vaccine targets for *Francisella tularensis*.

5.2 Genome-Based Vaccine Design Using Reverse Vaccinology and Immunoinformatics

Reverse vaccinology is an emerging and revolutionary vaccine development approach that starts with the prediction of vaccine targets by bioinformatics analysis of genome sequences. Predicted proteins are selected based on defined desirable attributes. Pioneered by Rino Rappuoli, reverse vaccinology was first applied to development of a vaccine against serogroup B Neisseria meningitidis (MenB), the major cause of sepsis and meningitis in children and young adults [2]. The complete MenB genome was screened using bioinformatic algorithms for ORFs coding for putative surface-exposed or secreted proteins, which are susceptible to antibody recognition and therefore the most suitable vaccine candidates. Out of approximately 600 novel vaccine candidates, 350 were expressed in *E. coli* and 28 were found to elicit protective immunity. It took less than 18 months to identify more vaccine candidates in MenB than had been discovered during the past 40 years by conventional methods [2]. The concept of reverse vaccinology has been successfully applied to many other pathogens such as *Streptococcus pneumoniae* [3], *Brucella* spp. [4], and *Cryptosporidium hominis* [5].

While the subcellular localization of proteins is the only criteria used in the MenB vaccine design based on the reverse vaccinology, many more criteria have been identified for efficient vaccine target prediction using reverse vaccinology. The key criteria considered today in reverse vaccinology are summarized below, together with a list of software programed useful for addressing these criteria.

5.2.1 Protein Subcellular Localization

Since the beginning of reverse vaccinology applications, subcellular location is one main criterion for vaccine target prediction. When an antibody response plays a major role in protecting host against infection of a pathogen (e.g., a pathogenic bacterium), secreted proteins and surface-exposed outer membrane proteins (OMPs) of the pathogen are ideal targets for vaccine development. Secreted proteins are often toxins or other virulence factors. Blocking the functions of these secreted proteins would stop the microbial pathogenesis. Similarly, allowing the host to generate antibodies against OMPs (e.g., adhesins) would inhibit the invasion, transfer, and function of the pathogen. For these pathogens, cytoplasmic or inner membrane proteins, however, may not be good vaccine targets due to the lack of close contact with the host cells. However, to develop vaccines against those pathogens against which T cell response is crucial, subcellular localization may not be an essential issue because a T cell response can be targeted to a pathogen protein in any location.

5.2.2 Transmembrane Helices

In the original paper of MenB vaccine discovery using reverse vaccinology, 250 out of 600 vaccine candidates from *N. meningitidis* B failed to be isolated and purified from recombinant *E. coli* strains, largely due to the presence of more than one transmembrane spanning region [2]. Therefore, it is wise to not consider those proteins with multiple transmembrane spanning regions as best vaccine candidates. In software development, a filter can be designed to remove the OMPs containing more than one transmembrane helix.

5.2.3 Adhesin Probability

An adhesin is typically an OMP that adheres to host cells and mediates the invasion of a host by a microbe pathogen. Adhesins are essential for bacterial colonization and survival. A blockage of adhesin functions by inducing adhesin-specific antibodies would prevent microbial invasion. Therefore, adhesins are ideal targets for vaccine development.

5.2.4 Pangenome Pathogen Sequence Conservation Prediction

With a large number of genomes available, it is imperative to conduct systematic comparative analysis of the whole genomes of different strains in a given bacterium to dissect their genetic conservation and variability. Specifically, a microbial species can be described by its pan-genome, which is composed of core genes present in all strains and dispensable (or accessory) genes present in two or more strains or unique to single strains. To develop a vaccine against infections of multiple virulent strains of a particular pathogen, it is important to identify those genes that are conserved core genes or at least dispensable genes that are present in as many virulent strains as possible. Therefore, a pan-genome analysis is important for genome-wide vaccine discovery.

Vaccine targets are likely those that exist in genomes of virulent pathogen strains, but are absent from attenuated or avirulent strains. Therefore, if one or more genomes from non-pathogenic strains of a pathogen (e.g., *E. coli* strain K-12) are available, we can exclude those proteins present in attenuated or avirulent strains from possible vaccine target list. However, this criterion may not be necessary. The proteins involved in attenuation of a virulent pathogen are called virulence factors. Many virulence factors are good vaccine targets. However, the vaccine targets to be identified are protective antigens. Protective antigens overlap with but are not equal to virulence factors [6]. Many protective antigens exist in attenuated and even avirulent strains. In addition, some virulence factors also exist in attenuated and even avirulent strains. The attenuation of a virulent pathogen may be due to mutation of one virulence factor instead of all virulence factors. Therefore, this criterion of excluding proteins present in attenuated or avirulent strains is subject to the vaccine designer's call and may not be necessary.

The sequence conservation problem is basically an issue to identify orthologs among strains. BLAST or BLAST-derived methods are typically used for this purpose. A reciprocal best-fit method is usually used. This method works by finding the best fit of a protein in one genome from another genome. If two proteins from two genomes are best-fit for each other, it means that these two proteins are orthologs.

5.2.5 Sequence Similarity to Host Proteome

Sequence similarity analysis has also been used to identify the homology between predicted vaccine targets from the pathogen side and the proteome from the host side (e.g., human). If a predicted vaccine target has high sequence similarity to a host protein, one of two extreme host responses may occur: (1) the vaccine target may induce autoimmunity, that is, the immune response induced by the vaccine target may be used against the homologous host protein and cause severe autoimmune disease; and (2) immune tolerance may occur, that is, the vaccine target may not induce any response to this target in host. Therefore, predicted vaccine targets are required not to have sequence similarity to proteins of hosts (e.g., human).

5.2.6 Prediction of MHC Class I and Class II Binding Epitopes Using Immunoinformatics Methods

Immunoinformatics is a research branch that studies immunology using informatics approaches. A major research area in immunoinformatics is the study of T cell epitope binding. T cells are activated by direct interaction with antigen presenting cells. The initial interaction occurs between the T cell receptor and antigen peptides bound in the cleft of MHC class I or II molecules. MHC class I molecules present peptides obtained from proteolytic digestion of endogenous proteins. MHC class I binding molecules are peptides 8–10 amino acids in length and are primarily recognized by CD8+ cytotoxic T lymphocytes. MHC class II molecules generally bind peptides derived from the cell membrane or extracellular proteins. Peptides presented by MHC class II molecules have more variable lengths (typically 11–25 amino acids) and more complex anchor motifs than class I binding epitopes. MHC class II molecules bind epitopes are recognized by CD4+ T helper (Th) cells.

Immunoinformatics tools were first used for vaccine design in the 1980s by pioneer researchers including DeLisi and Berzofsky [7]. Based on the fact that T cell epitopes are bound in a linear form to the MHC class I and II molecules, many T cell epitope-mapping algorithms have been developed [8, 9]. Our recent paper summarizes the lists of existing software programs for prediction of MHC class I and II binding epitopes [10].

By analyzing individual proteins in an entire proteome of a pathogen, these epitope prediction tools allow rapid identification and ranking of putative T cell epitopes from a whole genome.

5.3 The Vaxign Reverse Vaccinology Software Program

Vaxign is the first web-based vaccine design program utilizing the reverse vaccinology strategy [11, 12]. Vaxign predicts vaccine targets by bioinformatics analysis of genome sequences. Predicted features in the Vaxign pipeline include protein subcellular location, transmembrane helices, adhesin probability, conservation among pathogenic strains, sequence exclusion from genomes of nonpathogenic strains, sequence similarity to host proteins, and epitope binding to MHC class I and class II. Vaxign has been demonstrated to successfully predict vaccine targets for *Brucella* spp. [4, 12] and uropathogenic *E. coli* [11]. Currently, more than 200 genomes have been pre-computed using the Vaxign pipeline and available for query in the Vaxign website (http://www.violinet.org/vaxign) (23). Vaxign also performs dynamic vaccine target prediction based on input sequences.

Vaxign includes a list of criteria for vaccine design. Each criterion is addressed by independent program. A user can choose whether or not to use individual criteria and programs. Such module-based software is designed based on the observation that different researchers and vaccine developers often have different preferences in terms which criteria to use for their specific applications. The criteria and module programs used for Vaxign vaccine design are introduced as follows:

- *Subcellular Localization.* This feature is implemented by using optimized PSORTb 3.0 [13]. This program is the most precise bacterial protein subcellular localization predictor. For this to run smoothly, Vaxign automatically generates standard input data for PSORTb. After the execution of this program, Vaxign automatically parses and transfer the PSORTb output into the Vaxign MySQL database. Users do not need to worry about the tedious detail of how to process input and output data and how to execute PSORTb. Such a process makes seamless uses of PSORTb and other software programs in Vaxign.
- *Number of Transmembrane Helices.* The transmembrane helix topology analysis is performed using optimized HMMTOP [14]. A profile-based hidden Markov model implemented in PROFtmb is used in Vaxign for the prediction and discrimination of bacterial transmembrane β-barrels [15]. The execution of PROTtmb is time consuming. Thus, PROTtmb has not been used to pre-analyze all proteins in all genomes stored in the Vaxign database. However, a user can run individual proteins using PROTtmb dynamically.
- *Minimum Adhesin Probability* (0–1.0). Optimized SPAAN [16] is used to calculate adhesin probability. The default cutoff is 0.51. A probability of greater than 0.51 suggests that this protein is an adhesin or has adhesin-like characteristics.
- *Microbial Sequence Conservation by Ortholog Analysis.* This feature is used for finding conserved proteins among a selected list of strains. OrthoMCL is applied for the calculation [17]. The E-value of 10^{-5} is set as the default value.
- *Exclusion of Proteins having Orthologs in Selected Genome(s).* This is for excluding proteins that also exist in a non-pathogenic strain(s). A user may choose to use this feature depending on different scenarios.
- *No Similarity to Human Proteins.* Choose this selection to exclude those vaccine targets that also exist in humans.
- *No Similarity to Mouse Proteins.* Choose this selection to exclude those vaccine targets that also exist in mouse.
- *No Similarity to Pig Proteins.* Choose this selection to exclude those vaccine targets that also exist in pigs.
- *MHC Class I & II Epitope Prediction by Vaxitop.* The method used for the epitope prediction is based on Vaxitop, our internally developed program based on prediction of position-specific scoring matrices. Different from existing epitope prediction algorithms, Vaxitop relies on statistical *P*-value (instead of a percentage or top number) as the cutoff. A *P*-value of 0.05 provides a cutoff with high and balanced sensitivity and specificity [11]. Under this section, you can choose a *P*-value cutoff, host species, MHC allele, and epitope length.

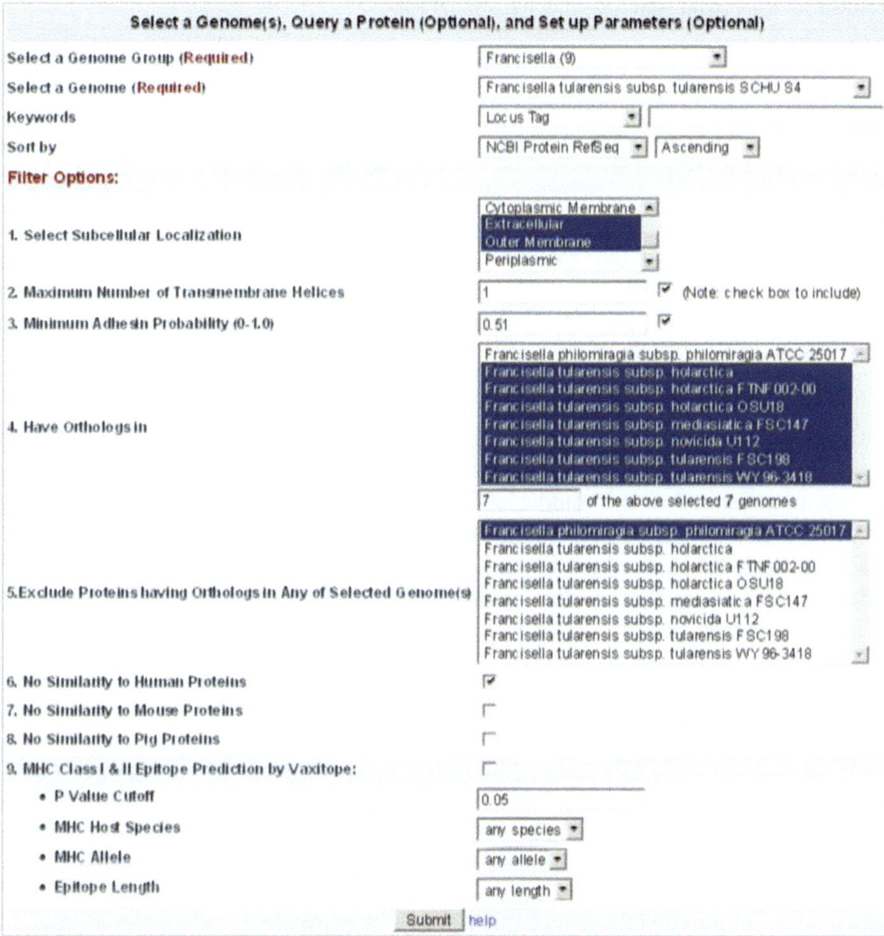

Fig. 5.1 Vaxign web interface for predicting tularemia vaccine targets

A screenshot of the Vaxign web interface for vaccine target prediction is shown in Fig. 5.1. Figure 5.1 can be used for analyzing vaccine targets for tularemia, caused by *F. tularensis*. This use case is described in detail below.

5.4 Vaxign Use Case: Prediction of *F. tularensis* Vaccine Targets

F. tularensis is a pathogenic species of Gram-negative, facultative intracellular bacteria. It is the causative agent of tularemia. Due to its ease of spread by aerosol and its high virulence, *F. tularensis* can be potentially used as a bioterrorism weapon. Although antibody response can protect against low virulence strains, an

Table 5.1 *Francisella* strains used in the Vaxign analysis

Francisella strains	Refseq Accession #	# of proteins
F. tularensis subsp. *tularensis* SCHU S4	NC_006570	1,603
F. tularensis subsp. *tularensis* FSC198	NC_008245	1,605
F. tularensis subsp. *tularensis* WY96-3418	NC_009257	1,634
F. tularensis subsp. *holarctica*	NC_007880	1,754
F. tularensis subsp. *holarctica* FTNF002-00	NC_009749	1,580
F. tularensis subsp. *holarctica* OSU18	NC_008369	1,555
F. tularensis subsp. *mediasiatica* FSC147	NC_010677	1,406
F. tularensis subsp. *novicida* U112	NC_008601	1,719
F. philomiragia subsp. *philomiragia* ATCC 25017	NC_010336, NC_010331	1,915

Note: In total 14771 proteins are present in these strains. NC_010331 is a plasmid pFPHI01 in *F. philomiragia* subsp. philomiragia ATCC 25017

antigen-specific memory T cell response is critical for protection against *F. tularensis* strain with high virulence [18]. An attenuated live vaccine strain LVS was generated in the middle of last century and has been successfully used to protect humans. However, LVS is not a licensed human vaccine due to its residual virulence and a lack of understanding of the basis of its attenuation. A safe and effective human vaccine against tularemia is desired. Here Vaxign is used to predict vaccine targets against *F. tularensis*.

5.4.1 Methods

Sequenced genomes of nine strains from four *F. tularensis* subspecies were downloaded from NCBI RefSeq database and used in this Vaxign data analysis. Human tularemia is caused by three *F. tularensis* subspecies: *tularensis* (type A), *holarctica* (type B), and *mediasiatica*. The first two subspecies are responsible for the majority of human tularemia cases reported worldwide. *F. tularensis* subspecies *novicida* has low virulence in humans at least partly due to its lack of a capsule, a virulence factor in *F. tularensis*. *F. philomiragia* subspecies *philomiragia* is an important pathogen of muskrats and fish, but it may occasionally infect humans [19]. In total, three *F. tularensis* subspecies *tularensis* strains, three *F. tularensis* subspecies *holarctica* strains, one *F. tularensis* subspecies *mediasiatica* strain, and one *F. philomiragia* subspecies *philomiragia* strain were used for this Vaxign prediction of tularemia vaccine targets (Table 5.1). The Vaxign analysis pipeline described above was implemented. The results were stored in the Vaxign database and are available for query and analysis.

5.4.2 Results and Discussion

Since different module programs used in Vaxign are independent from each other, different schemes can be used to query and analyze the results. The scheme used

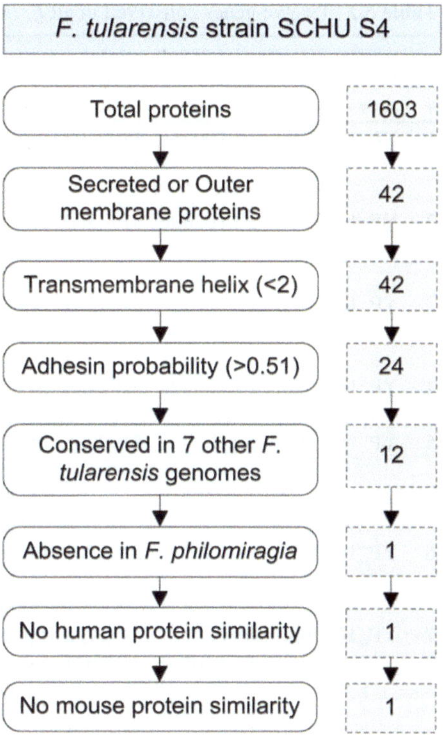

Fig. 5.2 Vaxign analysis of vaccine targets using *F. tularensis* strain SCHU S4 as seed genome. See the text for detailed explanation

here is outlined in Fig. 5.2. Basically, the genome of *F. tularensis* strain SCHU S4 was used as the seed genome. This genome contains 42 OMPs. None of these OMPs contains more than one transmembrane alpha helix. Among them, 24 proteins are predicted to be adhesins or have adhesin-like characteristics. Twelve of these 24 proteins are conserved among all other seven *F. tularensis* strains (Table 5.2). LpnA and FTT0382c are two lipoproteins in the list. Two OMPs OstA1 and OstA2 are organic solvent tolerance proteins. It is interesting that 5 out of the 12 proteins are hypothetic proteins. FTT1258 and FTT1573c are two other OMPs. Among the 12 proteins, LpnA and FopA have been found to be a protective antigen in *F. tularensis* [20]. However, it is unknown whether or not the other ten proteins are able to induce protective immunity.

A comparison between the 12 conserved proteins among 8 *F. tularensis* strains and the proteome of *F. philomiragia* strain ATCC 25017 shows that 11 of these proteins are also present in *F. philomiragia* strain ATCC 25017. The one protein that is absent from the *F. philomiragia* strain is an extracellular lipoprotein FTT0482c. While *F. philomiragia* (formerly *Yersinia philomiragia*) is able to cause human disease [21], *F. philomiragia* primarily infects muskrats and fish and is quite different from the three *F. tularensis* subspecies. How this gene plays a role in host specificity and induction of protective immunity is unclear and may deserve further investigation.

Table 5.2 Twelve genes conserved in all *F. tularensis* strains

#	Protein accession #	Gene symbol	NCBI Gene ID	Protein note	Localization (probability)	Adhesin prob.	Trans-membrane helices
1	YP_169101.1	FTT0025c	3192092	hypothetical protein FTT0025c	Extracellular (0.964)	0.586	1
2	YP_169339.1	FTT0289c	3191300	hypothetical protein FTT0289c	Extracellular (0.964)	0.620	0
3	YP_169505.1	ostA1	3191215	organic solvent tolerance protein	OMP (1)	0.651	0
4	YP_169520.1	FTT0482c	3191404	lipoprotein	Extracellular (0.964)	0.546	0
5	YP_169607.1	fopA	3192005	outer membrane associated protein	OMP (0.993)	0.679	0
6	YP_169751.1	ostA2	3191221	organic solvent tolerance protein	OMP (1)	0.538	0
7	YP_169898.1	lpnA	3191792	lipoprotein	OMP (0.992)	0.656	0
8	YP_170036.1	FTT1055c	3192031	hypothetical protein FTT1055c	Extracellular (0.964)	0.578	0
9	YP_170216.1	FTT1258	3191474	outer membrane efflux protein	OMP (1)	0.530	0
10	YP_170465.1	FTT1537c	3192317	hypothetical protein FTT1537c	OMP (0.949)	0.576	0
11	YP_170495.1	FTT1573c	3192167	outer membrane protein	OMP (1)	0.663	0
12	YP_170518.1	FTT1602	3191069	hypothetical protein FTT1602	Extracellular (0.965)	0.764	0

Note: *OMP*, outer membrane protein. The highlighted lipoprotein FTT0482c does not exist in *F. philomiragia* subsp. philomiragia ATCC 25017

Out of the initial 42 OMPs predicted, four of them (Gcp, Blc, Ndk, and FTT0610) have homologous proteins in humans and mouse. However, none of the 12 conserved proteins among *F. tularensis* strains have orthologs in human or mouse.

Vaxign includes an internally developed program Vaxitop that predicts MHC class I and II binding epitopes by calculating statistical *P*-value. Taking FTT0482c as an example, Vaxign predicts nine HLA-A*0201 immune epitopes in FTT0482c with the length of nine amino acids each (Fig. 5.3). As seen in Fig. 5.3, the current version of Vaxign also has an IEDB MHC class I prediction program [22]. A user

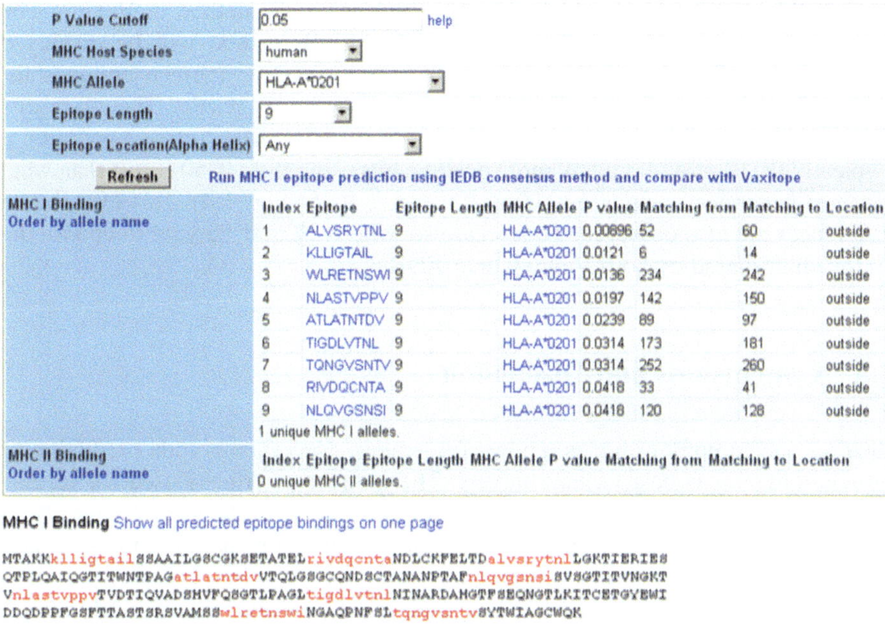

Fig. 5.3 HLA-A*0201 immune epitopes predicted by the Vaxitop program in Vaxign. The pre-defined epitope length for this analysis is 9

Index	Epitope	Epitope length	MHC allele	Matching from	Matching to	IC50 (IEDB consensus)	Vaxitope P-value
1	NLASTVPPV	9	HLA-A*0201	142	150	0.3	0.0197
2	KLLIGTAIL	9	HLA-A*0201	6	14	1.5	0.0121
3	TLATNTDVV	9	HLA-A*0201	90	98	2.8	>0.1
4	AMSSWLRET	9	HLA-A*0201	230	238	3.4	>0.1
5	ALVSRYTNL	9	HLA-A*0201	52	60	4.2	0.00896
6	LLGKTIERI	9	HLA-A*0201	60	68	5.2	>0.1
7	LVSRYTNLL	9	HLA-A*0201	53	61	5.3	>0.1
8	AILSSAAIL	9	HLA-A*0201	12	20	5.8	>0.1
9	WLRETNSWI	9	HLA-A*0201	234	242	6	0.0136
10	GTITWNTPA	9	HLA-A*0201	79	87	6.1	>0.1
11	TIGDLVTNL	9	HLA-A*0201	173	181	6.2	0.0314
12	NTVSYTWIA	9	HLA-A*0201	258	266	6.4	>0.1
13	ATLATNTDV	9	HLA-A*0201	89	97	6.7	0.0239
14	TQNGVSNTV	9	HLA-A*0201	252	260	6.9	0.0314
15	ITWNTPAGA	9	HLA-A*0201	81	89	7	>0.1
16	ISVSGTITV	9	HLA-A*0201	128	136	7.1	>0.1
17	KTVNLASTV	9	HLA-A*0201	139	147	7.2	>0.1
18	LLIGTAILS	9	HLA-A*0201	7	15	7.2	>0.1
19	QVGSNSISV	9	HLA-A*0201	122	130	7.5	>0.1
20	NLQVGSNSI	9	HLA-A*0201	120	128	8.3	0.0418
21	RIVDQCNTA	9	HLA-A*0201	33	41	9.2	0.0418

Fig. 5.4 Comparison of epitopes predicted by Vaxign/Vaxitop and IEDB. The epitopes are predicted to bind human HLA allele HLA-A*0201. The pre-defined epitope length is 9

can run this program with a default setting of consensus method in Vaxign. The comparative results between Vaxitop and the IEDB method will be displayed automatically. Comparative analysis of the HLA-A*0201 immune epitopes for FTT0482c indicates that the two programs have overlapped results. The top results from Vaxitop prediction are usually shown up in IEDB MHC class I prediction. Typically IEDB provides many more positive hits using their IC50 cutoff than what Vaxitop generates using a cutoff of P-value < 0.05 (Fig. 5.4). However, some differences are also observed. To increase specificity, it may be wise to choose the epitope hits shared by both Vaxitop and IEDB.

5.5 Conclusions and Discussion

Reverse vaccinology provides a powerful strategy for genome-wide prediction of protein antigens as best vaccine targets. The number of criteria used for reverse vaccinology vaccine design has dramatically increased in the past decade. With many genomes available for almost any pathogen, it is now possible to use a pan-genome approach to identify conserved proteins for the development of vaccines against multiple strains, subspecies, and even species. Immunoinformatics approaches for T cell epitope predictions can also be used in combination with genome-wide antigen prediction for ranking protein antigenicity and generating epitope vaccines. Vaxign is a user-friendly, publicly accessible tool for efficient implementation of genome-wide vaccine target prediction based on the reverse vaccinology strategy.

There are many more we can do to further develop the genome-wide vaccine discovery strategy and methods. For example, modeling of 3D structures of protein vaccine candidates would help us to predict the T and B cell epitopes and antibody response. Transcriptomic and proteomic gene expression data analyses will make our genome-wide prediction more effective. Advanced literature mining of existing knowledge from a large amount of literature publications also provides stronger evidences on our selections. In the future, it is even possible to make synthetic vaccines based on automatic vaccine target prediction results.

Acknowledgments This manuscript was supported by the NIH-NIAID grant R01AI081062.

References

1. Fleischmann RD, Adams MD, White O, Clayton RA, Kirkness EF, Kerlavage AR, Bult CJ, Tomb JF, Dougherty BA, Merrick JM et al (1995) Whole-genome random sequencing and assembly of *Haemophilus influenzae* Rd. Science 269(5223):496–512
2. Pizza M, Scarlato V, Masignani V, Giuliani MM, Arico B, Comanducci M, Jennings GT, Baldi L, Bartolini E, Capecchi B, Galeotti CL, Luzzi E, Manetti R, Marchetti E, Mora M, Nuti S, Ratti G, Santini L, Savino S, Scarselli M, Storni E, Zuo P, Broeker M, Hundt E, Knapp B, Blair

E, Mason T, Tettelin H, Hood DW, Jeffries AC, Saunders NJ, Granoff DM, Venter JC, Moxon ER, Grandi G, Rappuoli R (2000) Identification of vaccine candidates against serogroup B meningococcus by whole-genome sequencing. Science 287(5459):1816–1820
3. Wizemann TM, Heinrichs JH, Adamou JE, Erwin AL, Kunsch C, Choi GH, Barash SC, Rosen CA, Masure HR, Tuomanen E, Gayle A, Brewah YA, Walsh W, Barren P, Lathigra R, Hanson M, Langermann S, Johnson S, Koenig S (2001) Use of a whole genome approach to identify vaccine molecules affording protection against *Streptococcus pneumoniae* infection. Infect Immun 69(3):1593–1598. doi:10.1128/IAI.69.3.1593-1598.2001
4. He Y, Xiang Z (2010) Bioinformatics analysis of *Brucella* vaccines and vaccine targets using VIOLIN. Immunome Res 6(suppl 1):S5. doi:1745-7580-6-S1-S5 [pii]10.1186/1745-7580-6-S1-S5
5. Manque PA, Tenjo F, Woehlbier U, Lara AM, Serrano MG, Xu P, Alves JM, Smeltz RB, Conrad DH, Buck GA (2011) Identification and immunological characterization of three potential vaccinogens against *Cryptosporidium* species. Clin Vaccine Immunol 18 (11):1796–1802. doi:CVI.05197-11 [pii]10.1128/CVI.05197-11
6. Yang B, Sayers S, Xiang Z, He Y (2011) Protegen: a web-based protective antigen database and analysis system. Nucleic Acids Res 39:D1073–D1078. doi:gkq944 [pii]10.1093/nar/gkq944
7. DeLisi C, Berzofsky JA (1985) T-cell antigenic sites tend to be amphipathic structures. Proc Natl Acad Sci USA 82(20):7048–7052
8. De Groot AS, Berzofsky JA (2004) From genome to vaccine–new immunoinformatics tools for vaccine design. Methods 34(4):425–428. doi:S1046-2023(04)00123-9 [pii] 10.1016/j.ymeth.2004.06.004
9. De Groot AS, Moise L (2007) New tools, new approaches and new ideas for vaccine development. Expert Rev Vaccines 6(2):125–127. doi:10.1586/14760584.6.2.125
10. He Y, Rappuoli R, De Groot AS, Chen RT (2010) Emerging vaccine informatics. J Biomed Biotechnol 2010:218590. doi:10.1155/2010/218590
11. He Y, Xiang Z, Mobley HL (2010) Vaxign: the first web-based vaccine design program for reverse vaccinology and applications for vaccine development. J Biomed Biotechnol 2010:297505, 15 pages
12. Xiang Z, He Y (2009) Vaxign: a web-based vaccine target design program for reverse vaccinology. Procedia Vaccinol 1(1):23–29
13. Yu NY, Wagner JR, Laird MR, Melli G, Rey S, Lo R, Dao P, Sahinalp SC, Ester M, Foster LJ, Brinkman FS (2010) PSORTb 3.0: improved protein subcellular localization prediction with refined localization subcategories and predictive capabilities for all prokaryotes. Bioinformatics 26(13):1608–1615. doi:btq249 [pii]10.1093/bioinformatics/btq249
14. Kall L, Krogh A, Sonnhammer EL (2007) Advantages of combined transmembrane topology and signal peptide prediction–the Phobius web server. Nucleic Acids Res 35:W429–W432. doi:gkm256 [pii]10.1093/nar/gkm256 (Web Server issue)
15. Bigelow HR, Petrey DS, Liu J, Przybylski D, Rost B (2004) Predicting transmembrane beta-barrels in proteomes. Nucleic Acids Res 32(8):2566–2577. doi:10.1093/nar/gkh58032/8/2566 [pii]
16. Sachdeva G, Kumar K, Jain P, Ramachandran S (2005) SPAAN: a software program for prediction of adhesins and adhesin-like proteins using neural networks. Bioinformatics 21 (4):483–491. doi:10.1093/bioinformatics/bti028bti028 [pii]
17. Li L, Stoeckert CJ Jr, Roos DS (2003) OrthoMCL: identification of ortholog groups for eukaryotic genomes. Genome Res 13(9):2178–2189. doi:10.1101/gr.122450313/9/2178 [pii]
18. Oyston PC (2009) *Francisella tularensis* vaccines. Vaccine 27(suppl 4):D48–D51. doi:S0264-410X(09)01131-1 [pii]10.1016/j.vaccine.2009.07.090
19. Foley JE, Nieto NC (2010) Tularemia. Vet Microbiol 140(3–4):332–338. doi:S0378-1135(09)00339-3 [pii]10.1016/j.vetmic.2009.07.017
20. Savitt AG, Mena-Taboada P, Monsalve G, Benach JL (2009) *Francisella tularensis* infection-derived monoclonal antibodies provide detection, protection, and therapy. Clin Vaccine Immunol 16(3):414–422. doi:CVI.00362-08 [pii]10.1128/CVI.00362-08

21. Wenger JD, Hollis DG, Weaver RE, Baker CN, Brown GR, Brenner DJ, Broome CV (1989) Infection caused by *Francisella philomiragia* (formerly *Yersinia philomiragia*). A newly recognized human pathogen. Ann Intern Med 110(11):888–892
22. Zhang Q, Wang P, Kim Y, Haste-Andersen P, Beaver J, Bourne PE, Bui HH, Buus S, Frankild S, Greenbaum J, Lund O, Lundegaard C, Nielsen M, Ponomarenko J, Sette A, Zhu Z, Peters B (2008) Immune epitope database analysis resource (IEDB-AR). Nucleic Acids Res 36: W513–W518. doi:gkn254 [pii]10.1093/nar/gkn254 (Web Server issue)

Chapter 6
Computational Prediction of Protein Subcellular Localization, Genomic Islands, and Virulence to Aid Antigen Discovery

Bhavjinder K. Dhillon, Nancy Y. Yu, and Fiona S.L. Brinkman

Abstract Subunits of bacterial proteins involved in virulence, as well as bacterial cell surface and secreted proteins, may be prioritized as potential vaccine components warranting further study. Computational prediction of surface-exposed and extracellular bacterial proteins (that are more accessible to the host immune system) now exceeds the accuracy of most high-throughput "wet lab" methods and has improved markedly in recent years. Identification of proteins encoded within genomic islands is also now much more accurate than a decade ago and can provide insight on gene stability plus aid virulence gene identification. Identifying proteins/genes that are most likely involved in virulence is also desirable, but further improvements in bioinformatics tools for such predictions are needed. This chapter highlights such computational tools currently available to aid the discovery of new vaccine components, how they have improved in recent years, and summarize what is needed in the future to further accelerate vaccine discovery efforts. At minimum, researchers should consider that these recently improved computational methods can now predict more potential vaccine components, and so some bacterial genomes could benefit from reanalysis with these more accurate methods.

6.1 Introduction

Vaccine development has been transformed with the dawn of bacterial genomics and new sequencing technologies. The underlying sequence variability of pathogens may now be more easily examined and vaccines may be reverse-engineered to target proteins that are predicted to be the most suitable vaccine components. In the past, many studies have focused on classifying bacterial protein

---

F.S.L. Brinkman (✉)
Department of Molecular Biology and Biochemistry, Simon Fraser University, Burnaby, BC, Canada
e-mail: brinkman@sfu.ca

D.R. Flower and Y. Perrie (eds.), *Immunomic Discovery of Adjuvants and Candidate Subunit Vaccines*, Immunomics Reviews: 5, DOI 10.1007/978-1-4614-5070-2_6,

subcellular localization (SCL) to derive a list of surface-exposed or secreted proteins to identify candidate vaccine targets. One such study by Pizza et al. [1] explored group B *Neisseria meningitidis* for which they presented previously undiscovered surface proteins that were highly conserved across different strains. Follow-up studies confirmed that these surface proteins (e.g. factor H binding protein, fHBP) were in fact great targets for vaccines [2, 3]. They have since shown considerable promise, protecting against ten different strains of group B meningococcus with the development of chimeric proteins using genomic sequence data [4]. This has been followed by studies in other pathogens such as *Haemophilus influenzae* and *Helicobacter pylori* [5], *Streptococcus pneumoniae* [6], *Porphyromonas gingivalis* [7], *Bacillus anthracis* [8], and pathogens that are also of veterinary concern like *Leptospira interrogans* [9]. All of these studies follow a common theme of first scanning the genome for open reading frames, predicting protein localizations, manually comparing to genes with known functions in virulence, and including some comparative genomics to related strains. Accompanying proteomic analyses and further experimental validation helped narrow down the lists before testing proteins as vaccine components.

As important as it is to recognize secreted and cell surface proteins, it is additionally worthwhile to be aware of which of these proteins are found within genomic islands (GI's). GI's are classified as clusters of genes, typically 10–200 kb, acquired by means of horizontal gene transfer (HGT) [10]. These regions of the genome disproportionately encode virulence factors and are often key players in pathogen evolution [11, 12]. A classic example of pathogen evolution via HGT is the sharing of drug resistance genes. Recently, a multi-drug resistant strain of the common gut microbe *Proteus mirabilis* emerged, and upon genomic investigation revealed the presence of a *Salmonella*-derived GI containing multiple antibiotic resistance genes [13]. In this way, horizontally acquired genes of foreign origin can be passed on through lineages, evolving the drug resistance—and pathogenicity—of the organism [10, 14–17]. Thus, GI's are of particular interest for antigen discovery as they may encode proteins that are specific to pathogens or harbour components of pathogens that are key players in virulence or resistance. Conversely though, the subset of GI's that are plastic (not stable; seen only in some strains) are not desirable if they are missing in key strains, so GI characterization can identify proteins that are also less attractive as vaccine components. This chapter will highlight methods to aid in the discovery of candidate antigens by using computational tools predicting protein SCL, GIs of genes from foreign origin, and also proteins involved in virulence.

6.2 Protein SCL Prediction

One of the first critical steps to identify potential vaccine and drug targets for pathogens is the identification of surface-localized and secreted proteins [18]. Traditionally, such proteins are found by laboratory techniques, which is very time-consuming and expensive. Also, experimental identification of such proteins is not possible with unculturable bacteria. In recent years, the precision of computational predictors of protein SCL in bacteria has surpassed that of major high-throughput experimental SCL identification techniques [19]. Because of this, a multitude of different computational protein SCL predictors have been developed over the years for both eukaryotes and prokaryotes (visit www.psort.org for a comprehensive list).

Currently, the two most precise computational predictors of bacterial protein SCL prediction are PSORTb [20] and Proteome Analyst [21], both of which have an overall predictive precision of over 95 % (Precision defined as "TP/(TP + FP)" [20, 22];). PSORTb predicts SCL using a naive Bayesian network that combines several modules, each analyzing different sequence features that are characteristic of SCL. For instance, an SCL-BLAST module uses BLAST to search for homologs of proteins of known SCL, since proteins rarely evolve to change localization [22]. Similarly, support vector machines trained on sequences of known localizations also provides its own categorization of SCL. Additional modules include motif analysis for outer membrane beta barrels, transmembrane alpha helices, and cytoplasmic membrane signal peptides. The final prediction of SCL is then provided as an aggregated probabilistic likelihood based on the results of each module. Proteome Analyst features a machine learning classifier based on classifying homologous sequences of known localization found in the SWISS-PROT database of proteins. Proteome Analyst is comparable or exceeds PSORTb for predicting Gram-negative bacterial protein SCL's, and protein SCL for well-characterized bacteria or those similar to SWISS-PROT entries, while PSORTb is better at predicting SCL's for Gram-positive bacteria and many non-model organisms. PSORTb and Proteome Analyst use different approaches to make SCL predictions and complement each other if used together, generating even higher accuracy when used in concert [20].

PSORTb provides a user-friendly web server as well as a freely available standalone software version that allows users to enter protein sequences of interest as well as entire bacterial proteomes. The software provides SCL prediction if the prediction is above a certain cut-off and otherwise returns "Unknown" to minimize the number of false positive predictions. Pre-computed SCL prediction results for sequenced bacterial genomes are available at PSORTdb, an online database server (http://db.psort.org/; [23]). It is automatically updated regularly as newly sequenced bacterial genomes become available through NCBI (http://www.ncbi.nlm.nih.gov/genomes/lproks.cgi). Unfortunately, the web server for Proteome Analyst is no longer available so users cannot submit proteins for SCL prediction. However, pre-computed SCL prediction results for select Gram-negative bacteria; Gram-positive bacteria as well as a few other eukaryotic and archaeal species are still available.

The recent development of versions of SCL predictors with higher accuracy means that many more proteins that are cell surface or secreted can now be predicted from bacterial genomes. For example, on average, PSORTb version 3 (the current version, released in 2010) now predicts SCL for ~15 % more proteins in a Gram-negative bacterial genome than PSORTb version 2 did when it was released in 2005 [44]. So researchers who identified potential secreted or cell surface proteins using PSORTb, or PSORTdb, prior to 2010, may find they can identify more targets through re-analysis or review of precomputed genome result in the current version of PSORTdb.

Despite the high precision of PSORTb and Proteome Analyst prediction results, there is more work needed to further improve computational prediction of SCL. The prediction sensitivity of certain extracellular proteins is low compared to other SCLs, since some secreted proteins are often more unique/species-specific. Certain types of cell surface proteins, such as lipoproteins, are also not very well predicted. While signal peptide for proteins exported through the Sec secretion pathway is relatively well-predicted, the same cannot be said for effector proteins secreted through specialized secretion system such as Type III secretion system (T3SS), type IV secretion system (T4SS), and the more recently discovered type VI and type VII secretion systems. The secretion signals targeting effector proteins to these secretion systems are not well understood. Although there have been efforts at generating computational predictions for T3SS effectors [24, 25], the precision is not high for any of the available software. More efforts studying mechanism as well as the identification of more proteins secreted through these pathways are needed to serve as software training data. More species-specific proteomic studies identifying more of the less characterized surface and secreted proteins will greatly aid computational prediction for less well-studied bacteria.

6.3 GI Prediction

GIs are commonly defined as clusters of genes of potential horizontal origin in a bacterial genome that is usually >8 kb (the 8 kb cutoff primarily reflects limits of resolution of GI predictors). GIs display certain properties that can distinguish them from the rest of the genome since the origin of their genetic material is typically an unrelated species or prophage. They generally differ in sequence composition, as measured by GC content, dinucleotide bias, or codon usage, and are often found near tRNA genes or flanked by direct repeats (reviewed by [26]). These are sequence composition properties that can be exploited for computational prediction of GI's. Additionally, since whole genome sequences for many disease-causing pathogens and related avirulent strains are readily available in the public domain, other methods apply comparative genomics to identify GI's. Though this requires multiple genomes for analysis, using comparative genomics to identify GI insertions can greatly reduce the number of false predictions as well as provide insight on the stability of GI's across different lineages. The review by Langille et al. recommends using a combination of both sequence composition and comparative genomics methods for the best predictive coverage. In the future, it may become feasible to integrate population-level studies, including protein structures and common genes, to improve GI prediction. On the whole, by predicting GIs within the genomes of pathogens, we can quickly locate stable target genes for the design of effective vaccines or regions of particular interest for a given emerging pathogen. GI's have been shown to harbour disproportionately more virulence associated genes than the rest of a genome [12].

6.3.1 GI Prediction—Sequence Composition Methods

The typical strategy to detect GI's based on sequence composition involves calculating frequencies of variable lengths of nucleotide sequences (called *k*-mers, usually 2–9 bases) for segments of the genome and then comparing these to the frequencies over the entire genome. SIGI-HMM calculates the frequency of all codons (3-mers) to find genes with different codon usage bias than expected and to determine if it is more similar to another species. Clusters of these genes are then analyzed using a hidden Markov model (HMM) to statistically estimate if the region is a real GI ([27]; [43]). This approach works particularly well with reports of 92 % precision [26]. IslandPath-DIMOB is another GI predictor that predicts with the same precision but instead of codon usage bias it detects dinucleotide bias (2-mers) and the presence of mobility genes [28]. However, both programs only have 33 % and 36 % recall, respectively (recall as defined as "TP/(TP + FN)"; [26]). Centroid is a tool that examines regions of a specified size for sequence composition differences to the genome as a whole [29]. This program is more sensitive especially for larger insert sizes (>20 kb), but has the lowest recall (28 %) compared to the other programs. Alien_Hunter allows the user to specify variable lengths to compare sequence composition biases and is shown to have the highest recall (53 %), but has the lowest precision because of the sheer number of predictions made [30]. The overall precision, recall, and accuracy of all these programs were calculated by Langille et al. [26] by comparing GI predictions across 117 different strains of bacteria, using a dataset of GIs identified using completely unrelated methods.

Recently another algorithm, GIHunter, was developed to process Alien_Hunter predictions to improve its accuracy by incorporating additional gene information. GIHunter uses a decision tree model built upon differences in the types of genes and inter-genic distances in GIs compared to the rest of the genome [31]. This methodology increases the accuracy and precision compared to using Alien_Hunter alone. In evaluating this program against other previous sequence-based methods, GIHunter achieves comparable accuracy to that of SIGI-HMM and IslandPath-DIMOB. However, contrary to the claim by Wang et al., IslandPath-DIMOB is certainly able to predict one GI for *Streptococcus pyogenes* MGAS315. More robust accuracy calculations using the larger dataset used in comparing the earlier programs [26] is necessary to further assess GIHunter.

6.3.2 GI Prediction—Comparative Genomics Methods

Another approach, independent from the sequence composition-based approaches mentioned above, compares multiple-related genomes in order to find clusters of genes present in only one strain verses multiple-related strains. These tools depend on the input genomes, and if the selected genomes are too distantly or too closely related, this can lead to false or missed predictions. Because unstable GI's can randomly excise from the genome, some GIs can be found sporadically distributed among isolates from a given strain. Using comparative genomics, these unstable GI's can be easily recognized and avoided for vaccine design. IslandPick is a tool available through the web that automatically determines which genomes should be included in a GI analysis by evaluating their genome distances using CVTree [32, 33] to optimize GI prediction [34]. From these, whole genome alignments are performed using Mauve to determine regions of interest. It has been shown by Langille et al. that IslandPick has the highest concordance with known published GI's than predictions made by any of the sequence composition-based methods, highlighting the value of using a comparative genomics approach. Likewise, MobilomeFINDER is a comparative genomics approach that involves detecting GI's from Mauve alignments by focusing on regions of the genome upstream or downstream of tRNA genes [35]. Though a similar approach to IslandPick, this added flanking-tRNA constraint results in this program missing GI's that are not inserted near tRNA genes. While such comparative genomics methods can be more precise, the lack of comparative genomes suitable for analysis of some bacteria limits the utility of this method verses sequence composition approaches. However, as more and more genomes are sequenced, the utility of comparative genomics approaches will only increase, since they have the added benefit of being able to identify islands that have a similar sequence composition as the rest of a bacterial genome being analysed.

6.3.3 GI Prediction—Integrated Methods

IslandViewer (http://www.pathogenomics.sfu.ca/islandviewer/) is a web-based program developed to integrate the most precise GI prediction methods: SIGI-HMM, IslandPath-DIMOB, and IslandPick. All currently available sequenced genomes have pre-computed results accessible via the web interface. This, coupled with Alien_Hunter, the highest recall sequence composition-based method, allows most islands to be detected [36]. Figure 6.1 provides an example of IslandViewer output for the epidemic strain *Pseudomonas aeruginosa* LESB58. By hovering over each predicted GI, IslandViewer displays the genes encoded in that region (or one may simply obtain a table of all island predictions). The integrated predictions in this case correlate very well with known GI and prophage regions in *P. aeruginosa* LESB58 [37], with some additional novel predictions. Note that any one of these

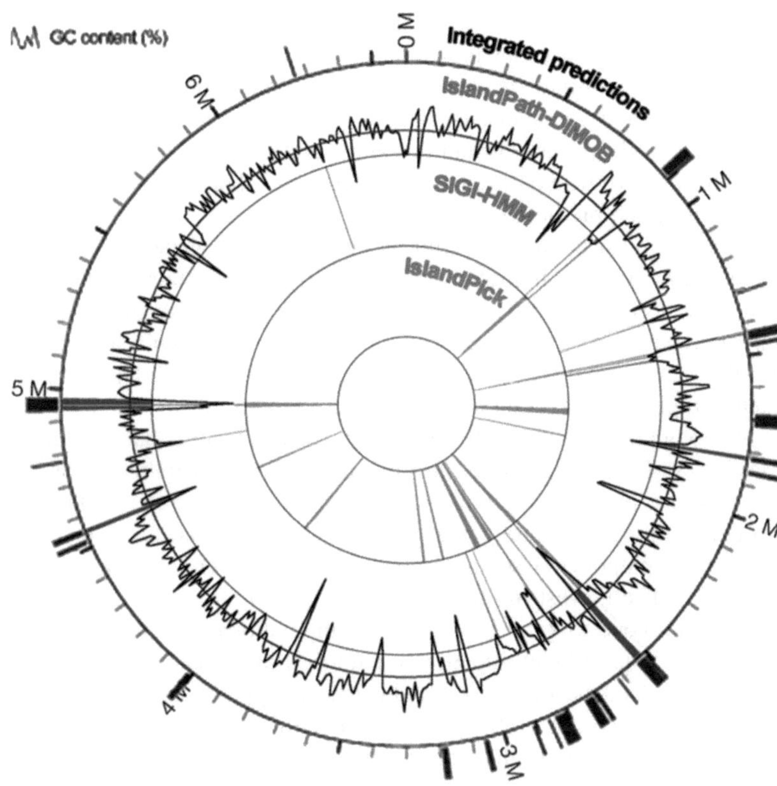

Fig. 6.1 IslandViewer results for *Pseudomonas aeruginosa* LESB58 epidemic strain. The black bars in the outer ring highlight all predicted GI regions integrated across the different methods. The gray bars within each consecutive inner ring highlight predicted GIs using IslandPath-DIMOB, SIGI-HMM, and IslandPick, respectively. The black line plot indicates the percentage GC content across the genome

methods alone did not predict all known GI's, so IslandViewer's integrative approach is particularly valuable.

6.4 Virulence Factor Prediction

Virulence factors are proteins that play a role in the pathogenesis of a microorganism. This can vary from host colonization, entry into host cells, nutrient usage, immune system evasion, and other functions. These proteins are often desirable vaccine components and many virulence factors have been used successfully as vaccine components in the past. For example, the vaccine for *Vibrio cholerae* contains recombinant subunits of the secreted cholera toxin [38]. In this case, the toxin gene is actually introduced into the genome via HGT of bacteriophage CTXφ [39]. Prediction of genes encoding virulence factors is very challenging because there is no one defining sequence or structural feature that all virulence genes exhibit. Manual review of genes is still necessary, thus advancements in virulence gene prediction are required. More large scale genome-wide analyses of virulence (e.g. signature-tagged mutagenesis screens or large scale knockout studies in suitable animal models) may expand our knowledge of novel proteins involved in pathogenesis and give us a dataset or virulence genes that may be large enough to enable more accurate predictive models to be made.

Currently, the most commonly used method to predict genes involved in virulence is to simply look for homology with known virulence factors. The virulence factor database (VFDB) [40–42] is a web resource containing information about experimentally verified virulence genes found in many pathogenic species of bacteria. It is fully searchable by genome, gene name, and via BLAST. There are also pre-computed comparisons of virulence factors between strains of the same genus or species. Although this is a valuable resource, virulence factors that are not found in databases like VFDB are otherwise entirely ignored. Because of this reason, it can be valuable to use a phyletic approach to identify potential virulence factors. This involves comparing genes among many species and/or strains at a given taxonomic level to identify pathogen-associated genes that are never found in related non-pathogens [12]. The newest implementation of VFDB allows this type of manual comparison on a gene to gene basis, but a computational tool to facilitate whole genome comparisons and identification of pathogen-associated genes, as well as an easily accessible database of genes found using this type of approach has yet to be developed. Overall, computation prediction of virulence factors is currently very limited and improvements in this area can not only advance our understanding of bacterial pathogenesis, but also enhance GI identification and vaccine design.

6.5 Concluding Comments

Bioinformatics methods have been developed that can predict proteins that are cell surface-accessible, stable in the genome, and play a role in virulence—qualities of interest when prioritizing potential vaccine components. The availability of the methods described here (summarized in Table 6.1), in particular web-based availability, allows researchers without a computational background to more easily utilize such tools. Most have been stably made available to researchers for years. However, and perhaps most importantly, all these computational tools have been recently updated (e.g., PSORTb for protein SCL, IslandViewer's integrated prediction tool for GIs, and the VFDB for virulence factor identification). So, if a researcher had previously identified potential vaccine components using even these specific methods, new targets may now be potentially identified due to the recently increased accuracy of such tools. As was summarized, there are improvements that can still be made in each of these bioinformatics predictors that should increase accuracy further. So even a regular re-running of new versions of such predictors against bacterial genomes should be performed, to not miss novel

Table 6.1 Location and accessibility of the programs described that predict (or provide data on) protein SCL, GI's, and virulence factors

	Tool	Accessibility	Website
SCL	PSORTdb	Web interface, downloadable	http://db.psort.org/
	PSORTb	Web interface, downloadable	http://www.psort.org/psortb
	Proteome Analyst	Pre-computed SCLs	http://webdocs.cs.ualberta.ca/~bioinfo/PA/GOSUB/
GI	IslandViewer	Web interface	http://www.pathogenomics.sfu.ca/islandviewer
	SIGI-HMM	Web interface	http://www.pathogenomics.sfu.ca/islandviewer
	IslandPath-DIMOB	Web interface	http://www.pathogenomics.sfu.ca/islandviewer
	IslandPick	Web interface	http://www.pathogenomics.sfu.ca/islandviewer
	GIHunter	Downloadable	http://www.esu.edu/cpsc/che_lab/software/GIHunter
	Centroid	Downloadable	By request from authors
	Alien_Hunter	Downloadable	http://www.sanger.ac.uk/resources/software/alien_hunter
	Mobilome FINDER	Web interface	http://db-mml.sjtu.edu.cn/MobilomeFINDER/
VF	VFDB	Web interface	http://www.mgc.ac.cn/VFs/

potential targets for vaccine discovery. In some cases, for example with PSORTb, there are pre-computed results regularly updated and made available through an associated database (i.e. PSORTdb). Combining such databases for SCL prediction, virulence factors, etc., together in the future, with updates noted, may help allow researchers to more easily note when particularly relevant new data is released. At a time when antimicrobial resistance is on the rise, it is critical that vaccine discovery efforts continue to move forward efficiently.

References

1. Pizza M, Scarlato V, Masignani V, Giuliani MM, Arico B, Comanducci M, Jennings GT, Baldi L, Bartolini E, Capecchi B (2000) Identification of vaccine candidates against serogroup B meningococcus by whole-genome sequencing. Science 287(5459):1816
2. Masignani V, Comanducci M, Giuliani MM, Bambini S, Adu-Bobie J, Aricò B, Brunelli B, Pieri A, Santini L, Savino S (2003) Vaccination against *Neisseria meningitidis* using three variants of the lipoprotein GNA1870. J Exp Med 197(6):789
3. Welsch JA, Rossi R, Comanducci M, Granoff DM (2004) Protective activity of monoclonal antibodies to genome-derived neisserial antigen 1870, a *Neisseria meningitidis* candidate vaccine. J Immunol 172(9):5606

4. Scarselli M, Aricò B, Brunelli B, Savino S, Di Marcello F, Palumbo E, Veggi D, Ciucchi L, Cartocci E, Bottomley MJ (2011) Rational Design of a Meningococcal Antigen Inducing Broad Protective Immunity. Sci Transl Med 3(91):91ra62
5. Chakravarti DN, Fiske MJ, Fletcher LD, Zagursky RJ (2000) Application of genomics and proteomics for identification of bacterial gene products as potential vaccine candidates. Vaccine 19(6):601–612
6. Wizemann TM, Heinrichs JH, Adamou JE, Erwin AL, Kunsch C, Choi GH, Barash SC, Rosen CA, Masure HR, Tuomanen E (2001) Use of a whole genome approach to identify vaccine molecules affording protection against *Streptococcus pneumoniae* infection. Infect Immun 69 (3):1593
7. Ross BC, Czajkowski L, Hocking D, Margetts M, Webb E, Rothel L, Patterson M, Agius C, Camuglia S, Reynolds E (2001) Identification of vaccine candidate antigens from a genomic analysis of *Porphyromonas gingivalis*. Vaccine 19(30):4135–4142
8. Ariel N, Zvi A, Makarova K, Chitlaru T, Elhanany E, Velan B, Cohen S, Friedlander A, Shafferman A (2003) Genome-based bioinformatic selection of chromosomal Bacillus anthracis putative vaccine candidates coupled with proteomic identification of surface-associated antigens. Infect Immun 71(8):4563
9. Gamberini M, Gómez RM, Atzingen MV, Martins EAL, Vasconcellos SA, Romero EC, Leite LCC, Ho PL, Nascimento ALTO (2005) Whole-genome analysis of *Leptospira interrogans* to identify potential vaccine candidates against leptospirosis. FEMS Microbiol Lett 244 (2):305–313
10. Hacker J, Kaper JB (2000) Pathogenicity islands and the evolution of microbes. Annu Rev Microbiol 54(1):641–679
11. Stephens C, Murray W (2001) Pathogen evolution: how good bacteria go bad. Curr Biol 11(2): R53–R56
12. Ho Sui SJ, Fedynak A, Hsiao WWL, Langille MGI, Brinkman FSL (2009) The association of virulence factors with genomic islands. PLoS One 4(12):e8094
13. Siebor E and Neuwirth C (2011) The new variant of Salmonella genomic island 1 (SGI1-V) from a *Proteus mirabilis* French clinical isolate harbours blaVEB-6 and qnrA1 in the multiple antibiotic resistance region. J Antimicrob Chemother
14. Boyd EF, Almagro-Moreno S, Parent MA (2009) Genomic islands are dynamic, ancient integrative elements in bacterial evolution. Trends Microbiol 17(2):47–53
15. Gal-Mor O, Finlay BB (2006) Pathogenicity islands: a molecular toolbox for bacterial virulence. Cell Microbiol 8(11):1707–1719
16. Dobrindt U, Hochhut B, Hentschel U, Hacker J (2004) Genomic islands in pathogenic and environmental microorganisms. Nat Rev Microbiol 2(5):414–424
17. Hacker J, Blum-Oehler G, Mühldorfer I, Tschäpe H (1997) Pathogenicity islands of virulent bacteria: structure, function and impact on microbial evolution. Mol Microbiol 23 (6):1089–1097
18. Relman DA (2011) Microbial genomics and infectious diseases. N Engl J Med 2011 (365):347–357
19. Rey S, Gardy J, Brinkman F (2005) Assessing the precision of high-throughput computational and laboratory approaches for the genome-wide identification of protein subcellular localization in bacteria. BMC Genomics 6(1):162
20. Yu NY, Wagner JR, Laird MR, Melli G, Rey S, Lo R, Dao P, Sahinalp SC, Ester M, Foster LJ (2010) PSORTb 3.0: improved protein subcellular localization prediction with refined localization subcategories and predictive capabilities for all prokaryotes. Bioinformatics 26 (13):1608
21. Lu Z, Szafron D, Greiner R, Lu P, Wishart D, Poulin B, Anvik J, Macdonell C, Eisner R (2004) Predicting subcellular localization of proteins using machine-learned classifiers. Bioinformatics 20(4):547
22. Gardy JL, Brinkman FSL (2006) Methods for predicting bacterial protein subcellular localization. Nat Rev Microbiol 4:741–751

23. Yu NY, Laird MR, Spencer C, Brinkman FSL (2011) PSORTdb—an expanded, auto-updated, user-friendly protein subcellular localization database for Bacteria and Archaea. Nucleic Acids Res 39(suppl 1):D241
24. Arnold R, Brandmaier S, Kleine F, Tischler P, Heinz E, Behrens S, Niinikoski A, Mewes HW, Horn M, Rattei T (2009) Sequence-based prediction of type III secreted proteins. PLoS Pathog 5(4):e1000376
25. Samudrala R, Heffron F, McDermott JE (2009) Accurate prediction of secreted substrates and identification of a conserved putative secretion signal for type III secretion systems. PLoS Pathog 5(4):e1000375
26. Langille MGI, Hsiao WWL, Brinkman FSL (2010) Detecting genomic islands using bioinformatics approaches. Nat Rev Microbiol 8(5):373–382
27. Waack S, Keller O, Asper R, Brodag T, Damm C, Fricke W, Surovcik K, Meinicke P, Merkl R (2006) Score-based prediction of genomic islands in prokaryotic genomes using hidden Markov models. BMC Bioinformatics 7(1):142
28. Hsiao WWL, Ung K, Aeschliman D, Bryan J, Finlay BB, Brinkman FSL (2005) Evidence of a large novel gene pool associated with prokaryotic genomic islands. PLoS Genet 1(5):e62
29. Rajan I, Aravamuthan S, Mande SS (2007) Identification of compositionally distinct regions in genomes using the centroid method. Bioinformatics 23(20):2672
30. Vernikos GS, Parkhill J (2006) Interpolated variable order motifs for identification of horizontally acquired DNA: revisiting the Salmonella pathogenicity islands. Bioinformatics 22(18):2196
31. Wang H, Fazekas J, Booth M, Liu Q, Che D (2011) An integrative approach for genomic island prediction in prokaryotic genomes. Bioinformatics Research and Applications 6674:404–415
32. Xu Z, Hao B (2009) CVTree update: a newly designed phylogenetic study platform using composition vectors and whole genomes. Nucleic Acids Res 37(suppl 2):W174
33. Qi J, Luo H, Hao B (2004) CVTree: a phylogenetic tree reconstruction tool based on whole genomes. Nucleic Acids Res 32(suppl 2):W45
34. Langille M, Hsiao W, Brinkman F (2008) Evaluation of genomic island predictors using a comparative genomics approach. BMC Bioinformatics 9(1):329
35. Ou HY, He X, Harrison EM, Kulasekara BR, Thani AB, Kadioglu A, Lory S, Hinton JCD, Barer MR, Deng Z (2007) MobilomeFINDER: web-based tools for in silico and experimental discovery of bacterial genomic islands. Nucleic Acids Res 35(suppl 2):W97
36. Langille MGI, Brinkman FSL (2009) IslandViewer: an integrated interface for computational identification and visualization of genomic islands. Bioinformatics 25(5):664
37. Winstanley C, Langille MG, Fothergill JL, Kukavica-Ibrulj I, Paradis-Bleau C, Sanschagrin F, Thomson NR, Winsor GL, Quail MA, Lennard N, Bignell A, Clarke L, Seeger K, Saunders D, Harris D, Parkhill J, Hancock RE, Brinkman FS, Levesque RC (2009) Newly introduced genomic prophage islands are critical determinants of in vivo competitiveness in the Liverpool Epidemic Strain of *Pseudomonas aeruginosa*. Genome Res 19(1):12–23
38. Ragot C, Garnotel E, Vedy S, Morillon M (2006) Dukoral, oral cholera vaccine. Med Trop (Mars) 66(3):237–239
39. Waldor MK, Mekalanos JJ (1996) Lysogenic conversion by a filamentous phage encoding cholera toxin. Science 272(5270):1910
40. Chen LH, Xiong ZH, Sun LL, Yang J, Jin Q (2012) VFDB 2012 update: toward the genetic diversity and molecular evolution of bacterial virulence factors. Nucleic Acids Res 40: D641–D645
41. Yang J, Chen L, Sun L, Yu J, Jin Q (2008) VFDB 2008 release: an enhanced web-based resource for comparative pathogenomics. Nucleic Acids Res 36(suppl 1):D539
42. Chen L, Yang J, Yu J, Yao Z, Sun L, Shen Y, Jin Q (2005) VFDB: a reference database for bacterial virulence factors. Nucleic Acids Res 33(suppl 1):D325
43. Merkl R (2004) SIGI: score-based identification of genomic islands. BMC Bioinformatics 5(1):22
44. Gardy JL, Laird MR, Chen F, Rey S, Walsh CJ, Ester M, Brinkman FS (2005) PSORTb v.2.0: expanded prediction of bacterial protein subcellular localization and insights gained from comparative proteome analysis. Bioinformatics 21(5):617

[illegible]

Chapter 7
On the Development of Vaccine Antigen Databases: Progress, Opportunity, and Challenge

Hifzur Rahman Ansari, Darren R. Flower, and Gajendra P.S. Raghava

Abstract The accumulation of relevant and appropriate data is the essential preliminary to any successful informatics-based exercise in prediction. Without quality data, meaningful prediction is impossible. This is as true in immunobiology as it is in any other branch of the natural sciences. Within the context of vaccine discovery, the accumulation, storage, and retrieval of immunological data within publically accessible repositories, typically web-based databases, is of overwhelming operational importance. Specifically, and with the special reference to the discovery of subunit vaccines, this chapter explores the current state and status of immunological databases focussed on immunogenic proteins, primarily pathogen antigens and environmental allergens. It sets this exploration firmly into context by simultaneously scoping out the rather more mature backdrop provided by epitope-orientated database systems.

7.1 Introduction

Vaccine antigen databases, which are typically compiled from numerous different varieties of resources, can lead, either directly or indirectly, to the facilitation of vaccine development. Vaccines are substances that train the host immune system to protect itself against the direct effects of pathogenic microorganisms mediating infectious disease, as well as symptoms of the disease itself. A vaccine is a molecular or composite supramolecular agent eliciting an enhanced adaptive immune response to subsequent infection or reinfection, primarily by potentiating immune memory. Vaccines evoke complex, system-wide immunity of various durations, engendering protection lasting year-long to life-long. The remarkable flexibility inherent in the concept of vaccination has prompted science to use it to

D.R. Flower (✉)
School of Life and Health Sciences, Aston University, Birmingham, UK
e-mail: d.r.flower@aston.ac.uk

D.R. Flower and Y. Perrie (eds.), *Immunomic Discovery of Adjuvants and Candidate Subunit Vaccines*, Immunomics Reviews: 5, DOI 10.1007/978-1-4614-5070-2_7,

attack infectious and contagious disease, allergy, addiction, and cancer, among many other targets.

Population-wide vaccination, which also subsumes the beneficial effects of herd immunity, is now commonly agreed to be the most effective prophylactic treatment for infectious disease. Such vaccination also now offers similar hope for many chronic diseases, including among others allergy and cancer. If you find such language dry, then we can further conceptualise how vaccines work in what follows, expressing things in more anthropomorphic terms. Vaccines offer the immune system the opportunity to encounter and respond to diverse structures on the molecular and mesoscopic scales, which are then memorised so that future immune responses are faster and more effective, and without themselves causing illness or disease. A variety of antigenic molecular structures, such as epitopes and PAMPs, can activate different arms of immune system including B-cells, T-cells, and various innate immune responses through the activation of pattern recognition receptors (PRRs), including the current pre-eminent PRR: Toll-like receptors.

Hitherto, vaccine development has been largely categorised by its doggedly empirical nature; as our understanding of immunology has increased, attempts have been made to give vaccine discovery a more explicable, mechanistic basis. With this sea change, has come the opportunity to introduce rational design supported by computational methods for analysis and prediction. Underlying attempts to predict key components of immunological systems are data capable of being understood, manipulated, and utilised, that is: quantitative molecular data and meaningful functional data. Immunoinformatics may reveal or elucidate recondite components of immunological or signalling pathways, or define protein function by establishing structural or sequence similarity to known proteins. Thus, what computational support of vaccinology can achieve is limited. Yet, there are also immense potential opportunities to exploit this technology for the benefit of vaccinology and thus for the benefit of human medicine and the prevention of infectious disease. It is of the greatest importance to understand fully what is useful and what is not.

By offering diverse tools and methods, immunoinformatics is able to support and facilitate experimental and clinical endeavour [1]. To be of value, information that we intend to model and predict must be properly accumulated, collated, annotated, and archived, before being analysed and dissected. This is surely the purpose of a database. Within immunology, such databases have a relatively extended history. Examples such as Kabat [2] and IMGT [3–5] focussed on compiling and annotating host-side sequences and structures. Indeed, for some time, the Kabat database was the only database containing protein sequence data.

In this chapter, we shall offer a succinct overview of immunological databases relevant to the design and discovery of vaccines, offering a concise yet synoptic outline which is comprised of several brief yet insightful descriptions of various publically accessible database systems, each of which impinges, directly or indirectly, upon vaccine design. See also Table 7.1.

Table 7.1 Immunoinformatic databases and servers for immunomics and vaccinomics

Host databases	
IMGT/HLA	http://www.ebi.ac.uk/imgt/hla/allele.html
IMGT/TR	http://imgt.cines.fr/textes/IMGTrepertoire
IPD Database	http://www.ebi.ac.uk/ipd/index.html
Kabat	http://www.kabatdatabase.com/
VBASE	http://www.vbase2.org/
ABG	http://www.ibt.unam.mx/vir/
V BASE	http://vbase.mrc-cpe.cam.ac.uk/
Pathogen databases	
APB	http://www.engr.psu.edu/ae/iec/abe/database.asp
APDD	http://psychro.bioinformatics.unsw.edu.au/pathogen/index.php
ARS	http://www.ars.usda.gov/research/projects/projects.htm?accn_no=406518
BROP	http://www.brop.org/
EDWIP	http://cricket.inhs.uiuc.edu/edwipweb/edwipabout.htm
FPPD	http://fppd.cbio.psu.edu/
LEGER	http://leger2.gbf.de/cgi-bin/expLeger.pl
ORALGEN	http://www.oralgen.lanl.gov/
Pathema	http://pathema.jcvi.org/Pathema/
ShiBASE	http://www.mgc.ac.cn/ShiBASE/
STDGen	http://www.stdgen.lanl.gov/
VBI	http://phytophthora.vbi.vt.edu/
VIDIL	http://insectweb.inhs.uiuc.edu/Pathogens/VIDIL/index.html
VFDB	http://zdsys.chgb.org.cn/VFs/main.htm
CandiVF	http://research.i2r.a-star.edu.sg/Templar/DB/CandiVF/
TVfac	http://www.tvfac.lanl.gov/
PRINTS	http://www.jenner.ac.uk/BacBix3/PPprints.htm
ClinMalDB-USP	http://malariadb.ime.usp.br/malaria/us/bioinformaticResearch.jsp
Fish Pathogen database	http://dbsdb.nus.edu.sg/fpdb/about.html
PHI-BASE	http://www.phi-base.org/
T-cell databases	
AntiJen	http://www.ddg-pharmfac.net/antijen/AntiJen/aj_tcell.htm
EPIMHC	http://bio.dfci.harvard.edu/epimhc/
FIMM	http://research.i2r.a-star.edu.sg/fimm/
HLA Ligand Database	http://hlaligand.ouhsc.edu/index_2.html
HIV Immunology	http://www.hiv.lanl.gov/immunology
HCV Immunology	http://hcv.lanl.gov/content/immuno/immuno-main.html
IEDB	http://epitope2.immuneepitope.org/home.do
JenPep	http://www.jenner.ac.uk/jenpep2/
MHCBN	http://www.imtech.res.in/raghava/mhcbn
MHCPEP	http://wehih.wehi.edu.au/mhcpep
MPID-T	http://surya.bic.nus.edu.sg/mpidt/
SYFPEITHI	http://www.syfpeithi.de
B-cell databases	
AntiJen	http://www.ddg-pharmfac.net/antijen/AntiJen/aj_bcell.htm
BCIPEP	http://www.imtech.res.in/raghava/bcipep

(continued)

Table 7.1 (continued)

CED	http://web.kuicr.kyoto-u.ac.jp/~ced/
EPITOME	http://www.rostlab.org/services/epitome/
IEDB	http://epitope2.immuneepitope.org/home.do
HaptenDB	http://www.imtech.res.in/raghava/haptendb/
HIV Immunology	http://www.hiv.lanl.gov/immunology
HCV Immunology	http://hcv.lanl.gov/immuno/
Innate immunity and evolution databases	
InnateDB	http://www.innatedb.ca/
ImmTree	http://bioinf.uta.fi/ImmTree
ImmunomeBase	http://bioinf.uta.fi/ImmunomeBase
Immunome Knowledge Base	http://bioinf.uta.fi/IKB/
PRRDB	http://www.imtech.res.in/raghava/prrdb

7.2 Immunoinformatics Databases

For a very long time, indeed rather longer than there has been such a discipline, a principal bed rock of immunoinformatics has been that collection of focussed molecular biology databases, christened IMGT [3–5]. IMGT, standing for the international ImMunoGeneTics information system (URL: http://www.imgt.org), describes itself as the world reference in immunogenetics and immunoinformatics, and was created in 1989 at the Laboratoire d'ImmunoGénétique Moléculaire LIGM (Université Montpellier 2 and CNRS, Montpellier, France). Rather than being a monolithic database system, IMGT instead comprises databases, interactive online tools, and Web resources; this database collective concentrates on the compilation and annotation of host-side nucleic acid and protein sequences and corresponding 3D structures. IMGT is an integrated resource encompassing the principal molecules of the adaptive immune system of humans and other vertebrate species: immunoglobulins (IGs) or antibodies, T-cell receptors (TR), and major histocompatibility (MH) complexes. IMGT also covers proteins of the immunoglobulin superfamily, proteins of the MH superfamily, and related proteins of the immune systems (RPI) from both vertebrates and invertebrates, together with therapeutic monoclonal antibodies and fusion proteins for immune applications.

The IMGT/HLA database (URL: http://www.ebi.ac.uk/imgt/hla/) is an independent and important self-contained component within the larger edifice of IMGT [6, 7]. The initial release of IMGT/HLA occurred in December 1998, being subsequently updated every 3 months, and includes all publicly available human major histocompatibility complex (MHC) sequences named by the WHO Nomenclature Committee. IMGT/HLA is a locus-specific database for human allelic sequences of the genes of the MHC or HLA system, which is found in the 6p21.3 region of chromosome 6, containing over 220 genes. More widely, the MHC is generally regarded as the most polymorphic of all proteins from higher vertebrates. Growth in the database reflects clinical interest in the MHC as a key mediator of host responses to infection and of tissue rejection in organ and stem cell transplants. The first version of IMGT/HLA included 964 alleles for 24 genes, while the April 2011 release contained in excess of 6,400 alleles for 34 genes. Another important database in the host area is VBASE2, which stores germ-line sequences of human and mouse IG variable (V) genes [8].

The Immuno Polymorphism Database (IPD) system (URL: http://www.ebi.ac.uk/ipd/), which covers data from important nonhuman species, including primates, as well as cattle, sheep, and other commercially important farm livestock, has emerged recently from IMGT's long shadow [9–12]. IPD comprises four specialist database systems. IPD-ESTDAB: a database of melanoma cell lines. IPD-KIR: a database of alleles of killer-cell IG-like receptors. PD-HPA: a database of human platelet alloantigens. IPD-MHC: a database of MHC sequences from different species.

A major omission to all extant immunoinformatics and immunogenetics database systems, including IMGT and IPD, is the requirement for a proper database of mouse MHC allele sequences equipped with and based upon a sound and solid consolidated system of nomenclature. The mouse MHC region is located on Chromosome 17, and for historical reasons is referred to *H-2*, for histocompatibility 2, with the different genes denoted by additional letters: D, L, K for Class I and A and E for Class II. Thus, a Class I mouse MHC allele will bear the somewhat inscrutable labels: H-2 Kb or H-2 Db. Within the context of understanding immunological mechanisms underlying vaccine development, the mouse is unarguably the most convenient and thus the most widely used model organism. In bred strains of mice thus provide the principal tool of empirical vaccinology. The albino laboratory strain Balb/c has the *d* haplotype comprising H2-Kd, H2-Dd H2-Ld, H2-IAd, and H2-IEd; the agouti lab strain C3H/He has the k haplotype comprising H2-Kk, H2-Dk, H2-IAk, H2-IEk; and the black mouse C57BL/6 has the *b* haplotype composed of H2-Kb, H2-Db, and H2-Iab. The agouti strain CBA also has the k haplotype. Outbred mice will obviously contain a greater variety of alleles and thus the need for a more extensible and flexible naming system. However, compilation of such a murine-orientated database, or even the formulation of a more overtly systematic and lucent nomenclature, has progressed little in the last 30 years.

For a long time now, there have been databases that focus upon properties of cellular immunology and look primarily at data pertinent to the discussion of the complexities of MHC processing, presentation, and subsequent T-cell recognition. Perhaps, the earliest such database [13, 14], and probably the first to gain any prominence, is SYFPEITHI (URL: http://www.syfpeithi.de/). This is still widely used database system is a high quality development, comprising a useful compendium of known T-cell epitopes. SYFPEITHI also comprises information on MHC ligands: peptides extracted ex vivo from MHCs on the cell surface. It does not include data on synthetic peptide "binders." "Binders" are peptides with experimentally measured affinity for MHCs. There are several well-used means to measure affinities: IC_{50} values [15–17]; BL_{50} values; association and dissociation equilibrium constants, and the half-life of radioisotope-labelled β_2-microglobulin–MHC complex [18–21]. No consensus has ever emerged on the most appropriate type of affinity measure.

MHCPEP [22–25], defunct database of some vintage, brought together epitope date from T-cells and peptide-MHC (p-MHC) binding data, subsequently making it available as a web-based database system [26]. Subsequently, MHCPEP was developed into a more sophisticated and ambitious database system, called FIMM [27–29]. This integrates data on MHC–peptide interactions: in addition to MHC–peptide binding data and T-cell epitopes, FIMM also includes sequence data on MHC proteins themselves and also information on the disease associations of MHC alleles. Other examples include EPIMHC (URL: http://imed.med.ucm.es/epimhc/), a database of T-cell epitopes and MHC-binding peptides [30]. At the time of writing, EPIMHC included 4,867 immunogenic sequences from a plethora of sources. The HLA Ligand Database is another, now defunct databank, with data from the area of T-cell epitology, including information on binding motifs and HLA ligands [31].

Another database of interest is MPID, and its successors: MPID-T and MPID-T2 [32–34]. Focussing primarily on TCR/pMHC interactions, MPID-T is a curated MySQL database which focusses on experimental structures of pMHC and TcR/pMHC complexes (URL: http://biolinfo.org/mpid-t2). Other related databases have emerged, each addressing data on different aspects of molecular immunology. Middleton and co-workers [35, 36] have described the Allele Frequency Database (URL: http://www.allelefrequencies.net/) which lists population frequencies of individual MHC alleles and haplotypes.

Let us now turn to databases that address the humoral, rather than the cellular, immune response. BciPep [37, 38] (URL: http://www.imtech.res.in/raghava/bcipep/): sourced from the primary scientific literature, it comprises 3,031 linear B-cell epitopes sequences, within a PostgreSQL database. Cross-referenced to the SWISS-PROT and PDB databases, epitopes are shown as sequences annotated with the host protein, the binding antibody, and the experimental method of immunogenicity determination. The Epitome database (http://www.rostlab.org/services/epitome/) consists of structurally inferred antigenic regions, as identified from X-ray protein structures. Together with a host of related information, including experimental methods, antibody, and antigen, the Discontinuous Epitope Database (CED) adumbrates experimentally determined discontinuous epitopes excised from the scientific literature (URL: http://immunet.cn/ced/index.php) [39].

Another interesting database, also targeting humoral immunology, is HaptenDB [40]. It presently comprises 2,021 entries for 1,087 haptens and 25 carrier proteins (URL: http://www.imtech.res.in/raghava/haptendb/). Entry details the nature of the hapten, as well as its 2D and 3D structures, and its associated carrier proteins. Data is also at present available for anti-hapten antibody production method, the coupling method, and the specificities of antibodies.

There also exist a number of combined databases which seek to cover both cellular and humoral immunology. The first such, and also arguably the best and most detailed and exhaustive, if not necessarily the broadest and most general, is the HIV Molecular Immunology Database (URL: http://www.hiv.lanl.gov/content/immunology/) [41]. It archives CD8+ and CD4+ T-cell epitopes, and also B-cell epitopes, derived from various strains of the HIV virus. The database features sequence alignments, viral protein epitope maps, drug-resistant viral protein sequences, and vaccine-trial data. At the time of writing, T-cell epitope data numbers 3,150 entries, describing 1,600 distinct MHC class I-epitopes. The HCV database comprises 510 entries describing 250 distinct MHC class I-epitope combinations [42]. Perhaps, in the future, all databases will be like the HIV Molecular Immunology Database.

AntiJen v2.0 [43] is another database system, somewhat more ambitious in its scope. It retains information on B- and T-cell epitopes, but also archives quantitative data on a variety of immunological interactions, thus making it both unique and useful. The database (URL: http://www.ddg-pharmfac.net/antijen/) contains more than 31,000 entries with 11 sub-databases. These interactions include peptide binding to transport-associated antigen processing (TAP), peptide binding to MHC, p-MHC binding to TCR, and protein–protein interactions in terms of molecular thermodynamic, kinetic, and biophysical data such as receptor copy number and diffusion coefficient

Updated version 4.0 of the MHCBN [44, 45] contains more than 25,000 experimentally characterised T-cell and MHC binding peptides with affinity and activity data compiled from 1,500 papers, as well as from diverse public databases (URL: http://www.imtech.res.in/raghava/mhcbn/). Coverage of 1,000 TAP and 4,000 MHC non-binder peptides put MHCBN at a position distinct from other similar immunological databases. Database covers all major hosts like human, mouse, rat, monkey, etc., and provide information of 20 major MHC-linked diseases. The database provides a user-friendly search interface which can be used for simple and customised queries. This also provides several tools for peptide searching, mapping, and BLAST search against MHCBN data.

However, the pre-eminent database of our age is doubtlessly the Immune Epitope Database (IEDB) [46–49]. It is the most comprehensive and progressive database yet available in the area of immunoinformatics. IEDB contains more than 75,000 experimentally characterised B- and T-cell epitopes, MHC binding and elution experiment data compiled from 10,500 literature sources, and data directly submitted by a series of labs (URL: http://www.immuneepitope.org/). They have covered 2,500 organisms based on the priority set by National Institute of Allergy and Infectious Diseases which includes allergens and auto-antigens. IEDB also provides useful complementary tools based on the latest algorithms for the analysis and prediction of epitopes and MHC binding. It provides improved user interface for general and advanced searching or browsing by source organism or MHC allele type.

7.3 Antigen and Virulence Factor Databases

Arguably, the clearest and least ambiguous example of an antigen is the so-called virulence factor (VF). Such antigenic proteins induce disease and/or undertake host colonisation. Analysis of known pathogenic species reveals recurrent "systems" of toxins and VFs. VFs have been categorised into several thematic groups: exotoxins, adherence/colonisation factors, transporters, invasins, iron-binding siderophores, and miscellaneous cell surface factors. A simpler yet more synoptic definition places VFs into three groups: (1) "true" virulence factors; (2) VFs associated with the expression and regulation of class 1 VF genes; and (3) VFs required for host colonisation [50].

Obviously, there is no absolute requirement for antigens to be VFs. Antigens do not need to be directly or indirectly implicated in mechanisms of infectivity; instead, they need only be available for immune surveillance. Thus, databases focussing solely on VFs are not enough and so other kinds of database are needed, capable of capturing and containing more and different relevant data. In the recent past, such a database has been created: AntigenDB [51]; it contains a compilation of in excess of 500 antigens drawn from other immunological resources, as well as the primary scientific literature. AntigenDB is a new stage in the development of immunoinformatics, signalling a switch away from the peptide epitope and towards the whole protein antigen. The AntigenDB database project commenced with the key objective of compiling all immunogenic antigens from all major pathogens for which epitope information is known. AntigenDB (URL: http://www.imtech.res.in/raghava/antigendb/) is intended to help researchers working on the development of antigen prediction algorithms; and also to aid vaccinologists who would like to use these antigens as a tool in the discovery of subunit vaccine candidates.

In AntigenDB, a database entry summarises a large amount of relevant information regarding antigens. It lists origin, structure, sequence, etc., with additional information such as MHC binding, T-cell and B-cell epitopes, gene expression, function, and post-translational modifications. Currently, AntigenDB contains more than 500 antigens coming from important pathogenic species. These antigens originate from 44 key pathogenic species. Entries comprise information pertaining to structure, origin, sequence, etc. They also hold information such as MHC binding data, B- and T-cell epitope, function, and gene expression information if available. A database can be searched by using simple keywords or browsing using pathogen names, after which data can be easily exported to an Excel file. AntigenDB also provides useful tools like BLAST for analysis of the antigenic similarity, epitope search to verify if similar epitopes exist in the database, and peptide mapping to determine the presence of previously known epitopes. AntigenDB also provides links to major internal and external databases. Data submission tool is also provided to submit data online which is included in the database after validation. AntigenDB will be updated on a continuous and continuing basis, with the regular, if infrequent, addition of new antigens and antigens from new organisms. AntigenDB should act as the kernel for future attempts to predict antigens accurately using sequence similarity or via more complex and subtle analysis.

A related database system has been christened VIOLIN (vaccine investigation and online information network) [52]: it allows straightforward curation, and the analysis and comparison of research data across diverse pathogens in the context of human medicine, animal models, laboratory model systems, and natural hosts. It contains 2,759 vaccines or candidates for 173 pathogens culled from 1,631 peer-reviewed papers, as well as 24,345 vaccine-related abstracts and 10,317 full-text articles. VIOLIN is a web-accessible resource (URL: http://www.violinet.org). Peer-reviewed vaccine-related literature has been downloaded into VIOLIN; and the database is searchable in various ways. Archived information includes vaccine preparation and characteristics, microbial pathogenesis, host-protective immunity, stimulated host responses post vaccination, and protection efficacy after challenge.

Vertebrates have developed an efficient immune system and pathogens need to adapt to this very hostile environment; therefore, they devise different counter strategies like antigenic drift and variation to evade a host immune system. Some pathogens mutate their antigens so that antibodies are no longer able to recognise them, while some hide themselves from the immune cells like malaria-causing pathogen plasmodium to reside in red blood cells. Genome-sequencing efforts revealed the existence of a large number of multi-copy gene families with suspected involvement in antigenic variation and virulence. The genomics and proteomics projects release a huge amount of sequence and phenotypic data. The varDB project [53–56] aims to produce a dedicated platform for the antigen variation, phenotypes, and clinical manifestations (URL: http://www.vardb.org/vardb/). So far, the varDB database has covered 42 gene families, accommodating 67,000 sequences from 27 species of organisms causing 19 different diseases. varDB has created a framework for automatic data download, processing, and annotation. Entries can be queried and sorted based on the UniProt ID, gene products, isolation source, host, locus tag, etc. varDB has implemented a user-friendly tool, a shopping cart where sequences can be added and analysed, and a correlation with disease outcome can be revealed, leading to the identification of functionally important residues and drug targets.

Several other databases targeting VFs have also been reported. They include TVFac (Los Alamos National Laboratory Toxin and Virulence Factor database; URL: http://www.tvfac.lanl.gov/). This has within it information on in excess of 250 organisms, with records for thousands of virulence genes. The *Candida albicans* virulence factor (CandiVF) is a fully searchable species-specific database containing diverse VFs [57]. The Virulence Factor Database (VFDB; URL: http://www.mgc.ac.cn/VFs/) targets 16 bacterial genomes; it focusses on functional and structural biology and is fully searchable in several ways [58, 59]. PHI-base integrates VFs from a veritable gallimaufry of plant and animal pathogens [60]. The Fish Pathogen Database (URL: http://www.fishpathogens.eu/vhsv/index.php), from the Bacteriology and Fish Diseases Laboratory, archives 500 VFs from fish.

7.4 Allergen Databases

Allergy is a complex pathological condition caused by allergenic proteins resulting from uncontrolled IgE antibody-mediated immune responses. Allergies of all types are escalating as the world moves inexorably towards a western lifestyle, with all its benefits and dangers. This gives rise to a reduction in the depth and breadth of immunity to microbial pathogens. As a consequence, the prevalence of atopy rises. Making inappropriate and immediate hypersensitivity reactions to harmless substances is the mark of atopy. Thus, significant exposure to pathogens, both viral and bacterial, during early life is vital to the proper regulation of allergen-specific immune responses. If such inappropriate and potentially catastrophic reactions are not the ransom to be delivered by certain populations for their freedom from microbial diseases, we must be prepared to continually train our immune systems, especially during infancy, in order to prevent allergic conditions. Allergy affects over 30 % of the population in developed countries, with a concomitant major economic health burden [61].

The aforementioned hypersensitivity reactions occur when allergens are bound by IgE tethered to the surface of basophils or mast cells. Allergenic proteins form a distinct class of antigens; they are able to induce specific production of IgE, which in turn leads to the secretion of inflammatory mediators. An individual sensitised to, say, pollen-derived allergens might additionally react to allergens also present in plant-based foods as a result of the intrinsic commonality of sequence and structure. This cross-reactive of distinct allergenic proteins from different sources can be problematic. Owing to the importance of allergens, a number of databases and analysis tools have been created. Fortuitously, a standard for the naming of allergens, maintained by Allergen Nomenclature Sub-committee of the World Health Organization and International Union of Immunological Societies (WHO/IUIS), has now been adopted, making construction of databases much more facile than hitherto. Major active databases in this area are adumbrated, limned, and otherwise outlined below.

The Structural Database of Allergenic Proteins, or SDAP, was released in 2001 and has been continuously updated [62, 63]. Currently, SDAP contains 1,396 allergens, 1,221 protein sequences and 28 IgE and IgG epitopes, 70 allergens with PDB structures, and 582 3D models. SDAP also provides information on a wide variety of relevant information, including: allergen name, IUIS nomenclature, type, source species, sequence, IgE epitopes, literature, family domain, and structure information when available (URL: http://fermi.utmb.edu/SDAP/). Database can be searched through a user-friendly interface. SDAP also hosts an array of computational tools for the prediction of allergenicity and cross-reactivity.

The Allergen Database for Food Safety [64, 65], or ADFS, was originally an initiative of the Japanese National Institute of Health Sciences (URL: http://allergen.nihs.go.jp/ADFS/). It was updated in February 2010, mainly deals with food safety, principally addressing Novel Foods and related immunochemistry. The database comprised 1,285 sequences, 77 molecular structures, and 91 epitopes. It also contains 88 sugar-attached allergens derived from air, pathogens, food, and venom/salivary allergens. ADFS provides domain information, links to other external databases, and tools for the allergen analysis and prediction.

Allergome [66, 67] is arguably the most complete resource for allergens produced to date and is updated on a daily basis; up-to-date statistics can be found at the Allergome statistics page (URL: http://www.allergome.org/script/statistic.php). The database comprises 173 biological functions, 1,759 allergen sources, 53 tissues, over 700 structures, 17,000 bibliographies, totalling 5,276 entries. Allergome entries contain information on allergen name, route of exposure, taxonomy, source tissue and organism, and cross-reactivity; as well as data on protein primary sequence, motifs, and post-translational modifications. Allergome introduced the concept of allergenicity score as a real-time characterisation status for a given allergen. This score can be visualised using a dedicated page using a 3-colour, 11-dot sequence. Dots represent data generation, sequence availability, and different functional/non-functional tests. Users can search the database for allergens matching these scores. The database also includes a user-friendly reference archive and an "allergome aligner" tool for the analysis of allergen sequences.

7.5 Discussion and Conclusion

The principal means of vaccine development remains largely empirical, although targets have moved away from an exclusive focus on live virulent or attenuated pathogens as candidate vaccines. Safety concerns have led to such entities being viewed as poor vaccine candidates despite their potent immunogenicity, although seasonal flu vaccines are still of this type. They are more likely to cause disease in children or immune-compromised individuals. Due to safety and availability of powerful adjuvants, the trend is shifting towards antigen, acellular, or subunit- and epitope-based vaccines. Approaches to antigen identification can include cumbersome assays for epitopes, antibodies, cytokine levels, as well as testing for extended survival within animal test groups. Most of the databases described in this chapter catalogue antigens for which B- and T-cell epitopes are known, other antigens, despite high intrinsic immunogenicity, are often lost in the literature. Yet, such antigens could be useful in the context of vaccine design and discovery, hence, the recent development of databases specifically target antigens as opposed to epitopes.

There remain many outstanding or unresolved challenges in the development of antigen database. We need immunology to assess antigens with the same rigour that it applies to the characterizing of epitopes, providing quantitative data on protein affinity measures for binding to B-cell receptors or soluble antibodies. All antigen databases should coordinate and define a universal format such as has been done for other protein sequence and structure databases. Terminology should be properly defined much as it has been done for vaccine ontology by the developers of IEDB. Lastly, and perhaps most importantly, updating should be a constant and consistent process, never stopping always progressing: this remains a remorseless, and thus challenging, task.

References

1. Flower DR (2007) Immunoinformatics and the in silico prediction of immunogenicity. An introduction. Methods Mol Biol 409:1–15
2. Wu TT, Kabat EA (1970) An analysis of the sequences of the variable regions of Bence Jones proteins and myeloma light chains and their implications for antibody complementarity. J Exp Med 132(2):211–250
3. Lefranc MP (2011) IMGT, the international ImMunoGeneTics information system. Cold Spring Harb Protoc 2011(6):595–603

4. Lefranc MP, Giudicelli V, Ginestoux C, Jabado-Michaloud J, Folch G, Bellahcene F, Wu Y, Gemrot E, Brochet X, Lane J et al (2009) IMGT, the international ImMunoGeneTics information system. Nucleic Acids Res 37:D1006–D1012, Database issue
5. Lefranc MP (2008) IMGT, the International ImMunoGeneTics Information System for Immunoinformatics: methods for querying IMGT databases, tools, and web resources in the context of immunoinformatics. Mol Biotechnol 40(1):101–111
6. Robinson J, Mistry K, McWilliam H, Lopez R, Parham P, Marsh SG (2011) The IMGT/HLA database. Nucleic Acids Res 39:D1171–D1176, Database issue
7. Robinson J, Waller MJ, Fail SC, McWilliam H, Lopez R, Parham P, Marsh SG (2009) The IMGT/HLA database. Nucleic Acids Res 37:D1013–D1017, Database issue
8. Retter I, Althaus HH, Munch R, Muller W (2005) VBASE2, an integrative V gene database. Nucleic Acids Res 33:D671–D674, Database issue
9. Robinson J, Marsh SG (2007) IPD: the immuno polymorphism database. Methods Mol Biol 409:61–74
10. Robinson J, Mistry K, McWilliam H, Lopez R, Marsh SG (2010) IPD–the immuno polymorphism database. Nucleic Acids Res 38:D863–D869, Database issue
11. Robinson J, Waller MJ, Fail SC, Marsh SG (2006) The IMGT/HLA and IPD databases. Hum Mutat 27(12):1192–1199
12. Robinson J, Waller MJ, Stoehr P, Marsh SG (2005) IPD–the immuno polymorphism database. Nucleic Acids Res 33:D523–D526, Database issue
13. Schuler MM, Nastke MD, Stevanovikc S (2007) SYFPEITHI: database for searching and T-cell epitope prediction. Methods Mol Biol 409:75–93
14. Rammensee H, Bachmann J, Emmerich NP, Bachor OA, Stevanovic S (1999) SYFPEITHI: database for MHC ligands and peptide motifs. Immunogenetics 50(3–4):213–219
15. Sette A, Sidney J, del Guercio MF, Southwood S, Ruppert J, Dahlberg C, Grey HM, Kubo RT (1994) Peptide binding to the most frequent HLA-A class I alleles measured by quantitative molecular binding assays. Mol Immunol 31(11):813–822
16. Sidney J, Oseroff C, del Guercio MF, Southwood S, Krieger JI, Ishioka GY, Sakaguchi K, Appella E, Sette A (1994) Definition of a DQ3.1-specific binding motif. J Immunol 152 (9):4516–4525
17. Kubo RT, Sette A, Grey HM, Appella E, Sakaguchi K, Zhu NZ, Arnott D, Sherman N, Shabanowitz J, Michel H et al (1994) Definition of specific peptide motifs for four major HLA-A alleles. J Immunol 152(8):3913–3924
18. DiBrino M, Parker KC, Margulies DH, Shiloach J, Turner RV, Biddison WE, Coligan JE (1994) The HLA-B14 peptide binding site can accommodate peptides with different combinations of anchor residues. J Biol Chem 269(51):32426–32434
19. Parker KC, Biddison WE, Coligan JE (1994) Pocket mutations of HLA-B27 show that anchor residues act cumulatively to stabilize peptide binding. Biochemistry 33(24):7736–7743
20. DiBrino M, Parker KC, Shiloach J, Turner RV, Tsuchida T, Garfield M, Biddison WE, Coligan JE (1994) Endogenous peptides with distinct amino acid anchor residue motifs bind to HLA-A1 and HLA-B8. J Immunol 152(2):620–631
21. Parker KC, Bednarek MA, Coligan JE (1994) Scheme for ranking potential HLA-A2 binding peptides based on independent binding of individual peptide side-chains. J Immunol 152 (1):163–175
22. Brusic V, Rudy G, Harrison LC (1998) MHCPEP, a database of MHC-binding peptides: update 1997. Nucleic Acids Res 26(1):368–371
23. Brusic V, Rudy G, Kyne AP, Harrison LC (1997) MHCPEP, a database of MHC-binding peptides: update 1996. Nucleic Acids Res 25(1):269–271
24. Brusic V, Rudy G, Kyne AP, Harrison LC (1996) MHCPEP–a database of MHC-binding peptides: update 1995. Nucleic Acids Res 24(1):242–244
25. Brusic V, Rudy G, Harrison LC (1994) MHCPEP: a database of MHC-binding peptides. Nucleic Acids Res 22(17):3663–3665

26. Hon L, Abernethy NF, Brusic V, Chai J, Altman RB (1998) MHCWeb: converting a WWW database into a knowledge-based collaborative environment. Proc AMIA Symp :947–951
27. Schonbach C, Koh JLY, Flower DR, Brusic V (2005) An update on the functional molecular immunology (FIMM) database. Appl Bioinformatics 4(1):25–31
28. Schonbach C, Koh JLY, Flower DR, Wong L, Brusic V (2002) FIMM, a database of functional molecular immunology: update 2002. Nucleic Acids Res 30(1):226–229
29. Schonbach C, Koh JL, Sheng X, Wong L, Brusic V (2000) FIMM, a database of functional molecular immunology. Nucleic Acids Res 28(1):222–224
30. Reche PA, Zhang H, Glutting JP, Reinherz EL (2005) EPIMHC: a curated database of MHC-binding peptides for customized computational vaccinology. Bioinformatics 21(9):2140–2141
31. Sathiamurthy M, Hickman HD, Cavett JW, Zahoor A, Prilliman K, Metcalf S, Fernandez Vina M, Hildebrand WH (2003) Population of the HLA ligand database. Tissue Antigens 61 (1):12–19
32. Khan JM, Cheruku HR, Tong JC, Ranganathan S (2011) MPID-T2: a database for sequence-structure-function analyses of pMHC and TR/pMHC structures. Bioinformatics 27 (8):1192–1193
33. Tong JC, Kong L, Tan TW, Ranganathan S (2006) MPID-T: database for sequence-structure-function information on T-cell receptor/peptide/MHC interactions. Appl Bioinformatics 5 (2):111–114
34. Govindarajan KR, Kangueane P, Tan TW, Ranganathan S (2003) MPID: MHC-Peptide Interaction Database for sequence-structure-function information on peptides binding to MHC molecules. Bioinformatics 19(2):309–310
35. Gonzalez-Galarza FF, Christmas S, Middleton D, Jones AR (2011) Allele frequency net: a database and online repository for immune gene frequencies in worldwide populations. Nucleic Acids Res 39:D913–D919, Database issue
36. Middleton D, Menchaca L, Rood H, Komerofsky R (2003) New allele frequency database: http://www.allelefrequencies.net. Tissue Antigens 61(5):403–407
37. Saha S, Raghava GP (2007) Searching and mapping of B-cell epitopes in Bcipep database. Methods Mol Biol 409:113–124
38. Saha S, Bhasin M, Raghava GP (2005) Bcipep: a database of B-cell epitopes. BMC Genomics 6:79
39. Huang J, Honda W (2006) CED: a conformational epitope database. BMC Immunol 7:7
40. Singh MK, Srivastava S, Raghava GP, Varshney GC (2006) HaptenDB: a comprehensive database of haptens, carrier proteins and anti-hapten antibodies. Bioinformatics 22(2):253–255
41. Kuiken C, Korber B, Shafer RW (2003) HIV sequence databases. AIDS Rev 5(1):52–61
42. Yusim K, Richardson R, Tao N, Dalwani A, Agrawal A, Szinger J, Funkhouser R, Korber B, Kuiken C (2005) Los alamos hepatitis C immunology database. Appl Bioinformatics 4 (4):217–225
43. Toseland CP, Clayton DJ, McSparron H, Hemsley SL, Blythe MJ, Paine K, Doytchinova IA, Guan P, Hattotuwagama CK, Flower DR (2005) AntiJen: a quantitative immunology database integrating functional, thermodynamic, kinetic, biophysical, and cellular data. Immunome Res 1(1):4
44. Lata S, Bhasin M, Raghava GP (2009) MHCBN 4.0: a database of MHC/TAP binding peptides and T-cell epitopes. BMC Res Notes 2:61
45. Bhasin M, Singh H, Raghava GP (2003) MHCBN: a comprehensive database of MHC binding and non-binding peptides. Bioinformatics 19(5):665–666
46. Peters B, Sidney J, Bourne P, Bui HH, Buus S, Doh G, Fleri W, Kronenberg M, Kubo R, Lund O et al (2005) The immune epitope database and analysis resource: from vision to blueprint. PLoS Biol 3(3):e91
47. Sette A (2004) The immune epitope database and analysis resource: from vision to blueprint. Genome Inform 15(2):299
48. Vita R, Zarebski L, Greenbaum JA, Emami H, Hoof I, Salimi N, Damle R, Sette A, Peters B (2010) The immune epitope database 2.0. Nucleic Acids Res 38:D854–D862, Database issue

49. Zhang Q, Wang P, Kim Y, Haste-Andersen P, Beaver J, Bourne PE, Bui HH, Buus S, Frankild S, Greenbaum J et al (2008) Immune epitope database analysis resource (IEDB-AR). Nucleic Acids Res 36:W513–W518, Web Server issue
50. Wassenaar TM, Gaastra W (2001) Bacterial virulence: can we draw the line? FEMS Microbiol Lett 201(1):1–7
51. Ansari HR, Flower DR, Raghava GPS (2010) AntigenDB: an immunoinformatics database of pathogen antigens. Nucleic Acids Res 38:D847–D853
52. Xiang Z, Todd T, Ku KP, Kovacic BL, Larson CB, Chen F, Hodges AP, Tian Y, Olenzek EA, Zhao B et al (2008) VIOLIN: vaccine investigation and online information network. Nucleic Acids Res 36:D923–D928, Database issue
53. Hayes CN, Diez D, Joannin N, Kanehisa M, Wahlgren M, Wheelock CE, Goto S (2009) Tools for investigating mechanisms of antigenic variation: new extensions to varDB. Genome Inform 23(1):46–59
54. Diez D, Hayes N, Joannin N, Normark J, Kanehisa M, Wahlgren M, Wheelock CE, Goto S (2010) varDB: a database of antigenic variant sequences–current status and future prospects. Acta Trop 114(3):144–151
55. Allred DR, Barbet AF, Barry JD, Deitsch KW (2009) varDB: common ground for a shifting landscape. Trends Parasitol 25(6):249–252
56. Hayes CN, Diez D, Joannin N, Honda W, Kanehisa M, Wahlgren M, Wheelock CE, Goto S (2008) varDB: a pathogen-specific sequence database of protein families involved in antigenic variation. Bioinformatics 24(21):2564–2565
57. Tongchusak S, Chaiyaroj SC, Veeramani A, Koh JLY, Brusic V (2005) CandiVF—Candida albicans virulence factor database. Int J Pep Res Ther 11(4):271–277
58. Yang J, Chen L, Sun L, Yu J, Jin Q (2008) VFDB 2008 release: an enhanced web-based resource for comparative pathogenomics. Nucleic Acids Res 36:D539–D542, Database issue
59. Chen L, Yang J, Yu J, Yao Z, Sun L, Shen Y, Jin Q (2005) VFDB: a reference database for bacterial virulence factors. Nucleic Acids Res 33:D325–D328, Database issue
60. Winnenburg R, Baldwin TK, Urban M, Rawlings C, Kohler J, Hammond-Kosack KE (2006) PHI-base: a new database for pathogen host interactions. Nucleic Acids Res 34:D459–D464
61. Kamble S, Bharmal M (2009) Incremental direct expenditure of treating asthma in the United States. J Asthma 46(1):73–80
62. Ivanciuc O, Mathura V, Midoro-Horiuti T, Braun W, Goldblum RM, Schein CH (2003) Detecting potential IgE-reactive sites on food proteins using a sequence and structure database, SDAP-food. J Agric Food Chem 51(16):4830–4837
63. Ivanciuc O, Schein CH, Braun W (2003) SDAP: database and computational tools for allergenic proteins. Nucleic Acids Res 31(1):359–362
64. Nakamura R, Teshima R (2009) Major revision of the allergen database for food safety (ADFS) and validation of the motif-based allergenicity prediction tool. Kokuritsu Iyakuhin Shokuhin Eisei Kenkyusho Hokoku 127:44–49
65. Nakamura R, Teshima R, Takagi K, Sawada J (2005) Development of Allergen Database for Food Safety (ADFS): an integrated database to search allergens and predict allergenicity. Kokuritsu Iyakuhin Shokuhin Eisei Kenkyusho Hokoku 123:32–36
66. Mari A, Scala E (2006) Allergome: a unifying platform. Arb Paul Ehrlich Inst Bundesamt Sera Impfstoffe Frankf AM 95:29–39, discussion 39–40
67. Chardin H, Peltre G (2005) Allergome: the characterization of allergens based on a 2D gel electrophoresis approach. Expert Rev Proteomics 2(5):757–765

Chapter 8
What Have Dendritic Cells Ever Done for Adjuvant Design? Cellular and Molecular Methods for the Rational Development of Vaccine Adjuvants

Alexander D. Edwards

Abstract Our new molecular understanding of immune priming states that dendritic cell (DC) activation is absolutely pivotal for expansion and differentiation of naïve T lymphocytes, and it follows that understanding DC activation is essential to understand and design vaccine adjuvants. This chapter describes how dendritic cells can be used as a core tool to provide detailed quantitative and predictive immunomics information about how adjuvants function. The role of distinct antigen, costimulation, and differentiation signals from activated DC in priming is explained. Four categories of input signals which control DC activation—direct pathogen detection, sensing of injury or cell death, indirect activation via endogenous proinflammatory mediators, and feedback from activated T cells—are compared and contrasted. Practical methods for studying adjuvants using DC are summarized and the importance of DC subset choice, simulating T cell feedback, and use of knockout cells is highlighted. Finally, five case studies are examined that illustrate the benefit of DC activation analysis for understanding vaccine adjuvant function.

8.1 Introduction

Bacterial lipopolysaccharide (LPS)—for decades, the scourge of the pharmacist due to potent toxicity when injected—is a common and abundant contaminant that is difficult to remove and notoriously expensive to measure, requiring an extract of horseshoe crabs more suited to witchcraft than modern pharmaceutical technology. Yet in the last few years, over 1.5 million schoolchildren [1] were deliberately injected with a synthetic analog of the core lipid A element of LPS to protect them

A.D. Edwards (✉)
Reading School of Pharmacy, Chemistry & Pharmacy, Whiteknights, Reading, UK
e-mail: a.d.edwards@reading.ac.uk

D.R. Flower and Y. Perrie (eds.), *Immunomic Discovery of Adjuvants and Candidate Subunit Vaccines*, Immunomics Reviews: 5, DOI 10.1007/978-1-4614-5070-2_8,

from cervical cancer, as an adjuvant component of the new human papillomavirus vaccine [2].

A simple PhD project—"start by screening some microbial extracts for their ability to activate dendritic cells in vitro"—led to the surprising discovery that boiled yeast induced IL-10 production without requiring the signaling microbial recognition receptors known at that time [3]. Further study revealed a new pathway of innate activation [4]—but the most startling discovery came when a pure agonist of this new pathway was shown to potently promote Th17 immunity—important for protection from fungal pathogens—when co-injected with protein antigen [5].

These examples are just two of many stories that illustrate the power of studying the cell biology and molecular genetics of dendritic cell activation for the rational development of vaccine adjuvants. This chapter will introduce the theoretical framework and practical methods for a systematic immunomics analysis of adjuvant components using dendritic cells, and finally discuss five case studies that illustrate the benefits of this approach.

8.2 A New Understanding of the Cellular and Molecular Mechanisms of Immune Response Priming

Ever since the basis for antigen recognition by T cells was discovered, immunologists have sought to understand how naïve T cells encountering new antigens for the first time are activated—a process termed priming. The last two decades have seen two major revolutions in our understanding of the molecular and cellular biology of priming. These have major implications both for our understanding of how vaccines work, and for the rational design of vaccine adjuvants. Firstly, a central role of activation of dendritic cells (DCs) for priming and controlling T cell activation was discovered [6]. Secondly, this was complemented by the discovery of the molecular pathways for innate DC activation by pattern recognition receptors (PRR) such as members of the toll-like receptor (TLR) family [7] and tissue injury or cell death [8]. In the light of these discoveries, it is now essential to re-assess the activity of vaccines and adjuvants in terms of their ability to activate DC, and determine which pathways they stimulate. Furthermore, fully synthetic adjuvants can now be rationally designed to deliberately target these pathways, allowing customized immune priming.

8.2.1 A Reductionist View Supports the Benefits of Quantifying Adjuvant Activity on Dendritic Cells In Vitro

Adjuvants are added to protein antigens to promote priming of protective and long-lived immune responses of the correct type and anatomical location against the antigen. Therefore, adjuvant design and engineering must take into account all of the factors that influence priming of a wide range of different types of adaptive immune response. Furthermore, an effective adjuvant must have other unrelated features: they must be safe; they must be simple to manufacture; they must be stable; and they must also be effective in a very wide range of different individuals, populations, and healthcare settings. The high complexity of the whole body immune system combined with these additional pragmatic restraints must always be kept in mind, but does not allow a rational, engineering approach.

A simplified reductionist approach based on two assumptions presents us with a more soluble problem: (1) The desired immune response primarily requires expansion of naïve T cells. Although antibody responses are vital for protective immunity to a large proportion of pathogens, long-lived antibody responses are usually T helper cell dependent. (2) To effectively prime long-lived immunity, naïve T lymphocytes must be driven to proliferate and differentiate by activated DC, the only cell able to initiate clonal expansion of naïve T cells [6]. Together, these assumptions suggest that the *most critical function of a vaccine adjuvant is to activate DC*. Critically, to facilitate a rational approach to adjuvant design, DC activation can rapidly be measured in vitro using robust cellular and molecular measurements.

Having made these assumptions, it becomes clear that two points of control must be studied. Firstly, the signals that drive naïve T cell activation must be measured on DC. Secondly, since these signals are only provided by *activated* DC, the input sensors on DC triggered by stimulatory components of an adjuvant must be studied.

8.2.2 Three Signals Provided by Activated DC to Prime Naïve T Cells

To measure the activity of candidate adjuvant components in vitro, the phenotypic markers of greatest interest should be those signals delivered by DC to activate naïve T cells and prime long-lasting new immune responses to vaccine antigens. DC provides three essential signals to naïve T cells: specific T cell receptor antigen, costimulatory molecules, and cytokines to promote differentiation.

8.2.2.1 Signal 1

Activated DC must present vaccine-derived protective antigens on both MHC class II to prime helper responses and MHC class I to prime cytotoxic T lymphocytes (CTL). DCs are characterized and defined by their highly specialized abilities to take up, transport, process, and present antigen, and all these processes are modulated by activation [9]. In the resting state, DCs are located in the periphery, have high antigen uptake capacity, but low levels of surface peptide:MHC complexes. Once activated, they rapidly migrate to secondary lymphoid tissues, downregulate antigen uptake, process antigens, and present high levels of peptide-loaded class I & II on their surface. In addition, some DCs have the unusual ability to present exogenous antigen on MHC class I—a process called "cross-presentation" which is vital to allow priming of antiviral cytotoxic CD8 T cells [10].

But what does measuring signal 1 mean for adjuvant function? Although effective vaccine formulations must deliver antigen to DC and allow presentation on the correct MHC molecules, two factors obscure the significance of using signal 1 to predict how effective a given DC stimulus will be for priming in vivo. Firstly, some DCs are tolerogenic and rather than promoting naïve T cell activation and immune response priming, antigen presented on these cells actually deletes or induces immunoregulatory differentiation [11]. Thus, increased antigen presentation does not automatically lead to immune priming. In other words, regulation of signals 2 and 3 may be more important than signal 1 for control of immunity. Secondly, T cells are exquisitely sensitive to antigen, and so the levels of antigen presented does not need to be very high to be sufficient for full T cell activation [12]. Thus, even if an adjuvant appears only to deliver low levels of antigen to DC, this level may be more than sufficient for efficient priming.

With these caveats, measuring signal 1 can still be highly informative. Firstly, alteration of simple characteristic signal 1 components—such as surface class II levels—is a potent measure of DC-stimulatory activity. Secondly, in some vaccines, specialized antigen presentation pathways must be targeted. For example, cross-presentation is essential to allow class I presentation of vaccine-derived peptides to prime cytotoxic immunity. In these cases, it is worth testing the ability of an adjuvant formulation to target that specific pathway.

8.2.2.2 Signal 2

Triggering of CD28 and other costimulatory receptors on naïve T cells plus T cell receptor provides proliferation and survival signals that together result in productive clonal expansion. Thus, activated DC must express high surface levels of the CD28 ligands CD80 and CD86 to promote priming [6]. The requirement for costimulation—combined with T cell receptor signaling—for successful naïve T cells priming represents a central dogma of immunology. Naïve T cells that encounter antigen in the absence of costimulation are deleted or inactivated in the process broadly know as peripheral tolerance. It follows that expression of costimulatory molecules is the simplest and clearest indicator of priming activity—and should be used as a primary marker of DC activation.

8.2.2.3 Signal 3

Finally, although signals 1 and 2 determine antigen specificity and clonal expansion, signal 3 is defined as the message that drives T cell differentiation, and thereby controls the *type* of immune response generated. Not all immune responses are equal, and different types of immune response are required to protect against a plethora of differing infectious challenges, including different antibody classes, different types of cellular responses including different T helper cells and cytotoxic cells, and responses located to different tissue sites. Many components of immune polarization are controlled by activated DC [13]. The type of immune response induced is strongly influenced by the nature of DC activation, both in terms of the subtype of DC activated, and the mechanism of DC activation—that is, what input sensors are triggered, because together these two factors determine the nature of signal 3 [13, 14].

Crucially to this reductionist approach to adjuvant development, the best known examples of signal 3 are cytokines secreted by DC, such as IL-12. Thus, although ultimately the type of immune response triggered by a given adjuvant must be measured in vivo, DC cytokine production can be rapidly measured in vitro to estimate the type of immunity likely to be triggered. In practical terms, measurement of these cytokines is the most powerful indicator of the pathway of DC activation induced by a given stimulus even when the exact function of many cytokines is not yet clear.

In summary, provision of signal 1 on DC stimulated with a given adjuvant formulation is essential but not sufficient to promote immune priming. Signal 2 is essential and sufficient to prove an adjuvant component can activate DC. Signal 3 signifies the quality of priming and thereby indicates the type of DC activation.

8.2.3 Mechanisms of DC Activation

In order to design an adjuvant that optimally primes immunity by inducing these three signals for T cells, we must understand what stimuli activate DC. These can be classified by the origin of the stimulus (external or endogenous). External stimuli are either microbial in origin, or represent cell death or tissue damage. Endogenous stimuli are either an indirect signal that external stimuli have been detected by other cells, or they are feedback signals from T lymphocytes.

8.2.3.1 Direct Innate Recognition of Pathogens

The mechanisms of DC activation by direct sensing of microbial components—termed pathogen-associated molecular patterns (PAMPs)—have been the subject of intense study for the last decade (reviewed in [7, 15]). Inflammatory activation by pathogen components (such as LPS) and many receptors (such as CD14) involved in binding and uptake of these components have been studied for many decades. However, the discovery of the specific transmembrane-signaling receptors for pathogens, such as TLR4 [16], that are evolutionarily conserved in molecular structure from man to fly has led to a major paradigm shift in our understanding of immunity. A range of cellular Pattern Recognition Receptors (PRR) including TLR, Nod-like Receptors (NLR), and C-type lectins (CLEC) have been discovered, which are essential for the activation of DC by a corresponding range of viral, bacterial, and fungal pathogen components, such as bacterial cell wall components (e.g., LPS, peptidoglycan) or viral nucleic acids (e.g., dsRNA). Some of the earliest identified and most potent DC stimuli act via TLR, such as LPS [17] and CpG DNA [18].

8.2.3.2 Direct Sensing of Cell Death and Tissue Injury

As well as sensing pathogens directly, several mechanisms have been identified, whereby DC are able to directly sense tissue injury and abnormal (as opposed to programmed) cell death. Examples of danger associated molecular patterns include inappropriate release of cell contents such as ATP [19], and also injury-induced factors such as heat-shock proteins [20]. Less is known about innate injury sensing than microbial sensing, and new pathways are rapidly being identified such as the recently discovered signaling CLEC receptor, named DNGR-1, which detects uptake of necrotic cells by the $CD8\alpha^+$ subset of mouse DC [21]. An early criticism of some of these studies is that experimental stimuli were contaminated by microbial agents (such as mycoplasma or LPS), especially when activation is found to be dependent on PRR such as TLR4. However, it has become very clear that inappropriate cell death and tissue injury is sensed directly via several distinct non-PRR pathways, and the molecular pathways of "danger" detection by the immune system are finally becoming clear [8].

8.2.3.3 Indirect Activation by Endogenous Proinflammatory Mediators

In addition to direct sensing of microbes and injury, DC are exquisitely sensitive to "indirect" activation by endogenous inflammatory signals produced by other cell types, which can be thought of as endogenous messages of ongoing inflammation. These can be divided into innate microbial, innate injury, and adaptive inflammatory signals. Classic endogenous proinflammatory signals released on innate microbial recognition that potently activate DC include TNFα, IL-1 and type I interferon, which can be produced by other innate sentinel cells such as macrophages or mast cells, but also by nonimmune tissue cells. To further complicate matters, DC subsets also signal to each other [14]. Other important endogenous proinflammatory signals include the chemokines that promote DC migration to secondary lymphoid tissues and subsequently recruit them to T cell areas [22]. DC also sense injury via acute inflammatory mediators involved in coagulation, including via the PAR1 and S1P3 receptors [23]. Finally, as well as innate microbial and injury signals, DCs sense ongoing adaptive immunity. For example, Th1-cell derived IFNγ released after antigen recognition can promote increased IL-12 production from DC [24].

8.2.3.4 Endogenous Feedback Signals from Activated T Cells

The interaction between an activated DC and a naïve T cell that has recognized antigen not only involves signals from the DC to the T cell, but also returns signals from the T cell. These ensure that the activated DC can respond to the presence of an antigen-specific T cell—for example, by secreting signal 3 cytokines.

The first of these T cell feedback signals to be clearly identified was CD154, which is upregulated on T cells in response to antigenic stimulation, and triggers the CD40 receptor expressed on DC. Initially identified alongside TNFα and LPS simply as a stimulus for DC activation, the breakthrough in understanding came with the realization that CD40 triggering acts synergistically with microbial activation to promote signal 3, that is, secretion of differentiation cytokines [25]. Furthermore, in spite of potent augmentation of cytokine responses by CD154 from microbially activated DC, it cannot induce IL-12 alone, but only when combined with microbial stimuli. This is in part because microbial activation of DC results in upregulation of CD40, which is expressed only at low levels on nonactivated DC. However, even when CD40 is expressed, ligation does not always lead to IL-12 production. Instead, the nature of cytokine produced in response to CD40 stimulation depends on the stimulus that induced CD40—thus CD154 can promote secretion of high levels of IL-12, IL-10, or other cytokines from DC activated with different microbial agents [3].

8.3 In Vitro Methods to Determine the Dendritic Cell Stimulatory Activity of Adjuvant Components

Section 8.1 outlined theoretical grounds for measuring three priming signals induced on activated DC, and identified four categories of stimuli that DC sense. But what exactly should be measured to determine the activity of a novel adjuvant component or formulation, and how? In vitro studies can be used to answer the following important questions:

(1) *Does the adjuvant or component activate DC?* Any activation marker provides *evidence of stimulatory activity*; the first sign of priming activity however is typically upregulation of signal 2.
(2) *How active is the component?* Once evidence of signal 2 upregulation is detected, a dose–response comparison to standard stimuli, such as classic TLR agonists (e.g., CpG oligos) and endogenous proinflammatory stimuli (e.g., TNFα) should be conducted. This will give an indication of the *relative potency* of the adjuvant component, and may allow prediction of possible in vivo adjuvant activity by comparison to published data.
(3) *What type of activation is seen, and what signals do stimulated DC deliver?* Crucially, the *activation phenotype* can be fully characterized of DC stimulated with suitable doses of the test agents. Production of signal 3 cytokines may

indicate in vivo polarization; for example, IL-12 production might predict Th1 priming.

(4) *Which DC types does it act on?* Similarly, screening activation of different *DC subsets* will provide information on possible polarization.

(5) *What receptors are triggered?* Again, if well-characterized microbe or injury sensing pathways such as TLRs are triggered by a test formulation or agent, activity in vivo may be predicted based on published data on the type of immunity typically induced by other known agonists of that receptor family.

(6) Last but not least, *what is the fate of antigen formulated with the adjuvant?* Although activation is vital for adjuvant activity, protective antigen must also be delivered and presented by activated DC.

This section introduces the methods used to address these questions, and highlights some additional essential considerations for experimental design.

8.3.1 General Principles of DC Culture

The sensitivity of DC to a wide range of exogenous and endogenous stimuli presents several general experimental challenges. Firstly, most DC types studied are primary cells, which require very carefully controlled culture conditions, specialized media, and expensive recombinant growth factors such as GM-CSF. Different experimental conditions are used by different researchers, and there are no standardized methods for DC culture, leading to variable results. Furthermore, they have limited life spans and differentiate over time; thus, experimental work must be carefully planned to ensure DCs are tested at the correct timepoint. Secondly, many potent microbial stimuli—the most obvious of which is endotoxin, LPS—are also common lab contaminants, and are also widely present in commercial cell biology reagents (including fetal calf serum). If microbial contaminants are present in culture, all DCs will have a high degree of activation without addition of test agents, and assays will have a limited dynamic range. The only way to guarantee the absence of DC-stimulatory contaminants is constant monitoring of all reagents. Lab glassware is also frequently contaminated with LPS; thus, exclusive use of tissue-culture grade, pyrogen-free disposable plasticware is vital.

8.3.2 Measuring DC Activation

8.3.2.1 Measuring Costimulatory Molecules

Costimulatory molecules are induced at high levels on the surface of DC after activation by a wide array of exogenous and endogenous stimuli, and thus the original and still the most direct method for measuring DC activation is by antibody staining for CD80 and CD86 [17]. Additional costimulatory signals have been described and can be monitored alongside CD28 ligands [26].

The kinetics of surface costimulatory molecule expression—with maximal upregulation typically seen after around 14 h of culture with stimuli—are highly suited to overnight stimulations. Direct staining using fluorescently labeled monoclonal antibodies (mAbs) allows the simultaneous measurement of multiple costimulatory molecules that can be differentially regulated. Vast catalogues of directly conjugated mAbs are available conjugated to a wide array of different fluorophores, and the widespread use of multiparameter flow cytometers allows the measurement of four or more markers on a single sample of DC. Use of microtitre plates, multichannel pipettors and autosamplers has increased throughput, allowing hundreds of conditions to be tested in a single experiment. This methodology allows multiple doses of adjuvant components to be titrated into microwell plates and compared to dose ranges of "classical" DC stimuli to determine relative potency. Measuring potency is vital since changing the formulation of DC stimuli when engineering adjuvants can directly influence specific activity; for example, covalent conjugation of a small-molecule TLR7 agonist to mouse serum albumin increased potency by 10–100-fold [27].

8.3.2.2 Measuring Cytokine Secretion

In theory, induction of signal 3, typically in the form of a select group of cytokines, is a far more informative measure of DC activation than measuring signals 1 or 2, because signal 3 controls the *type* of immune response. Ideally, a panel of "standard" signal 3 cytokines should be presented that would correspond to pathways all known classes of immunity. Unfortunately, in spite of extensive study of polarization paradigms, such as innate IL-12 production leading to Th1 induction [28], this is a complex and evolving field; the discovery of Th17 cells, probably at least as important as Th1 and Th2 cells, as recently as 2005, illustrates how rapidly the field is changing [29]. Importantly, even if the exact role of many DC-derived cytokines is not certain, what is absolutely clear is that measuring these cytokines reveals *clear and informative activation patterns*. Thus, more important than their theoretical role in polarization is the fact that these signals are characteristically stimulus-specific. Thus, while costimulatory molecules that are induced by many stimuli are excellent screening tools, signal 3 provides vital additional clues about the mechanism of activation.

Several cytokines, such as IL-1, TNFα and IL-12p40, are secreted in response to a wide range of different stimuli, others are selectively secreted in response to only very specific stimuli; examples include type I interferon, IL-2, IL-10, IL-12p70, and IL-23. Depending on the nature of the adjuvant in question, the DC subset studied, and the desired class of immunity, a panel should be selected, including both broad-stimulus and selective cytokines. By screening multiple cytokines and matching with previously identified patterns of cytokine production, the likely composition of a given adjuvant may be identified.

On a practical level, DC-derived cytokines are easy and rapid to measure; when cells are harvested for flow cytometric analysis after overnight culture, supernatants can be frozen and then assayed when convenient by ELISA or microbead immunoassays. When microwell supernatants are assayed for cytokines, the cellular origin of secreted factors cannot be confirmed unless only a pure preparation of a single DC subset is cultured. If necessary, to ensure that the expected cell type is producing a given cytokine, intracellular staining or cytokine capture reagents can be used [3].

Although many stimuli (typically PRR agonists) induce signal 3 cytokines, the absence of these factors after stimulation by an agent that clearly induces activation measured by signal 1 and/or 2 upregulation can be very informative. It could indicate indirect activation by endogenous stimuli such as TNFα or stimulation through non-PRR pathways, rather than direct activation via PRR such as TLRs that are known to be potent inducers of signal 3 cytokines such as IL-12.

Although they may not directly induce cytokine secretion, endogenous signals can certainly influence the level and type of cytokine secreted in response to other (usually microbial) stimuli. T cell feedback signals such as CD40L are discussed in detail in Sect. 3.3. In addition, recombinant cytokines or growth factors such as GM-CSF can be included in culture medium to "reveal" low-level signal 3 production in response to stimuli such as PRR agonists [30].

Note that some cell surface molecules have also been shown to deliver differentiation signals—rather than proliferation signals—and should thus be classed and measured as signal 3, alongside surface costimulatory molecules measured as signal 2. For example, different Notch ligand families were found to be induced on DC by T helper polarizing stimuli and instruct T cell differentiation via Notch family receptors [31].

8.3.2.3 Measuring Antigen Processing and Presentation

Unlike cell surface molecules and cytokines that can be simply measured by FACS and ELISA using specific mAbs, the antigen recognized specifically by T cells—that is, a particular peptide:MHC complex—is difficult to directly measure. As discussed in Sect. 2.2.1, antigen presentation can also be difficult to interpret. Nevertheless, no adjuvant can function without antigen being delivered and presented.

Although mAbs that selectively bind the same epitope as T cell receptor have been made and characterized, these exist for only a very few specific peptide–MHC complexes. The mAb 25D.1 recognizes the ovalbumin $CD8^+$ T cell epitope formed when the SIINFEKL peptide binds to K^b MHC class I [32]. Similarly, the mAb C4H3 specifically recognizes a specific hen egg lysozyme peptide bound to A^k MHC class II [33]. Typically, these mAbs also bind to some degree to other MHC: peptide complexes, leading to background staining that changes after DC activation even in the absence of specific antigen. A further limitation of these antibodies is their sensitivity, which is typically an order of magnitude lower than T cells [12]. For the majority of T cell epitopes, measurement using mAbs is not feasible and epitope-specific T cells must be used instead. This can be achieved using T cell clones, with T cells derived from TCR transgenic mice, and also using primary cells taken from previously immunized mice. When T cells cocultured with a DC preparation recognize antigen, T cell activation markers are upregulated, allowing antigen measurement. Depending on the type of T cells used and the activation marker studied, the presence of signal 2, that is, costimulatory molecules on DC may also influence levels of T cell activation. Therefore, to measure "pure" signal 1, differentiated effector T cells (such as clones) should be used, and early markers of TCR triggering (such as CD69) measured.

An informative alternative to measuring levels of specific surface MHC:peptide complexes is to measure related mechanisms involved in antigen presentation. Total surface MHC class II, which rises rapidly following DC activation, can be as useful as signal 2 for detecting DC stimuli. It can be rapidly measured using surface staining alongside signal 2. Similarly, antigen uptake—rather than presentation—can be very simple to measure, making it a useful screening tool. Antigen uptake is measured using fluorescently labeled antigens or formulations (e.g., microparticles); binding is detected simply by FACS. Antibodies or competitive unlabelled agents can then be screened to identify the mechanism of antigen uptake. For example, studies using soluble polysaccharides and mAbs to block binding of fluorescent zymosan were used to identify the contribution of surface β-glucan receptors in zymosan uptake by DC [4]. Finally, measurement of specialized DC-specific mechanisms of antigen processing—such as cross-presentation—can have great significance for developing some types of vaccine. The identification of molecular mechanisms required for cross-presentation is beginning to allow more precise measurement of cross-presentation [34].

8.3.3 *Use of CD40L to Simulate T Cell Activation and Reveal Signal 3 Cytokine Secretion*

Given their importance in driving differentiation, it is essential that signal 3 cytokines are selectively delivered only to antigen-specific T cells; thus, they must only be maximally secreted during cognate DC–T cell interactions. Thus, to measure signal 3, it is vital to simulate the presence of antigen-specific T cells to DC during in vitro stimulation with adjuvant components. This is achieved by providing appropriate feedback signals—usually CD40 triggering—during stimulation.

8.3.3.1 Methods for Triggering CD40 on DC

A range of methods have been shown to be effective in triggering CD40 on DC to synergize with microbial stimulation. The simplest is the use of agonistic antibodies to CD40; however, the natural ligand CD154 may deliver a qualitatively different and more potent signal, and is preferred to mAbs. Monomeric CD154 is not agonistic, and thus engineered forms of recombinant CD154 that are agonistic have been developed that are either trimeric or oligomeric [35]. The closest recombinant mimic of T cell-expressed CD154 is the full trimeric ligand expressed on cell lines such as fibroblasts, which can be conveniently grown in microwell plates prior to adding DC and stimuli—with the caveat that additional cells are present in cultures, raising the possibility that these cells may modulate DC responses or respond to adjuvant components themselves. Finally, T cells can be used to provide genuine feedback signals, by coculturing with DC and adding specific antigen [12, 25]. In this final method, additional signals beyond CD40 are clearly delivered, as blocking antibodies to CD154 do not completely block synergistic cytokine secretion [25].

8.3.4 Choice of DC Source and Subset

Given the range of subsets of DC with clear phenotypic, transcriptional, and functional differences, it is vital that the correct type of DC is used to study adjuvant function. For example, in mouse, early expression profiling studies identified broad transcriptome differences between subsets of CD11c$^+$ splenic DC distinguished by surface CD8α and CD4 levels [36]; notably, differences in PRR expression on these subsets are responsible for major functional differences such as the absence of TLR7 on CD8α$^+$ DC, resulting in unresponsiveness to the small-molecule TLR7 agonist R848 [30]. These differences in input sensors found on DC subsets are coupled to different priming outputs to T cells. Thus, CD8α$^+$ DC have a specialized capacity to deliver signal 1, with a major role in cross-presentation, and plasmacytoid DC (pDC) are important sources of the signal 3 cytokine IFNα [14]. The three best-studied functionally distinct mouse splenic DC subtypes thus comprise CD8α$^+$ CD11c$^+$, CD4$^+$ CD11c$^+$ DC, and pDC; however, new subsets with special function are regularly identified in this fast-moving field [14]. A notable addition are skin DC such as Langerhans Cells—one of the earliest DC types to be studied, but recently receiving attention due to their role in responses to advanced vaccine delivery systems such as microneedle patches [37].

8.3.4.1 Methods for Obtaining DC

The two dominant methods for obtaining DC for in vitro study are direct isolation, and differentiation from precursors using recombinant growth factors. Most immunology research is conducted in mice and man, and although a wide range of DC have been identified in most tissues studied, the majority of research focuses on either DC directly isolated from mouse spleen or DC differentiated in vitro from precursors found in mouse bone marrow or human peripheral blood.

Magnetic separation using antibody-conjugated paramagnetic nanoparticles that are too small to affect DC function is the standard method for direct isolation from tissues. Thus, early mouse studies focused on CD11c-bright DC, of which there are 1–3 million per spleen. When primary DCs are purified from tissues, cell purity is vital because of their sensitivity to indirect activation—thus magnetic cell sorting should ideally be followed by flow cytometric sorting.

The alternative to direct isolation of DC is to use growth factors such as GM-CSF and FLT3L that drive expansion and eventually differentiation of precursor cells found in mouse bone marrow [38, 39] and human blood [40]. The advantage of in vitro differentiated DC is the large number of uniform cells generated; one disadvantage is that the phenotype and function of these cells is determined by the growth factors used, and may therefore not reflect in vivo function.

Once activated, DCs change irreversibly and rapidly; thus most studies require a short-lived culture of primary quiescent DC. An alternative is to use cell lines with some characteristics of DC [41]; furthermore, DCs have been differentiated from ES cells, allowing generation of primary-like cells without a tissue source [42].

8.3.5 Use of Knockout Mice to Determine the Molecular Mechanisms of Adjuvant Activity

Given the long history of study, measurement, and control of levels of LPS and other potent proinflammatory microbial biomolecules, it is perhaps surprising how immunologists have recently become so excited about the study of such agents. Of course, the reason for this renewed focus is the insight gained from the study of knockout mice lacking specific—and often highly evolutionarily conserved—molecules. The importance of these tools must not be underestimated. Notable examples include PRR knockouts such as TLRs. Mice lacking components of PRR signaling pathways such as MyD88 or Syk that are unresponsive to many PAMPs are also useful screening tools, but these knockouts can be misleading because of their role in signaling by receptors for endogenous stimuli such as IL-1.

8.3.5.1 Sources of Knockout, Knockdown, and Transduced DC

Although most knockout DCs are taken directly from mouse tissues or cultured from freshly isolated bone marrow, bone marrow cells can be cryopreserved, then differentiated in vitro into DC after thawing, allowing cost-effective storage of stocks of knockout cells. Furthermore, many tissue DCs repopulate from bone marrow stem cells with rapid turnover: stored or internationally transported bone marrow can be used to make radiation chimeras, and then knockout primary DC purified, allowing rapid evaluation of DC function without breeding new colonies of knockout mice [3]. Radiation chimeras can also be generated using fetal liver cell-derived stem cells, allowing study of embryonic lethal knockouts such as *Syk* [4]. This approach cannot be used with DC subsets derived from radio-resistant precursors, such as those found in the dermis of mice and humans [43].

Retroviral transduction and siRNA knockdown have been used for gain- and loss-of-function experiments in DC. Given the exceptional sensitivity of this class of cells to viral components such as abnormal nucleic acids, this approach does present additional problems compared to similar experiments in most other cell types. Thus, pDC are activated via RNA sensing PRR after transfection with siRNAs [44], and likewise, retrovirally transduced DC can be activated via TLR9 [45].

8.4 Case Studies: Examples Where Study of DC Activation Has Informed Rational Adjuvant Development

The following five case studies illustrate how study of DC activation within the framework presented above has given us valuable insight into vaccine function and provided clues about how to rationally design more effective adjuvants.

8.4.1 Current Vaccines Activate DC Through PRR and Non-PRR Pathways

We cannot hope to design new vaccines without first understanding how current effective vaccines induce protective immunity. So what has the study of DC activation taught us about tried and tested human vaccines?

Case study 1: what have DC taught us about current human vaccines?

Most conventional human vaccines are attenuated or inactivated pathogens and therefore contain a similar array of PAMPs to the microbes they derive from. It is not surprising to find that many potently activate DC via PRR. Indeed, rather than DC teaching us about vaccine function, inactivated and attenuated pathogens—closely related to many vaccines—have been vital tools for understanding DC activation and subsequently identifying PRR. Microbial extracts were used to demonstrate that signal 2 is induced—not constitutive—on DC [17] and to identify DC as a major source of the signal 3 cytokine IL-12 [46]. Proinflammatory cell wall components (LPS) of whole killed bacteria and heat-killed yeast particles (zymosan) were used to identify proinflammatory signaling through TLR4, TLR2, and Dectin-1 [4, 16, 47]. Attenuated and inactivated viruses have likewise been vital for the identification of PRR involved in sensing viral nucleic acids. For example, heat-inactivated influenza virus was used to identify TLR7 as a receptor for viral ssRNA required for interferon induction from pDC [48], and the eponymous vaccinia virus has been utilized to identify DC activation via TLR2/6, MDA-5, and most recently mouse TLR8 [49, 50].

So if attenuated and inactivated vaccines contain microbial PAMPs, is PRR triggering actually required for their immunogenicity? Just as PRR knockout mice have illustrated a vital function for TLRs in resistance to infection, knockouts show reduced responses to many vaccines. Again, influenza is a clear example; without TLR7, whole inactivated influenza virus vaccine loses immunogenicity [51]. Furthermore, this study highlighted the importance of TLR7 in driving a particular class of immune response—specifically Th1 immunity—reinforcing the notion that direct microbial recognition can control immune polarization. In contrast to whole inactivated virus vaccine, split virus or subunit vaccines are less potent and show little TLR7 dependence [51]. Both processing whole inactivated virus to produce split virus and purifying particular antigens to produce subunit vaccine result in loss of the packaged viral ssRNA that potently stimulates TLR7 on DC. Whole inactivated bacterial vaccines can likewise trigger PRR on DC and some require microbial sensing for optimal immune priming; for example, TLR4 knockout mice mount impaired immunity to whole-cell pertussis vaccine [52]. Even some subunit vaccines comprising protective antigens purified from microbial sources can contain PAMPs and require PRR triggering; thus outer membrane vesicles purified from *Neisseria meningitides* make effective human vaccines against type B meningitis, contain LPS that activate DC via TLR4, and induce reduced immune priming in TLR4 knockouts [52].

Equally important have been studies that demonstrate that PRR are not required for immunity to all vaccines. A pure protein antigen formulated in a sterile PAMP-free adjuvant such as alum should not trigger PRR, and PRR-deficient mice mount long-lived immunity to such vaccines [53]. Even some adjuvants that clearly contain PAMPs can be effective even without PRR. Detailed study of alum and other PRR-independent adjuvants has proved highly informative about mechanisms of direct and indirect sensing of injury and cell death, and the influence of such sensing on immune priming [8, 54].

In summary, studies of direct microbe- and injury-sensing mechanisms using knockout mice and by measuring signal 3 cytokine production from different subsets of DC have identified what components of current human vaccines and adjuvants are responsible for priming which types of protective immunity. Conversely, vaccines have proved useful tools for understanding DC activation and its role in adaptive immune priming.

8.4.2 *Synthetic Agents that Directly Activate DC Can Increase Adjuvant Potency and Polarize Immunity*

Although many of our oldest and most effective vaccines comprise live attenuated or inactivated pathogens, there are disadvantages of these formulations. For example, each one has to be produced using highly specific and challenging biomanufacturing methods, and the resulting formulations are complex mixtures of unstable biomacromolecules. In the age of next-generation recombinant biologics, these vaccines seem rather old-fashioned; ideally, they could be replaced by highly defined, fully synthetic vaccines comprising pure recombinant protein antigens formulated with customized synthetic adjuvants.

As rapidly as PRRs have been discovered, a range of synthetic compounds or purified microbial components which selectively trigger PRR and potently activate DC have been identified. Deliberately incorporating these synthetic PRR agonists into adjuvants should offer a number of benefits, such as increased potency compared to PAMP-free adjuvants, simpler manufacturing and simpler composition compared to attenuated or inactivated microbial vaccines, and finally should induce priming of a range of different classes of immunity, by selectively triggering different forms of DC activation and targeting different DC subsets.

The most clinically relevant demonstration of the benefits of adding synthetic PRR agonists to adjuvants is GSK's adjuvant AS 04, which combines the synthetic TLR4 agonist monophosphoryl lipid A (MPLA) with alum [2]. The human papillomavirus vaccine Cervarix is formulated with AS 04, which may account for its increased potency compared to Gardasil, a similar vaccine formulated with alum alone [55]. Ironically, this adjuvant was not the product of DC and PRR research; instead, credit lies with the microbiologists who identified MPLA and the decades of development work that followed [56].

So can study of DC activation in vitro tell us anything about this rational approach to engineering synthetic adjuvants?

Case study 2: DCs reveal non-TLR pathways to Th17 polarization

Although TLRs are the best studied family of signaling PRR, an ever-expanding array of pathogen sensors has been identified mostly by studying DC activation. One of the first hints of a TLR-independent signaling pathway for DC activation by microbial recognition came from the study of signal 3 (DC cytokine secretion) in response to panels of pathogen extracts. In contrast to many microbial stimuli that—when combined with CD40L (see Sect. 3.3)—induce high levels of IL-12 production from mouse splenic DC, stimulation with the yeast particle zymosan plus CD40L triggers high-level IL-10 production but no IL-12 [3]. At the time, although a number of phagocytic yeast receptors were known, zymosan and yeasts were thought to signal for cellular activation through TLR2 [47]. Other known TLR agonists such as CpG oligos and LPS all triggered IL-12 and no IL-10 production. This hint of an alternative non-TLR pathway of cellular activation resulting in different signal 3 cytokine production became a powerful indication when it was found that neither TLR2 nor MyD88 were required for IL-10 production in response to zymosan [3]. At the time, this excluded all known molecular signaling mechanisms for DC activation by yeasts.

Blocking experiments suggested that zymosan particle uptake was partially mediated by beta-glucan binding via the Dectin-1 receptor, a CLEC family yeast receptor recently identified on macrophages [57]—however, at the time, this receptor had no known transmembrane signaling activity. The breakthrough came from the prediction that if an atypical ITAM motif identified in the cytoplasmic tail of Dectin-1 could signal, it must utilize the tyrosine kinase Syk. This led to the breakthrough experiment of stimulating Syk−/− DCs with zymosan—these showed a dramatic absence of IL-10 production, but still produced IL-12 in response to TLR triggers [4]. But what is the consequence of DC activation via Dectin-1 signaling? Further study identified a selective Dectin-1 trigger, curdlan, that when combined with protein antigen and injected into mice promoted induction of Th17 responses via Syk and another adaptor called CARD9 [5]. More recently, another potent Th17-inducing adjuvant, trehalose 6,6-dibehenate (TDB), a synthetic mimic of a mycobacterial cell wall component, was shown to signal via the same Syk/CARD9 pathway [58], suggesting that this pathway represents an alternative axis of microbial recognition comprising ITAM-containing transmembrane microbial recognition receptor, coupled via Syk/CARD9 to DC activation that leads to Th17 priming.

Thus, the systematic study of cytokine production by DC, the use of CD40 triggering to reveal signal 3 cytokines, and the use of PRR knockout DC led to the discovery of a new PRR signaling pathway with a corresponding potent synthetic agonist—curdlan—which primes an important class of immune polarization.

Case study 3: Lessons about formulation from adjuvants incorporating TLR agonists

Although synthetic PRR agonists offer hope of producing "designer" adjuvants, a number of formulation challenges remain, some of which can be tackled using DC. These challenges include their toxicity if released systemically (many TLR agonists can trigger lethal toxic shock), and their wide range of physiochemical properties—with the exception of small-molecule TLR7/8 agonists, they vary in size, charge, and hydrophobicity and include extremely hydrophobic and highly charged agents that are difficult to formulate.

A third challenge is to understand how to combine antigens with PRR agonists. It has become increasingly clear that TLR agonists may need to be physically linked with the target protein antigen within a vaccine to most effectively increase potency. Thus, direct covalent coupling of CpG oligos to antigen improves immune responses to antigen, especially CD8 T cell responses; however, conjugates still induce better cytotoxic responses in TLR9 knockout mice, by promoting TLR9-independent antigen uptake and cross-presentation [59], highlighting the fact that many TLR agonists are biomacromolecules that interact with a range of signaling and non-signaling receptors. TLR9-deficient mice do show reduced Th1 differentiation in spite of enhanced antigen delivery and priming. Surprisingly, a similar benefit was seen of covalently conjugating a small-molecule TLR7 agonist to antigen over co-injection of antigen plus TLR7-agonist, even though the small-molecule TLR7 agonist did not directly promote antigen uptake [60]. Another method to link antigen to PRR agonists is to immobilize both on a particulate scaffold. Crucially, when antigen and CpG oligonucleotides were co-encapsulated with a TLR9 agonist using the biodegradable polymer PLGA, only when both were present in the same PLGA microsphere, was an effective cytotoxic T cell response achieved [61]. Further benefits of microparticle formulation became clear when they were shown to directly activate DC via the NALP3 inflammasome [62]. To prevent precipitation or aggregation, hydrophobic PRR agonists can be incorporated into liposomes; again, study of TDB liposome adjuvants highlighted that they must retain antigenic peptide at the site of injection to retain adjuvant activity, supporting the idea that PRR agonists must be linked to antigen [63].

Thus, studies of levels of signal 1 alongside DC activation via PRR and injury sensors have identified several essential parameters for effective formulation of synthetic PRR agonists into adjuvants.

8.4.3 Endogenous Immunostimulatory Signals Can also Be Added to Adjuvants

Possible disadvantages of targeting direct DC activation via PRR and injury sensors include undesirable responses such as pain and localized or systemic inflammation. So why not design adjuvants that target downstream pathways and shortcut direct DC activation? As the host-derived signals responsible for T cell priming are more clearly defined, it should become possible to develop effective adjuvants that deliberately trigger pathways downstream of DC activation and thereby prime T cells. Targeting inflammatory pathways to promote immunity has long been an aim in adjuvant design. A classic example was the fusing of C3d to antigen, simulating complement activation during acute inflammation, which covalently "tags" proteins and targets them to B cells, thereby reducing the dose required to promote antibody responses [64].

More recently, two distinct approaches to the use of endogenous signals—as opposed to pathogen-associated or injury signals—in adjuvants can be identified. Firstly, the discovery of chemokines and cytokines combined with advances in recombinant protein manufacturing has resulted in prolonged interest in using endogenous DC activation signals in adjuvants. Secondly, given the potent effects of feedback signals (such as CD40) on DC activation, deliberately targeting this endogenous pathway offers the hope of priming cytotoxic responses without requiring CD4 T cell help. The last two case studies explore the use of DC to understand how to use synthetic endogenous signals to prime immunity.

Case study 4: Blinding DC to microbial stimulation: can endogenous proinflammatory signals replace direct DC activation?

As rapidly as proinflammatory cytokines such as TNFα, IL-1, and IL-12 were identified, they have been produced using recombinant technology and explored for augmenting adjuvant activity [65]. In addition to incorporating recombinant cytokine proteins, they have been genetically engineered into live attenuated viral and bacterial vectors and DNA vaccines. But can endogenous signals replace direct DC activation? Although DCs are potently influenced by endogenous signals including inflammatory cytokines, how effective are indirectly activated DCs for T cell priming?

An elegant experiment designed to answer this question made use of MyD88 knockout mice as a source of DCs that are "blind" to direct TLR stimulation, and therefore can only respond to indirect activation signals. Bone marrow chimeras were made containing both MyD88-sufficient and MyD88-deficient DC, each with different MHC classes and thus able to present antigen to different sets of T cells. By immunizing these mice with protein antigen plus synthetic PRR agonist, the phenotype of T cells primed by direct vs. indirectly activated DC could be simultaneously monitored in the same mouse. Although indirectly activated "blind" DC promoted CD4 expansion, Th1 differentiation was only seen by T cells activated by PRR-sufficient DC that produced IL-12 after direct TLR stimulation [66].

Although triggering inflammation at the site of vaccine injection is sufficient to enhance immunity to vaccine antigens—for example by promoting DC and lymphocyte recruitment—studies like this one suggest that the immune system has highly sophisticated methods to distinguish antigens that are directly linked to PRR triggers from other antigens also present at an inflamed site. This has implications for the formulation of synthetic PRR agonists with antigen; specifically, antigen should be delivered to the same DC as PRR triggers, otherwise the DC that present antigen will only be indirectly activated. This may explain the observations about formulation of PRR agonists discussed in case study 3.

Study of direct injury sensing has also revealed an essential role for indirect DC activation in T helper polarization following immunization with the PRR-independent adjuvant alum. Priming by alum induction requires not only $CD11c^+$ APC [67] and DC activation via the NLRP3 inflammasome [68, 69] but also recruitment of eosinophils that produce IL-4 and drive Th2 polarization [70].

These studies illustrate the importance of understanding the different effects of direct and indirect DC activation for correct design of adjuvants, and reinforce the power of knockout mice for unpicking complex responses.

Case study 5: Short circuiting T cell help: Promoting cytotoxic responses using synthetic T cell feedback signals

The importance of revealing signal 3 cytokine production using CD40 agonists was highlighted in Sect. 3.3, and the benefits of this approach illustrated by case study 3. However, CD154 feedback signals are not only vital to indicate the presence of T cells to the DC; they are also pivotal for the provision of CD4 help to license DC for priming naïve $CD8^+$ T cells, and thereby promote new cytotoxic responses [71–73]. It follows that synthetic CD40 agonists can be utilized in vaccine adjuvants to circumvent the need for CD4 help and thereby directly promote cytotoxic immunity. Once again, the study of DC proves to be highly informative to this approach. Although CD40-agonistic antibodies can be used to promote CTL responses when co-injected with antigen [74], detailed study of the biology of CD40 on DC was required to unpick the requirement for microbial activation before CD40 is expressed on DC [25]. This observation predicted that deliberately triggering CD40 to license DC for priming CD8 responses would require microbial activation; and indeed it was subsequently demonstrated that agonistic CD40 antibodies promote cytotoxic immunity far more potently when combined with TLR agonists [75].

In summary, in vitro study of signal 3 cytokines produced by DC in response to microbial and T cell feedback stimuli was required to understand how best to directly target endogenous pathways that promote cytotoxic immunity.

8.5 Conclusions

It is disappointing that given our deep understanding of the complex mammalian immune system, we are still unable to rapidly develop "designer" vaccines against emerging or existing infectious diseases. Our existing vaccines are made using old-fashioned and unwieldy methods. A stark reminder of this is the fact that we still make influenza vaccine—a vital tool to protect thousands of at-risk individuals from seasonal epidemics every year—in fertilized chicken eggs. The study of cellular and molecular biology of DCs and pattern recognition receptors has provided a strong theoretical and experimental foundation for the rational design of vaccine adjuvants. However, in common with other biomedical disciplines, clinical uptake typically lags behind scientific discovery. This is particularly apparent in vaccine development due to the unusual features of vaccines—namely, the large number of recipients, and the low tolerance of adverse effects in vaccinees, who are typically healthy individuals that may not individually benefit from immunization. The recent widespread use of the TLR4 stimulatory adjuvant AS04 suggests an immediate impact of the study of TLRs on adjuvant design. However, it is in fact nearly 30 years since MPLA was first reported [56]. Hopefully, as our understanding of immunology advances, translation will be accelerated, and we will eventually establish an "adjuvant toolkit" that will allow rapid and safe development of new effective vaccines to order.

One element of this toolkit should be the measurement of DC activation, the use of known DC stimuli, and study of DC lacking pathways such as PRR, for rapid in vitro adjuvant development. This chapter has described, with examples, the three signals to be measured, and the four classes of stimuli that DC sense. Although the in vitro DC stimulatory activity of a given adjuvant formulation will have a significant bearing on in vivo performance, a large number of additional factors are also critical, including the injection site and method, the kinetics and distribution of antigen and adjuvant components after injection, the involvement of other cells (e.g., B cells, eosinophils) and tissue responses, potential for causing local and systemic adverse affects, and finally the practical details of the ultimate vaccine formulation. Pragmatic considerations include the stability of the fully formulated vaccine, the cost, speed and scalability of manufacture, and of course the purpose of the vaccine will influence many of these factors.

Disclaimer The effectiveness of your adjuvant can go down as well as up. The complexity of both the innate and adaptive immune systems should never be underestimated. In this chapter, one antigen presenting cell, three T cell priming signals, and four input signals are discussed. Although DCs take a central role in controlling immune priming and polarization, other cell types have an equally important role in both sensing antigen and controlling immunity. Similarly, classification of DC–T cell signals into three categories is helpful; however, in reality, the interaction between these cells is so complex that it is termed the immune synapse, and many signals fall into more than one category. Although signal 3 is conceptually vital, and study of cytokines in this class such as IL-12 has proven highly informative, much is still unknown about what signals lead to which immune responses. Worse, for many important pathogens, the class of immunity required for protection is still unclear. DC studies are only a simple starting point and all adjuvants must ultimately be tested in vivo to determine efficacy.

References

1. Department of Health. (2011). Annual HPV vaccine coverage in England in 2009/2010. Retrieved August 2011, 2011, from http://www.dh.gov.uk/prod_consum_dh/groups/dh_digitalassets/documents/digitalasset/dh_123826.pdf.
2. Didierlaurent AM, Morel S et al (2009) AS04, an aluminum salt- and TLR4 agonist-based adjuvant system, induces a transient localized innate immune response leading to enhanced adaptive immunity. J Immunol 183(10):6186–6197
3. Edwards AD, Manickasingham SP et al (2002) Microbial recognition via toll-like receptor-dependent and -independent pathways determines the cytokine response of murine dendritic cell subsets to CD40 triggering. J Immunol 169(7):3652–3660
4. Rogers NC, Slack EC et al (2005) Syk-dependent cytokine induction by Dectin-1 reveals a novel pattern recognition pathway for C type lectins. Immunity 22(4):507–517
5. LeibundGut-Landmann S, Gross O et al (2007) Syk- and CARD9-dependent coupling of innate immunity to the induction of T helper cells that produce interleukin 17. Nat Immunol 8(6):630–638
6. Banchereau J, Steinman RM (1998) Dendritic cells and the control of immunity. Nature 392 (6673):245–252
7. Takeuchi O, Akira S (2010) Pattern recognition receptors and inflammation. Cell 140 (6):805–820
8. Kono H, Rock KL (2008) How dying cells alert the immune system to danger. Nat Rev Immunol 8(4):279–289
9. Guermonprez P, Valladeau J et al (2002) Antigen presentation and T cell stimulation by dendritic cells. Annu Rev Immunol 20:621–667
10. Heath WR, Belz GT et al (2004) Cross-presentation, dendritic cell subsets, and the generation of immunity to cellular antigens. Immunol Rev 199:9–26
11. Reis e Sousa C (2006) Dendritic cells in a mature age. Nat Rev Immunol 6(6):476–483
12. Sporri R, Reis e Sousa C (2002) Self peptide/MHC class I complexes have a negligible effect on the response of some CD8+ T cells to foreign antigen. Eur J Immunol 32(11):3161–3170
13. Kapsenberg ML (2003) Dendritic-cell control of pathogen-driven T-cell polarization. Nat Rev Immunol 3(12):984–993
14. Pulendran B, Tang H et al (2008) Division of labor, plasticity, and crosstalk between dendritic cell subsets. Curr Opin Immunol 20(1):61–67
15. Beutler BA (2009) TLRs and innate immunity. Blood 113(7):1399–1407
16. Poltorak A, He X et al (1998) Defective LPS signaling in C3H/HeJ and C57BL/10ScCr mice: mutations in Tlr4 gene. Science 282(5396):2085–2088
17. De Smedt T, Pajak B et al (1996) Regulation of dendritic cell numbers and maturation by lipopolysaccharide in vivo. J Exp Med 184(4):1413–1424
18. Sparwasser T, Koch E-S et al (1998) Bacterial DNA and immunostimulatory CpG oligonucleotides trigger maturation and activation of murine dendritic cells. Eur J Immunol 28(6):2045–2054

19. Schnurr M, Then F et al (2000) Extracellular ATP and TNF-α synergize in the activation and maturation of human dendritic cells. J Immunol 165(8):4704–4709
20. MacAry PA, Javid B et al (2004) HSP70 peptide binding mutants separate antigen delivery from dendritic cell stimulation. Immunity 20(1):95–106
21. Sancho D, Joffre OP et al (2009) Identification of a dendritic cell receptor that couples sensing of necrosis to immunity. Nature 458(7240):899–903
22. Randolph GJ, Ochando J et al (2008) Migration of dendritic cell subsets and their precursors. Annu Rev Immunol 26(1):293–316
23. Niessen F, Schaffner F et al (2008) Dendritic cell PAR1-S1P3 signalling couples coagulation and inflammation. Nature 452(7187):654–658
24. Snijders A, Kalinski P et al (1998) High-level IL-12 production by human dendritic cells requires two signals. Int Immunol 10(11):1593–1598
25. Schulz O, Edwards AD et al (2000) CD40 triggering of heterodimeric IL-12 p70 production by dendritic cells in vivo requires a microbial priming signal. Immunity 13(4):453–462
26. Sharpe AH (2009) Mechanisms of costimulation. Immunol Rev 229(1):5–11
27. Wu CC, Hayashi T et al (2007) Immunotherapeutic activity of a conjugate of a Toll-like receptor 7 ligand. Proc Natl Acad Sci USA 104(10):3990–3995
28. Trinchieri G (2003) Interleukin-12 and the regulation of innate resistance and adaptive immunity. Nat Rev Immunol 3(2):133–146
29. Korn T, Bettelli E et al (2009) IL-17 and Th17 cells. Annu Rev Immunol 27:485–517
30. Edwards AD, Diebold SS et al (2003) Toll-like receptor expression in murine DC subsets: lack of TLR7 expression by CD8 alpha(+) DC correlates with unresponsiveness to imidazoquinolines. Eur J Immunol 33(4):827–833
31. Amsen D, Blander JM et al (2004) Instruction of distinct CD4 T helper cell fates by different notch ligands on antigen-presenting cells. Cell 117(4):515–526
32. Porgador A, Yewdell JW et al (1997) Localization, quantitation, and in situ detection of specific peptide-MHC class I complexes using a monoclonal antibody. Immunity 6 (6):715–726
33. Zhong G, Sousa CRe et al (1997) Production, specificity, and functionality of monoclonal antibodies to specific peptide–major histocompatibility complex class II complexes formed by processing of exogenous protein. Proc Natl Acad Sci USA 94(25):13856–13861
34. Amigorena S, Savina A (2010) Intracellular mechanisms of antigen cross presentation in dendritic cells. Curr Opin Immunol 22(1):109–117
35. Haswell LE, Glennie MJ et al (2001) Analysis of the oligomeric requirement for signaling by CD40 using soluble multimeric forms of its ligand, CD154. Eur J Immunol 31(10):3094–3100
36. Edwards AD, Chaussabel D et al (2003) Relationships among murine CD11c(high) dendritic cell subsets as revealed by baseline gene expression patterns. J Immunol 171(1):47–60
37. Giudice EL, Campbell JD (2006) Needle-free vaccine delivery. Adv Drug Deliv Rev 58 (1):68–89
38. Brawand P, Fitzpatrick DR et al (2002) Murine plasmacytoid pre-dendritic cells generated from Flt3 ligand-supplemented bone marrow cultures are immature APCs. J Immunol 169 (12):6711–6719
39. Inaba K, Inaba M et al (1992) Generation of large numbers of dendritic cells from mouse bone marrow cultures supplemented with granulocyte/macrophage colony-stimulating factor. J Exp Med 176(6):1693–1702
40. Romani N, Gruner S et al (1994) Proliferating dendritic cell progenitors in human blood. J Exp Med 180(1):83–93
41. Girolomoni G, Lutz MB et al (1995) Establishment of a cell line with features of early dendritic cell precursors from fetal mouse skin. Eur J Immunol 25(8):2163–2169
42. Fairchild PJ, Brook FA et al (2000) Directed differentiation of dendritic cells from mouse embryonic stem cells. Curr Biol 10(23):1515–1518
43. Bogunovic M, Ginhoux F et al (2006) Identification of a radio-resistant and cycling dermal dendritic cell population in mice and men. J Exp Med 203(12):2627–2638

44. Hornung V, Guenthner-Biller M et al (2005) Sequence-specific potent induction of IFN-alpha by short interfering RNA in plasmacytoid dendritic cells through TLR7. Nat Med 11 (3):263–270
45. Pichlmair A, Diebold SS et al (2007) Tubulovesicular structures within vesicular stomatitis virus G protein-pseudotyped lentiviral vector preparations carry DNA and stimulate antiviral responses via Toll-like receptor 9. J Virol 81(2):539–547
46. Sousa CRe, Hieny S et al (1997) In vivo microbial stimulation induces rapid CD40 ligand–independent production of interleukin 12 by dendritic cells and their redistribution to T cell areas. J Exp Med 186(11):1819–1829
47. Underhill DM, Ozinsky A et al (1999) The Toll-like receptor 2 is recruited to macrophage phagosomes and discriminates between pathogens. Nature 401(6755):811–815
48. Diebold SS, Kaisho T et al (2004) Innate antiviral responses by means of TLR7-mediated recognition of single-stranded RNA. Science 303(5663):1529–1531
49. Delaloye J, Roger T et al (2009) Innate immune sensing of modified vaccinia virus Ankara (MVA) is mediated by TLR2-TLR6, MDA-5 and the NALP3 inflammasome. PLoS Pathog 5 (6):e1000480
50. Martinez J, Huang X et al (2010) Toll-like receptor 8-mediated activation of murine plasmacytoid dendritic cells by vaccinia viral DNA. Proc Natl Acad Sci USA 107 (14):6442–6447
51. Geeraedts F, Goutagny N et al (2008) Superior immunogenicity of inactivated whole virus H5N1 influenza vaccine is primarily controlled by Toll-like receptor signalling. PLoS Pathog 4 (8):e1000138
52. Fransen F, Stenger RM et al (2010) Differential effect of TLR2 and TLR4 on the immune response after immunization with a vaccine against Neisseria meningitidis or Bordetella pertussis. PLoS One 5(12):e15692
53. Gavin AL, Hoebe K et al (2006) Adjuvant-enhanced antibody responses in the absence of toll-like receptor signaling. Science 314(5807):1936–1938
54. De Gregorio E, D'Oro U et al (2009) Immunology of TLR-independent vaccine adjuvants. Curr Opin Immunol 21(3):339–345
55. Einstein MH, Baron M et al (2009) Comparison of the immunogenicity and safety of Cervarix and Gardasil human papillomavirus (HPV) cervical cancer vaccines in healthy women aged 18–45 years. Hum Vaccin 5(10):705–719
56. Qureshi N, Takayama K et al (1982) Purification and structural determination of nontoxic lipid A obtained from the lipopolysaccharide of Salmonella typhimurium. J Biol Chem 257 (19):11808–11815
57. Brown GD, Gordon S (2001) Immune recognition: a new receptor for [beta]-glucans. Nature 413(6851):36–37
58. Werninghaus K, Babiak A et al (2009) Adjuvanticity of a synthetic cord factor analogue for subunit Mycobacterium tuberculosis vaccination requires FcRgamma-Syk-Card9-dependent innate immune activation. J Exp Med 206(1):89–97
59. Heit A, Maurer T et al (2003) Cutting edge: Toll-like receptor 9 expression is not required for CpG DNA-aided cross-presentation of DNA-conjugated antigens but essential for cross-priming of CD8 T cells. J Immunol 170(6):2802–2805
60. Oh JZ, Kedl RM (2010) The capacity to induce cross-presentation dictates the success of a TLR7 agonist-conjugate vaccine for eliciting cellular immunity. J Immunol 185(8):4602–4608
61. Schlosser E, Mueller M et al (2008) TLR ligands and antigen need to be coencapsulated into the same biodegradable microsphere for the generation of potent cytotoxic T lymphocyte responses. Vaccine 26(13):1626–1637
62. Sharp FA, Ruane D et al (2009) Uptake of particulate vaccine adjuvants by dendritic cells activates the NALP3 inflammasome. Proc Natl Acad Sci 106(3):870–875
63. Henriksen-Lacey M, Christensen D et al (2010) Liposomal cationic charge and antigen adsorption are important properties for the efficient deposition of antigen at the injection site and ability of the vaccine to induce a CMI response. J Control Release 145(2):102–108

64. Dempsey PW, Allison ME et al (1996) C3d of complement as a molecular adjuvant: bridging innate and acquired immunity. Science 271(5247):348–350
65. Nohria A, Rubin RH (1994) Cytokines as potential vaccine adjuvants. Biotherapy 7 (3):261–269
66. Sporri R, Reis e Sousa C (2005) Inflammatory mediators are insufficient for full dendritic cell activation and promote expansion of CD4+ T cell populations lacking helper function. Nat Immunol 6(2):163–170
67. Kool M, Soullié T et al (2008) Alum adjuvant boosts adaptive immunity by inducing uric acid and activating inflammatory dendritic cells. J Exp Med 205(4):869–882
68. Eisenbarth SC, Colegio OR et al (2008) Crucial role for the Nalp3 inflammasome in the immunostimulatory properties of aluminium adjuvants. Nature 453(7198):1122–1126
69. Kool M, Pétrilli V et al (2008) Cutting edge: alum adjuvant stimulates inflammatory dendritic cells through activation of the NALP3 inflammasome. J Immunol 181(6):3755–3759
70. Jordan MB, Mills DM et al (2004) Promotion of B cell immune responses via an alum-induced myeloid cell population. Science 304(5678):1808–1810
71. Bennett SR, Carbone FR et al (1998) Help for cytotoxic-T-cell responses is mediated by CD40 signalling. Nature 393(6684):478–480
72. Ridge JP, Di Rosa F et al (1998) A conditioned dendritic cell can be a temporal bridge between a CD4+ T-helper and a T-killer cell. Nature 393(6684):474–478
73. Schoenberger SP, Toes RE et al (1998) T-cell help for cytotoxic T lymphocytes is mediated by CD40-CD40L interactions. Nature 393(6684):480–483
74. Diehl L, den Boer AT et al (1999) CD40 activation in vivo overcomes peptide-induced peripheral cytotoxic T-lymphocyte tolerance and augments anti-tumor vaccine efficacy. Nat Med 5(7):774–779
75. Ahonen CL, Doxsee CL et al (2004) Combined TLR and CD40 triggering induces potent CD8 + T cell expansion with variable dependence on type I IFN. J Exp Med 199(6):775–784

Chapter 9
Towards the Systematic Discovery of Immunomodulatory Adjuvants

Darren R. Flower

Abstract Adjuvants potentiate immune responses, reducing the amount and dosage of antigen needed for protective immunity. Adjuvants are particularly important when considering subunit, epitope-based, or other more exotic vaccine formulations that lack significant inherent immunogenicity. While innumerable adjuvants are known, only a handful are licensed for human use: principally alum, and squalene-based oil-in-water adjuvants. Alum, the most commonly used, is suboptimal. There are many varieties of adjuvant: proteins, oligonucleotides, drug-like small-molecules, and liposome-based delivery systems with adjuvant activity being perhaps the most prominent. Like poisons, adjuvants function via several mechanisms. Many plausible alternatives have been proposed. Focussing in particular on the discovery of small-molecule adjuvants, in the following we give a brief and fairly synoptic overview of adjuvants and their discovery.

9.1 Introduction

An underexplored approach for maximising the efficacy, effectiveness, and efficiency of vaccines is the discovery, development, and optimisation of efficacious adjuvants. Adjuvants can be defined as any molecule or complex molecular or supramolecular assembly significantly able to augment an immune response when administered simultaneously with a vaccine. It is thought that many adjuvants mediate their effects by acting as immune potentiators, eliciting early innate immune responses which enhance vaccine effectiveness by greatly exacerbating the overall vaccine responses.

D.R. Flower (✉)
School of Life and Health Sciences, Aston University, Aston Triangle, Birmingham, UK
e-mail: d.r.flower@aston.ac.uk

D.R. Flower and Y. Perrie (eds.), *Immunomic Discovery of Adjuvants and Candidate Subunit Vaccines*, Immunomics Reviews: 5, DOI 10.1007/978-1-4614-5070-2_9,

This review focuses on adjuvants within vaccinology. As is so often the case, the word Adjuvant has many meanings: as an adjective, it means assisting or aiding, and its use in this context can be traced at least as far as the early seventeenth century; as a noun Adjuvant can mean "A person or thing helping or aiding; a help, helper, or assistant", which again appears first at the start of the seventeenth century. The Oxford English Dictionary traces the etymology or derivation of the word adjuvant through the sixteenth century French word adjuvant to the Latin *adjuvant*, the present participle of *adjuvare*, meaning *to assist*; which is itself derived from *juvare*, meaning *to help*. More specifically within medicine, adjuvant has the following meaning: "A substance added to a prescription to assist the action of the principal ingredient or base". This use of adjuvant appears first in the mid seventeenth century.

More specifically still, within the disciplines of vaccinology and vaccination, adjuvants are chemical substances of various types that, when added to weakly immunogenic vaccines, typically greatly augment or modify any concomitant immune response, thus inducing protection. Almost all currently available commercial subunit vaccines targeted for human use will incorporate adjuvants, additional to any antigenic molecules derived from pathogens. Indeed, adjuvants—acting as either immunomodulators or as immune potentiators—have been widely utilised for many decades. Adjuvants also improve vaccination by enhancing and modifying the depot effect, principally by slowing the diffusion of antigens from the site of infection in order that antigen assimilation proceeds over a much longer time.

This contrasts with other medical uses of the word adjuvant. An adjuvant can be any substance that modulates the effects caused by other agents, particularly drugs, while having little effect if administered alone. Adjuvant therapy, also known as adjuvant care, is defined as a treatment given additional to a primary, principal, or incipient treatment. Over time, this terminology has come to mean almost exclusively supplementary treatment regimens used in cancer therapy. Adjuvant therapy is used to refer to treatment occurring after treatment, neoadjuvant therapy occurs before it, and concomitant systemic therapy for treatment after. Adjuvant therapy—which may take many forms, including radiotherapy or systemic therapy, such as chemotherapy, immunotherapy, or hormone therapy—is typically used where a statistical risk of relapse remains.

Within the context of vaccinology, adjuvants bring with them two principal benefits. First, the use of an adjuvant typically allows the dose of administered antigen or antigens to be decreased, thus reducing the overall cost of any deploying vaccine. Secondly, the exacerbated immune response engendered by adjuvants can augment, hasten, and lengthen specific immune responses made to vaccine antigens and thus provide a better and longer-lasting protection against target pathogens. The main adjuvants currently licensed for human use include alum salts and—albeit to a lesser extent—oil-in-water emulsions.

The use of aluminium-based adjuvants in vaccinology has a long history, at least comparatively so. Such adjuvants have been used since the 1920s, when Glenny et al. found that diphtheria toxoid, when precipitated on alum, was successful when used as a vaccine [1]. Aluminium-precipitated human vaccines, principally tetanus and diphtheria toxoid, were shown to be significantly more immunogenic than the corresponding soluble toxoid during the 1930s [2, 3]. Subsequently, the use of such adjuvants in diverse vaccines has become common, being widely used in the preparation of vaccines. The properties of such vaccine products were studied intensely in terms of their in vivo immunogenicity, although the aluminium hydroxide carrier habitually took a standard form. Despite the success of alum-based adjuvants, the successful development of other adjuvant systems has by contrast been stymied.

Several hundred adjuvants have been tested for their ability to exacerbate immunity in the last decade or so. Such adjuvants have included: mineral salts and emulsions, as well as adjuvants derived from microorganisms; nucleic acids; proteins, such as cytokines; and polysaccharides; amongst many others. Very few such adjuvants have proved commercially successful, with limitations such as lack of efficacy, prohibitive cost, unacceptable toxicity, problematic manufacture, poor adsorption, or poor stability [4–6]. Thus there remains an imperative need for new substances that can act as adjuvants.

Adjuvant discovery is a particular focus of modern biopharmaceutical vaccine research. There is clear interest from vaccine companies of all sizes in identifying novel adjuvants able to enhance (either qualitatively or quantitatively) protective immune responses to specific pathogens. This has translated into some significant recent commercial transactions, such as the acquisitions of Corixa (which developed the MPL adjuvant) by GlaxoSmithKline (GSK) for $300M and of Coley Pharmaceutical Group (which developed CPG) by Pfizer for $164M. Currently, the vaccine market is valued at greater than $12 billion; it is projected to exceed $40 billion in 2015. The vaccine industry has recently been commercially re-invigorated by the release of blockbuster vaccines such as Wyeth's paediatric vaccine, Prevnar (subunit vaccine based on pneumococcal bacteria), with annual sales of $1.5 billion. It is said, that over 400 vaccines against infectious diseases and cancer are on the market or currently in development.

Until the recent past, adjuvant development was largely empirical; yet now newly emergent concepts in our understanding of the way innate and adaptive immune responses begin have transformed the development of new adjuvants, making such discovery, optimisation, and formulation fundamentally more rational. In this review, we explore the nature of adjuvants, their physical and functional properties, and, to some extent at least, the mechanism and nature of their discovery, within the wider context of vaccine discovery. Our tacit intention is also to highlight the potential of a neglected area of research in this area: the identification of synthetic, quasi-drug-like small molecule immunomodulatory adjuvants. However, we will specifically exclude reference to delivery systems, which are dealt with at great length elsewhere in this book; such delivery systems often also possess significant adjuvant properties.

9.2 Extant Adjuvants

While a bewilderingly complex variety of different adjuvants have been investigated experimentally, only a handful are currently licensed and commercially available for use in humans. While the number of adjuvants that are used routinely in the lab is rather higher, it is still small when compared to the number of putative adjuvants that have been evaluated over the last few decades. This dearth represents, in part at least, the natural conservatism of the working scientist keen to pursue their own limited scientific goals rather than engaging widely with the cutting-edge of technology on all fronts. Yet, it is also a measure of the degree to which the field of adjuvant research has lagged behind other areas of vaccinology.

Nonetheless, the argument for the use of adjuvants is and remains compelling, and strongly so: adjuvants can heighten the immunogenicity of antigens; they can modify the mechanism of immune responses; they can decrease the quantity of antigen necessary for vaccination to be successful; they can reduce the requirement for, or the frequency of, booster immunisations; and they can increase appropriate immune responses in immune-compromised or elderly patients. When selecting an adjuvant, one in general wants at least the following properties: high efficacy and efficiency; low toxicity, and thus few-if-any side effects; adjuvanticity with multiple antigens; and, of course, ease of use and low unit cost.

An additional area of particular interest is the rational selection of adjuvants to help steer or direct the course of an immune response, targeting desired responses, which partly dependent on the disease being targeted. Thus we may wish our adjuvant to favour one or more type of response—Th1, Th2, antibodies, or CTL—over another; or to promote specific cellular or organ target, such as stimulating antibody responses at mucosal surfaces; or to select a particular immunoglobulin class.

Identifying a possibly extensive set of adjuvants, each capable of directing immune responses to vaccines in an appropriate direction, and thus facilitating optimal protection against each infection, should be a highly desirable goal for vaccine research. Thus, a key challenge for adjuvant discovery is to induce particular types of immune response against particular infections. Yet, as stated before and elaborated hereafter, only three classes of adjuvant have actually been licensed thus far for human vaccine formulations: alum-based adjuvants, adjuvants based on squalene oil-in-water emulsions, and an monophosphoryl lipid A (MPL) containing adjuvant.

Aluminium compounds, including aluminium phosphate ($AlPO_4$), aluminium hydroxide ($Al(OH)_2$), and alum-precipitated vaccines, historically known as protein aluminate, are, for human and animal hosts, the most used vaccine adjuvants [7, 8]. These adjuvants are often incorrectly denoted as "alum" in the immunological literature: strictly speaking alum is potassium aluminium sulphate ($KAl(SO_4)\cdot 12H_2O$). This substance has never been utilised as an adjuvant per se. For convenience sake, we shall nonetheless adopt the term alum here, but acknowledge its inexactitude.

Alum has, overall, a good, even an excellent, safety record. For infections that can be prevented by antibody induction, aluminium adjuvants remain the de facto adjuvants of choice, with the rapid development of long-lasting, high-titered antibody responses. Many, many studies in human and animal hosts ably show the apparent superiority of aluminium-adsorbed diphtheria and toxoids tetanus, when compared to soluble equivalents, particularly after the initial dose [9, 10].

Careful selection of aluminium adjuvant is vital; as is optimisation of adsorption conditions for every antigen, as both depend upon the physic-chemical character of both antigen and adjuvant. Adsorption onto alum depends primarily on electrostatic interactions: two well-used aluminium adjuvants—aluminium hydroxide and aluminium phosphate—are oppositely charged at physiological pH.

Thus, alum is an imperfect, suboptimal adjuvant. It provides inadequate antibody induction to protein subunits; and it is a poorly immunogenic adjuvant in the context of cellular immune responses, particularly CTL immunity [11]. It primarily induces increases in IgG1, though not IgG2a or IgG2b, signifying the so-called Th2-driven immune response [12]. Alum can also induce and/or augment IgE antibody responses, typical of human allergic reactions [13]. Other limitations of alum include local inflammatory reactions and its perplexing ineffectiveness with particular antigens.

There are several adjuvants which can be bracketed together as the so-called oil-in-water emulsions; several or these are licensed for human and veterinary use, and others—such as Freund's adjuvant—which are widely used in laboratory or animal studies. Freund's adjuvant, named after Jules T Freund (1890–1960), a Hungarian-born American immunologist [14, 15], comes as either Freund's complete adjuvant (FCA) or Freund's incomplete adjuvant (FIA). The complete formulation comprises dried, inactivated mycobacteria (such as *Mycobacterium tuberculosis*), while the incomplete form is by contrast a simple oil-in-water emulsion, lacking mycobacterial components [16]. FCA stimulates cell-mediated immunity leading to the potentiation of antibody production. Its use in human hosts is prohibited, due principally to safety concerns over toxicity. Even in animals, the use of FCA and FIA is deprecated due to induced pain and tissue damage.

Many alternatives to FCA have been proposed and marketed. These include: Ribi Adjuvant System or RAS, an oil-in-water emulsion comprises MPL endotoxin and mycobacterial cell wall components in 2 % squalene [17]; TiterMax, a stable, metabolisable oil-in-water adjuvant [18]; Syntex Adjuvant Formulation or SAF [19], an oil-in-water emulsion stabilised by a combination of polyoxyethylene/polyoxypropylene block copolymer L121 and Tween 80 [20], which activates complement and may also bias humoral immune responses towards IgG2a; Elvax 40W, an ethylene-vinyl acetate copolymer; and AdjuPrime, a carbohydrate polymer; among many more.

There are two main oil-in-water adjuvants licensed for human use: MF59 [21, 22] and AS03 [23, 24]. They are both emulsions containing the natural product Squalene. See Fig. 9.1. Squalene has no intrinsic adjuvant activity, but has been combined with surfactants in certain adjuvant formulations. Various other squalene-based adjuvants are being investigated.

Initially developed in the 1990s through collaboration between Ciba-Geigy and Chiron, MF59 was the first commercially available, oil-in-water adjuvant to be

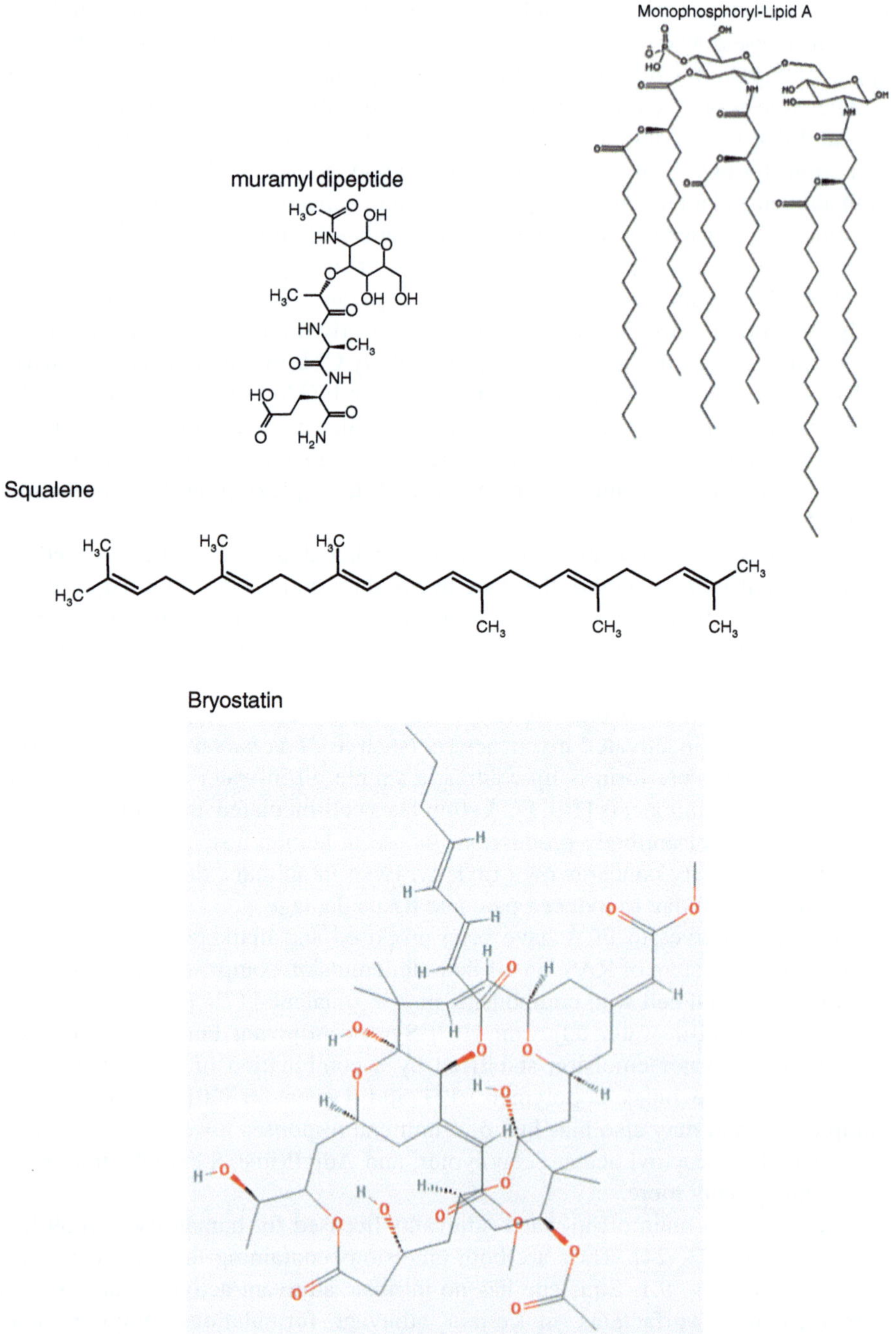

Fig. 9.1 (continued)

Bis-(3',5')-cyclic dimeric adenosine monophosphate

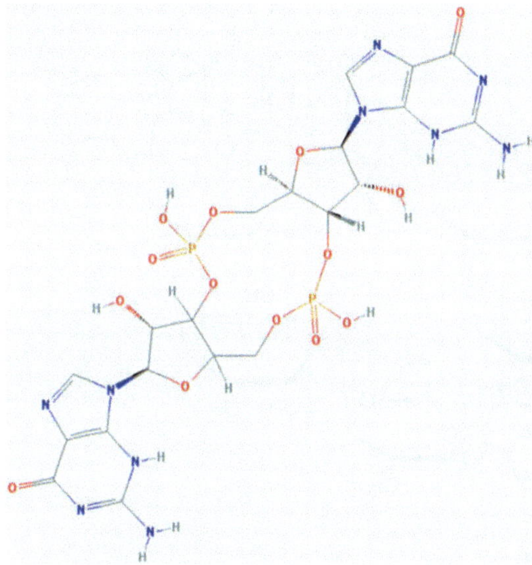

mannide monooleate (Montanide ISA 720)

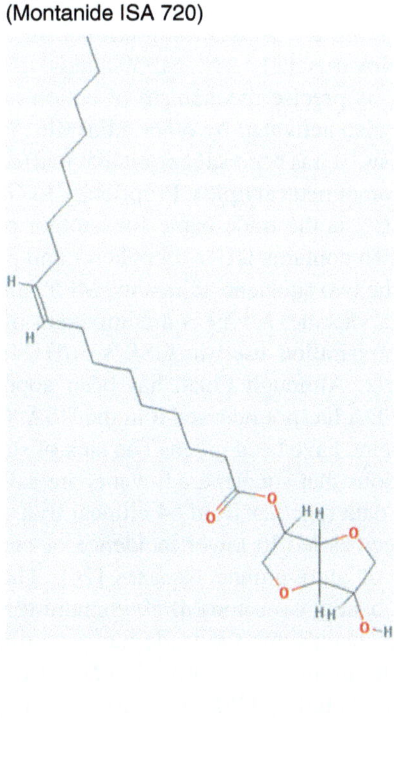

Fig. 9.1 (continued)

QS21

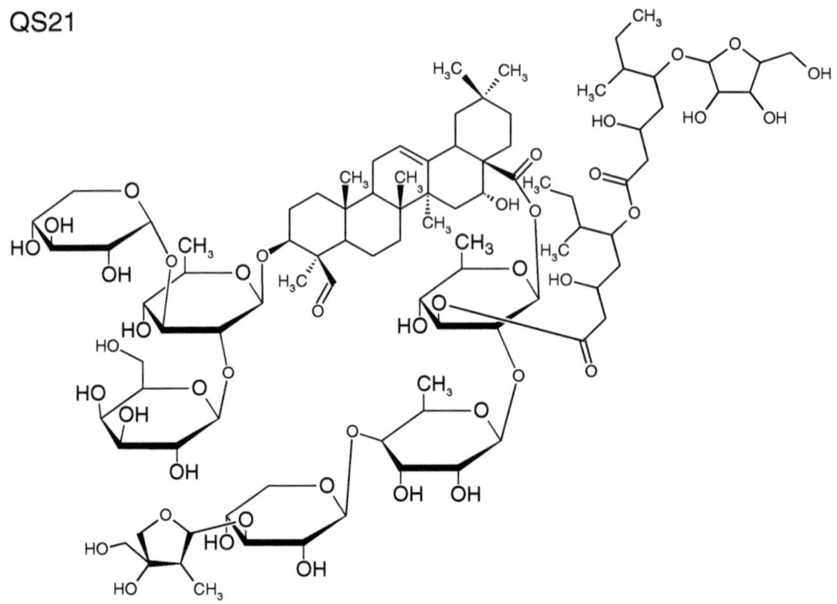

Fig. 9.1 (continued)

licensed in humans. Its main use is as an adjuvant of the seasonal influenza virus vaccine marketed by Novartis [21, 22]. MF59 tends to favour a Th2 immune response [25], although its precise mechanism of action is not known. MF59 can switch on several genes also activated by other adjuvants. No receptors specific for MF59 have been found, and it has been suggested that it affects cellular behaviour by inducing the accumulation of neutral lipids. Proprietary to GSK, AS03, which stands for "Adjuvant System 03", is the trade name for another predominantly squalene-based adjuvant, which also contains DL-α-tocopherol and polysorbate 80 [23, 24].

As indicated above, the two squalene adjuvants, MF59 and AS03, have found use as adjuvants in influenza vaccine. MF59 is a component of Novartis' Fluad, while AS03 is the adjuvant preparation used in GSK's A/H1N1 pandemic flu vaccine Pandemrix and Arepanrix. Although Fluad has been approved for human use in Europe since 1997, the FDA has not licensed it in the USA. Over 22 million doses of squalene-containing vaccine have been given. The lack of subsequent adverse events is consistent with assertions that squalene adjuvants are safe. Indeed, a 2009 meta-analysis, which brought data together from 64 clinical trials, seemed to indicate that squalene-adjuvanted vaccines led to lower incidence of chronic disease, while not altering the prevalence of autoimmune diseases [26]. The report concluded that "there may be a clinical benefit over non-MF59-containing vaccines".

Finally, AS04, which stands for the trade-name "Adjuvant System 04", is a combination of MPL and aluminium hydroxide [27]. It has been licensed for use with the HPV vaccine marketed by GSK: Cervarix. See Fig. 9.1.

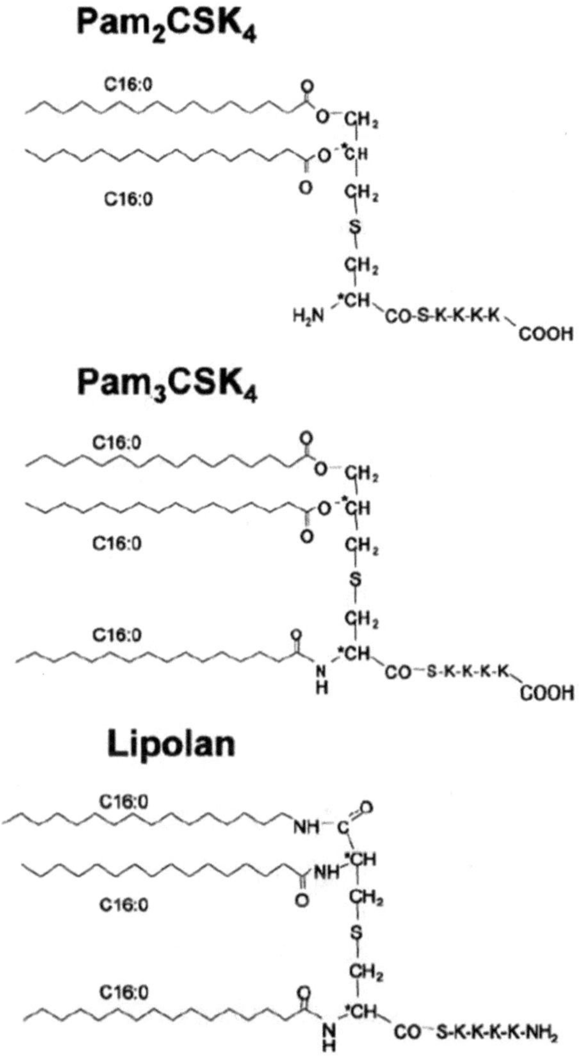

Fig. 9.1 (continued)

9.3 Mechanisms of Adjuvant Action

Adjuvants form a disparate group much like poisons, in that they work via several distinct mechanisms and take many forms. Adjuvants have been thought to work via a restricted set of defined mechanisms [28, 29]. First, adjuvants can act through the presentation of, and the physical form taken by, vaccine-formulated antigens, and thus altering the duration of antigen availability. Secondly, adjuvants can alter antigen and adjuvant uptake, changing the cellular compartments that an antigen

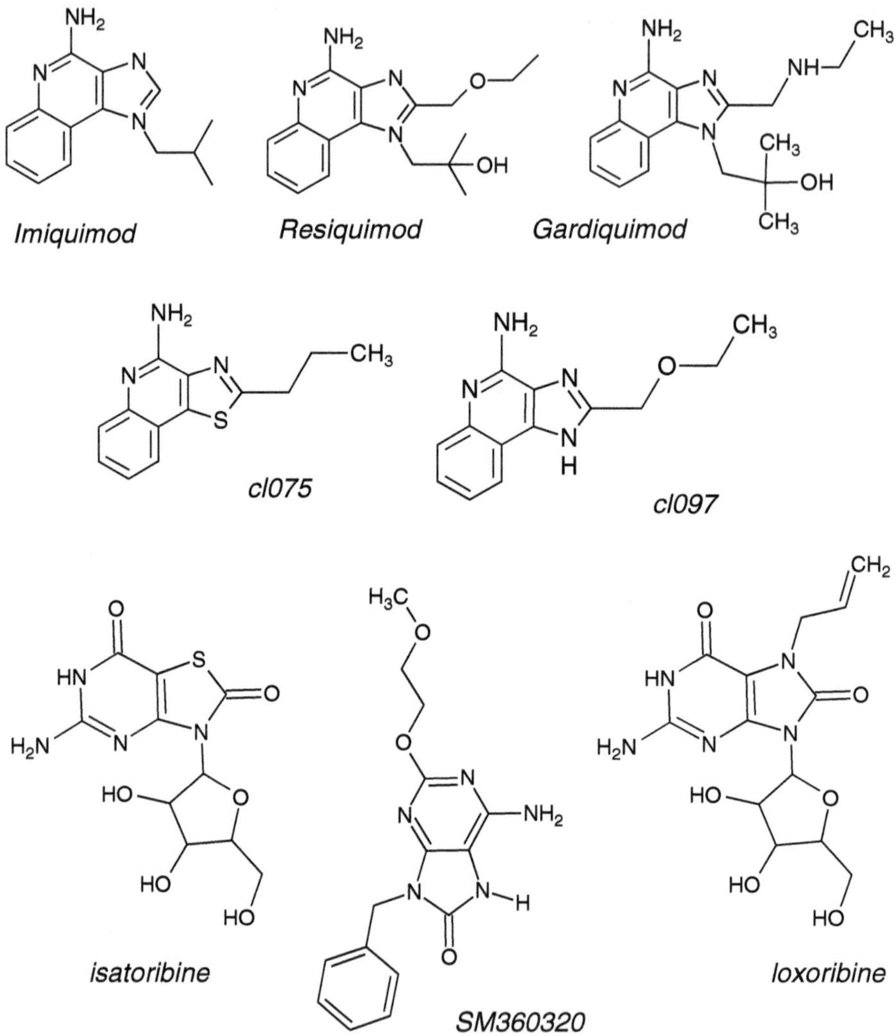

Fig. 9.1 (continued)

enters, which in turn alters the nature and magnitude of resulting immune responses. Thirdly, adjuvants can function via the targeting of antigen to specific cells and/or organs. Fourthly, adjuvants can work to prevent the elimination of antigens through proteolytic degradation or other catabolic mechanism. Finally, adjuvants can work via specific immune potentiation and/or immune modulation, including regulation of both qualitative and quantitative aspects of the immune response.

Many adjuvants seem to act via several mechanisms simultaneously. For example, aluminium-based adjuvants can act via several routes [30]: firstly, through the formation of a vaccine depot; secondly, by enhancing the productive uptake by

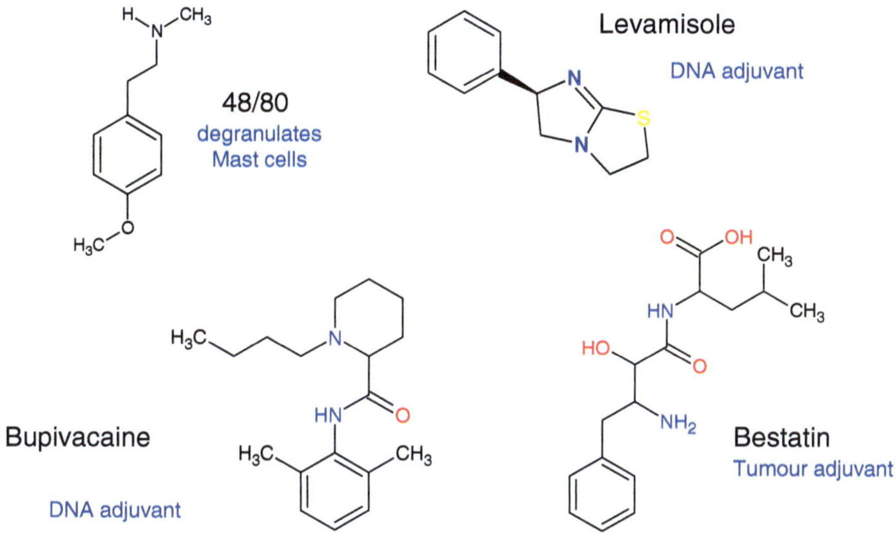

Fig. 9.1 Structure of various small-molecule adjuvants

antigen-presenting cells (APCs) of optimally sized (<10 μm) antigen particles adsorbed onto aluminium; and thirdly by direct stimulation of immune cells through activation of complement, induction of eosinophilia, and also via macrophage activation.

The mechanism underlying the action of mineral salt adsorbents and particulate adjuvants relies primarily on appropriate antigen presentation to the immune system [28–30]. Certain adjuvants, such as alum, may enhance vaccination in several ways: by magnifying the depot effect; through the co-sequestration of antigen and immune potentiators; by slowing the diffusion of antigen material away from the vaccination site, such that absorption and assimilation happens over a long timescale. Emulsions, on the other hand, may promote gradual antigen release and help deter rapid antigen elimination, since stable, resident antigens are of intrinsically greater immunogenicity than are unstable antigens.

The features of adjuvants adumbrated in the preceding paragraphs synergise with the effects mediated by the physical form and the intrinsic temporal stability of antigens. The physical form exhibited by antigens, particularly those of aggregated antigens [31], can help determine the nature and the magnitude of immune responses, primarily by affecting the interaction of antigens with APCs, and thus moderating the duration of antigen presentation. Soluble antigens typically elicit antibody responses while particulate or aggregated antigens are thought to enter the cytosol of APCs, generating or enhancing CTL responses via mechanisms otherwise associated with cross-presentation. Microbial, synthetic, and endogenous adjuvants may, by contrast, function primarily by directly stimulating and/or modulating any response mounted by the immune system. Such adjuvants may act as direct potentiators or modulators of the innate immune system, triggering early innate responses that in turn increase the vaccine effectiveness by increasing uptake.

However, it is now emerging that such simple categorisation masks more complex mechanisms. As we have said above, alum was long thought to act via the depot effect, as well as stimulating the IgG1 and IgE antibody production, and by triggering interleukin-4 secretion [30]. However, within the last 5 years or so, it has been found that alum helps activate caspase 1 and enhances the release of IL-1β and IL-18 from mammalian APCs [32]. Several subsequent reports indicated that alum-induced inflammasome activation depended on ASC and NLRP3 [33, 34]. Eisenbarth et al. showed that alum uptake, followed by tubulin polymerisation, and the release of potassium were all required for inflammasome activation [35]. The inflammasome is an increasingly well-studied supramolecular protein complex: inflammasome-activated caspase-1 cleaves proinflammatory cytokines IL-1β and IL-18 into biologically active forms and also triggers release of HMGB1 into the extracellular environment. Inflammosome activation appears to underlie many inflammatory responses. Other events, such as lysosomal disruption and cathepsin B activity, have also all been implicated in alum-induced NLRP3 inflammasome activation.

In part, adjuvants act by mimicking specific evolutionarily conserved molecules—the so-called Pathogen Associated Molecular Patterns, also known as PAMPs—including lipopolysaccharide (LPS), liposomes, and bacterial cell wall components; as well as certain nucleic acids that are structurally distinct from host RNA and DNA: unmethylated CpG dinucleotide-containing DNA, double-stranded RNA (dsRNA), and single-stranded DNA (ssDNA) [36]. PAMPs are typically features of whole classes of organisms: LPS is a common constituent of Gram-negative bacteria. The effect of PAMPs is made manifest through their interaction with pattern recognition receptors (PRRs), which are expressed on cells characteristic of the innate and adaptive systems. PRRs recognise PAMPs, such as LPS, that are demonstrably different in structure from host molecules, and are thus capable of being readily identified as non-host in origin [37].

PAMPs can be viewed as a subtype of *danger signals*: a concept delineated and conceived by Matzinger [38, 39]. She views innate immune receptors as evolving to recognise damage to the host organism not simply to identify pathogens. Such danger or damage signals include free RNA or DNA, as well as a multitude of subcellular components released in the course of necrotic rather than apoptotic cell death. The necrosis of cells induces inflammatory responses which in turn foments, fosters, and facilitates adaptive immune responses. The ubiquitous metabolite uric acid, which is generated in large amounts by cellular injury, is another interesting example of the so-called danger signal: it is able to exacerbate immune responses even when microbial stimulation is absent [40]. Uric acid crystals can trigger interleukin-1β-mediated inflammation through activation of the NLRP3 inflammasome [41].

The innate immune system has vital role in modulating and moderating the adaptive immune system. The overall activation of the innate immune system, the primary initial bulwark against invading pathogens, is essential if a strong adaptive immune response is to be engendered, and thus through this the eventual development of immune memory. Development of immunological memory that is protective against infection and reinfection is the ultimate aim and principal *raison detre* of vaccination. Adjuvants should in modern era possess well-defined target receptors, and through such interaction with these modulate in a rational and explicable manner the course and intensity of any immune response generated by vaccination. We need to target, and target specifically, such innate immune receptors, identifying molecular adjuvants with agonistic properties. Alternatively, for inhibitory or regulatory immune receptors, antagonists are needed in order to nullify the suppressive or inhibitory effects of these receptors on the innate or adaptive immune systems.

Indeed, and as we have intimated above, many extant adjuvants may act solely or partially by stimulating PRRs present on innate immune cells. PAMPs, either in purified form or synthetic PAMP-analogues, can exert potent effects through this receptor-mediated mechanism-of-action [42]. PRRs targeted by adjuvants are many, yet three classes are paramount [43]: Toll-like receptors, or TLRs, which bind a range of diverse ligand molecules; nucleotide-binding oligomerisation domain (NOD)-like proteins, which bind the muramyl dipeptide component of peptidoglycan (PGN); and retinoic acid-inducible protein-related proteins, or RIGs, which detect dsRNA.

There are, of course, many other PRRs; the list includes scavenger receptors and C-type lectin-like receptors, such as mannose receptors, which detect mannosylated lipoarabinomannans; β-glucan receptors; and dendritic cell-specific intercellular adhesion molecule 3-grabbing non-integrin, or DC-SIGN, which detects protein-ligated carbohydrate moieties.

Another route by which adjuvants may exert their effects is by altering the regulation of the adaptive immune response. There are many such mechanisms. One of the most pertinent, and thus exciting, targets for adjuvants are regulatory T-cells (Tregs) [44]. These dampen immune responses, preventing excessive responses against infection and helping maintain self-tolerance.

9.4 Large Molecule Adjuvants: Proteins

In a review published in 2006, Kornbluth and Stone proclaimed a nascent golden age of rational vaccine discovery [45]. Their particular focus was the growing potential for the exploitation of immunomodulators adjuvants capable of enhancing the observed immunogenicity of subunit and other vaccines. They grouped adjuvants into stimulatory and suppressive immunomodulators. In this context, several different proteins have been shown to possess adjuvant properties. Such large molecule or protein adjuvants are clearly detectable via both sequence-based methods and potentially also by the so-called alignment-free approaches. In this way we can conceive of "adjuvant hunting", and see it as an analogous process to "reverse vaccinology", however with adjuvants not antigens as our target.

Immunostimulatory adjuvants include a wide variety of putative protein adjuvants. These include agonists of CD40, which can induce dendritic cell activation and maturation [46]. Other members of the TNF receptor superfamily, such as OX40L, CD30L, CD27L/CD70, 4-1BBL, LIGHT, and GITRL, also show promise as protein adjuvants [47], as do protein agonists of the NLR system [48]. Immunosuppressive protein adjuvants include antagonist antibodies and IFN-γ.

It is also apparent that, within the context of immunovaccinology, protein adjuvants may be either endogenous or exogenous; having either a self- or non-self-origin. The first, endogenous alternative is typified by the use of cytokines [49, 50]. Recombinant human Interleukin-12 (IL-12) has been extensively explored for its adjuvant properties [51, 52], demonstrating efficacy in pneumococcal vaccination amongst others [53]. Proteins of microbial origin have also been shown to act as adjuvants [54, 55]. Other studies have also highlighted the potential for synergistic effects from combining proteins adjuvants with distinct molecular adjuvants, such as those of natural product origin or synthetic small-molecule adjuvants (SMAs), both classes of which are described more completely below.

It is also possible to combine both endogenous or exogenous proteins into a single molecular adjuvant through the auspices of protein engineering. For example, Gupta et al. evaluated two CD40 mimics, one the EBV gene product LMP1 and the other an LMP1-CD40 chimaera [56]. Overall, SIV expressing both LMP1 and LMP1-CD40 induced a wide, potent Th1-biased response in both macrophages and DC in both human and rhesus macaque. SIV-LMP1 also improved antigen presentation by lentiviral vector vaccines, which is suggestive that immune activation mediated by LMP1 may be able to enhance anti-HIV-1 lentiviral vaccines.

Thinking more widely, the ability to engineer protein adjuvants using the techniques of site-directed mutagenesis and/or by generating chimerical or fusion proteins allows for the exciting prospect of modulating and moderating the biological effects of such adjuvant molecules, in a rational and efficient manner. We can conceive of enhancing the affinity of a protein adjuvant for its target receptor by introducing point mutations into the protein sequence which target suboptimal intermolecular interactions, increasing hydrophobic complementarity, optimising potential hydrogen bonds, or improving the energetic balance of charge–charge pairs. Likewise, we can use the same approach to try to design out ADMEt problems with their origin in disadvantageous pharmacokinetics or safety concerns over toxicity or immunogenicity.

9.5 Adjuvants Based on Natural Products

Many molecules of natural origin have also been investigated and evaluated for their adjuvant properties [57]. Such putative or extant adjuvants include QS21 [58–61], muramyl dipeptide [62], and mannide monooleate formulated as an oil-in-water adjuvant, as marketed by Seppic in various guises, of which the best known are Montanide ISA 720 and Montanide ISA-51 [63]. Muramyl dipeptide is known to act through the nucleotide-binding oligomerisation domain 2 (NOD2); while another, somewhat similar, natural product with adjuvant-like properties is MurNAc-L-Ala-γ-D-Glu-mDAP (M-TriDAP), also known as DAP-containing muramyl tripeptide [64]; this molecule is a PGN degradation product from Gram-negative bacteria, which is again recognised by the intracellular NOD1 and NOD2 system. Purely for the purposes of classification, we shall also class CpG oligonucleotides as natural products.

Several putative adjuvants are related, at least structurally speaking, to the prevalent microbial compound known colloquially as LPS: these include MPL, which acts as an adjuvant via a TLR4-mediated mechanism [65, 66]. There are in addition a variety of other semi-synthetic molecules, which are, as a class, all derived ultimately from biological molecules, and that all act with adjuvant-like properties [67]: these include an extensive group of lipopeptides including glucopyranosyl lipid A (GLA) [68, 69]; Pam2CSK4 (acting via the TLR2/TLR6-activated signalling pathway); Pam3CSK4; and lipolan [70].

As these molecules are natural in origin, being predominantly derived from plants and microbial sources, and share much of the chemical complexity which other biosynthesised molecules possess, there is a clear connection in terms of perceived mechanism to known PAMPS, including bacterial cell wall components, double-stranded and single-stranded nucleic acids, and unmethylated CpG dinucleotide-containing DNA.

The triterpene squalene, which was discussed at length above, is a natural product obtained originally from shark oil [71, 72], though now plant sources (including amaranth seed, rice bran, wheat germ, and olives) are used [73]. Another purified plant extract, QS-21, a mixture of water soluble triterpene glucoside compounds, also exhibits adjuvant activity [58–60, 74, 75]. It is a saponin, derived from the Chilean Soap bark tree (*Quillaja saponaria*). Despite high toxicity, haemolytic effect, aqueous instability, limiting their potential use as human adjuvants, several commercial animal vaccines have been prepared from quillaja saponins: rabies, foot-and-mouth disease, bovine mastitis, and feline leukaemia. Principal saponin-based adjuvants are Quil A and QS-21 [59]. They have been used as adjuvants in vaccines against HIV in guinea pig and human [61], human cancer [76], primate and murine malaria [77], RSV [78], and murine visceral leishmaniasis [79]. Saponin-based adjuvants stimulate both Th1 responses and generate CTLs against exogenous antigens; making them suitable for a variety of vaccines, including subunit vaccines, vaccines vs. intracellular pathogens, and therapeutic cancer vaccines [80].

Another molecule with interesting adjuvant properties, including dendritic cell activation, is the natural product Bryostatin-1 [81]; a potent activator of protein kinase C [82]. It is one of the several macrocyclic lactones isolated from Bugula neritina [83], a species of Bryozoa, Ectoprocta, or "moss animals", a phylum of marine invertebrates. Bryostatin-1 is believed to exacerbate the antigen-presenting ability and general maturation of DCs, via the NF-κB pathway, inducing expression of various co-stimulatory molecules [84]. Bryostatin-1 also induces augmented T-bet and IFN-γ mRNA levels [85].

Another distinct category of molecular adjuvant, again with a natural product origin, is that based around nucleotide structures. Examples include bis(3′,5′)-cyclic diguanylic acid [86, 87] and Bis-(3′,5′)-cyclic dimeric adenosine monophosphate [88, 89]. Bis-(3′,5′)-cyclic dimeric adenosine monophosphate (c-diAMP) is a second messenger within archaea and bacteria, that has strong Th1/Th2/Th17 promoting adjuvant activities when delivered mucosally, inducing significantly higher serum antigen-specific IgG titres, as well as by increasing local antigen-specific secretion of IgA.

Another set of adjuvants based around a nucleotide core is the last set of molecules we will look at in this section; these are the so-called synthetic CpG oligodeoxynucleotides or CpG-ODN, which activate TLR9 [90–92]. These have been widely investigated as a class, and upon the subject of which much has been written; rather too much to even true to summarise in these few pages. Examples of CpG ODN include several notable commercial entities: CPG-1826 [93] and CPG-7909 [94]. CpG7909 is an agonist of B cells and plasmacytoid dendritic cells that exacerbates antibody generation, stimulates B-cell proliferation, secretion of interleukin-10 and interferon-α. Polyinosinic:polycytidylic acid (poly I:C) is another immuno-stimulant, often used as an adjuvant, which interacts with TLR3, expressed on dendritic cells, macrophages, and B-cells [95]. Synthetic poly I:C is structurally analogous to double-stranded viral RNA, with one strand of polymerised inosinic acid and the other of polymerised cytidylic acid. From the vaccine design perspective, one of the most exciting, and potential productive, aspects of CpG-ODNs is that there exists currently sufficient structure–activity data to suggest that we can undertake iterative design of such compounds [96], using QSAR technology to guide the synthesis of novel ODNs that are optimised for activity, selectivity, and toxicity.

9.6 Small-Molecule Adjuvants

There is another, and often neglected, type of molecular adjuvant: one which we shall term small-molecule adjuvants (SMA), for want of a more apposite term. We have enforced a rather artificial distinction here between adjuvants that are natural products and those which are synthetically derived, drug-like small molecules. Many drugs are themselves natural products, or are derived by synthetic modification from natural products, possessing that level of structural and chiral complexity characteristic of molecules produced by long, bifurcating enzymatic pathways. Natural products and SMAs also share common features, principally size. They differ primarily in terms of their complexity, with natural products typically being rather more complex, and thus synthetically intractable, than the majority of synthetic drug, derived via serial synthesis and/or reagent coupling via parallel synthesis.

It may be argued that SMAs are the class which have been most obviously under-explored, despite this many exist: apart from the well-studied imidazoquinolines, and the variety of natural products described previously, such as QS21 or MPL, there are a number of distinct other well-studied small molecules which act as general purpose adjuvants: Bestatin (Ubenimex or UBX) [97–99], Levamisole [100–102], and Bupivacaine [99, 103, 104]. See Fig. 9.1. Another example of a promising SMA is 2-(4-methoxyphenyl)-*N*-methylethanamine also known as compound 48/80 [105], a compound previously known to degranulate mast cells; this molecule has been shown to be a mast cell-dependent non-toxic nasal adjuvant capable of inducing protective humoral immunity in mice.

The apparent activity of small molecules as adjuvants is incidental to their original discovery, and coincidental to any other bioactivities they display. For example, Levamisole was developed originally as an anti-helminthic [106]; Bestatin is an inhibitor of aminopeptidase N [107, 108]; Bupivacaine is a local anaesthetic [109]; and the Imidazoquinolines were originally discovered as nucleoside analogues with anti-tumour and antiviral activity [110–112].

However, by far and away the best explored group of SMAs are the so-called Imidazoquinolines [111, 113], which target specific TLRs: TLR7 and/or TLR8, inducing IFN, TNF, and IL-12 secretion. There are numerous imidazoquinoline compounds available, of which the best known are Imiquimod, Resiquimod, and Gardiquimod [112–114]. See Fig. 9.1. A variety of other molecules based around guanine have shown potential as adjuvants, for example loxoribine [115] and isatoribine [116].

The realisation that PAMPs stimulate and activate defined PRRs has provided a strong rational impetus to the systematic discovery and development of SMAs; despite this, many current SMAs were discovered serendipitously. Most, if not all, drug molecules show significant, or at least measurable, off-target activity: on the one hand, this is the cause of inconvenient and unwanted side-effects and toxicity, and, on the other, the basis for burgeoning area of drug repurposing. While it may be a step-too-far to equate adjuvant discovery with drug repurposing, per se, there is no reason to suppose that we cannot significantly increase the celerity of the life-cycle of adjuvant discovery and licensing by seeking to identify SMAs directly, using the same techniques that have proven to be successful tools in drug discovery. By combining virtual screening, with in vitro assays, and in vivo validation it should be more than possible to discover novel small molecules that can act in vivo as adjuvants in a plethora of experimental settings.

There is a pressing need properly to explore in whole animals the biological mechanisms exhibited by these compounds and simultaneously elaborate the structure–activity relationships of such compounds using a combined virtual screening and parallel synthesis approach to both extrapolate and interpolate within exist structure–activity data. Combining an understanding of structure–activity and property–activity relationships with an understanding of detailed biological mechanisms will enable us fully to capitalise on the potential of SMAs. We discuss this below.

9.7 Computational Approaches to the Discovery of Small-Molecule Adjuvants

If the preceding discussion tells us anything, it says the following: that several small-molecules exist—and exist in sufficient numbers—which display significant potential as adjuvants, and seemingly do so via a variety of mechanistic routes. In many cases, SMA molecules have displayed toxic properties or poor adsorption, or have otherwise proved unsatisfactory. Thus, there is a continuing and as yet largely unmet need for new candidate adjuvants, much as there is an ongoing requirement for new vaccines. One of the main failings of adjuvant research has been its overwhelmingly haphazard and unsystematic nature. The identification of SMAs requires instead the application of various innovative and systematic methods for molecular discovery.

Techniques used routinely by the pharmaceutical industry can also be used to discover SMAs. Three-dimensional or structure-based virtual screening (SB-VS), which utilises automated protein docking (APD), is an effective means of identifying ligands with high celerity [117–119]. APD-based SB-VS docks enormous numbers of ligand molecules into a defined binding site [120]. In this way, large small-molecule databases are screened rapidly and accurately; particularly if we can target collections that contain specific molecular subsets, enriched by pre-selection for a specific target or set of related targets.

SB-VS is exceptionally logistically efficient, saving time, labour, and resource. Months, years, or decades of robotically mediated experimentation, bedevilled as it is by signal-to-noise issues, are replaced by weeks of computational analysis, albeit complemented by a mere handful of reliable, hand-crafted assays. By using SB-VS, tens or hundreds of thousands of molecules can be reduced in number by several orders of magnitude, principally via extensive pre-screening; the tiny number left is then docked against a PRR structure. This yields at most a few hundred molecules that can be readily tested [120]. This handful is put through a hierarchical cascade of highly specific and informative assays in vitro, with actives then tested for their whole system adjuvant properties in vivo. In this way, lead adjuvant molecules are found without the need for highly expensive and often misleading HTS.

Databases, as typified by ZINC [121], contain literally millions of molecules available commercially. Developing many of these proves pointless, since many hits from HTS do not act as drugs should: they are poorly or non-selective, possess counterintuitive structure–activity relationships, and are non-competitive binders. Screening protocols—both computational and experimental—which identify reactive groups, promiscuous inhibition, and non-competitive-inhibition are widely available [122–126]. Screens exists for bioavailability, cytochrome P450 binding (such as 3A4, 2C9, 2D6), and cytotoxicity [127, 128]. More explicit screens also exist for diverse inconvenient activities, such as hERG channel inhibition, $\alpha 1$ adrenergic binding leading to orthostatic hypotension effects, and, inter alia, 5-HT2 cholinergic activity leading to obesity [129]. Screens for lead- or drug-likeness are now also in wide use [123].

The pre-processing compounds for VS also requires the preparation of multiple candidates for each de facto molecular structure [120], since each structure may possess one or several stereo centres, or exist as a racemate, or exist as an ensemble of tautomers, or require the construction of all potential protomers. However, many examples of VS have shown even the simplest, most parsimonious, most unsophisticated approaches may prove successful: this is a key strength of the VS technology.

We can justifiably reflect that despite present technical limit, virtual screening is an unequivocal, undisputed success. As a method, it works: not perfectly, but it delivers real results. VS can identify real, high-affinity ligands with unmatched cost-effectiveness and efficiency. In the context of adjuvant discovery, we exemplify such assertions by echoing our recent application of VS to the discovery of antagonists of the CCR4 chemokine receptor. These molecules function as effective adjuvants, acting via the regulatory mechanisms of the cellular arm of the adaptive immune system.

Chemokine receptors are a large and important subfamily, comprising 18 distinct proteins, of the G-protein coupled receptors or GPCRs, which transduces leukocyte chemo-attractant chemokines, which are secreted by cells when activated by inflammatory stimuli [130, 131]. Chemokines can be partitioned into the CXC and CC family, the latter containing two adjacent cysteines while in the former they are separated by an extra amino acid. Activation of chemokine receptors induces an inflammatory response by triggering migration of leukocytes from circulation to the point of injury or infection. GPCRs are a well-known and well-understood superfamily of transmembrane proteins that transduce a variety of extracellular but endogenous signals into an intracellular response [132, 133].

CCR4 is a chemokine receptor which is expressed by Th2-type CD4+ T cells. It has been linked to allergic inflammation conditions including allergic rhinitis, atopic dermatitis, and asthma. CCL22 and CCL17 are two chemokines which bind the CCR4 receptor exclusively [134]; their inhibition reduces T-cell migration to sites of inflammation. This suggests that CCR4 antagonists might provide effective treatments for allergy and asthma; a speculation consistent with the behaviour of anti-CCL17 and anti-CCL22 antibodies in mouse models of asthma.

Inhibiting CCR4 receptors may give rise to adjuvantism as the receptor is expressed by Tregs that normally suppress immune responses, inhibit maturation of DCs, and down-regulate co-stimulatory molecule expression. Inhibiting CCR4 function, and thus blocking interaction of DC with Tregs at vaccination, is anticipated to exacerbate vaccine responses, and thus an effective CCR4 antagonist should prove to be an effective adjuvant. By combining experimental validation with VS, we have identified several potential adjuvants, acting through the apparent inhibition of Treg proliferation [44, 135]. These molecules behave appropriately in a variety of in vitro assays, and increase the levels of various correlates of protection in vaccinated mice, and even show some enhancement in related challenge models observations supported by independent analysis [136]; and also shows activity against potential cancer antigens [137].

9.8 Discussion and Conclusions

Our purpose here has not been to encapsulate all knowledge of all adjuvants, and we have certainly not included reference to every known adjuvant, not yet even to every class, but rather our purpose has been to highlight some of the darker recesses of the adjuvant discovery landscape, particularly SMAs. Adjuvants are key to eliciting robust and protective immune responses from many vaccines, yet their underlying mechanisms remain to be fully and properly elaborated [138–141].

Vaccine adjuvants primarily target the so-called professional APCs, activating innate immunity through several PRR pathways [43], predominantly those linked to TLRs. To protect against viruses and other intracellular pathogens, adjuvants must stimulate Th1 responses, which is required to optimise B-cell and CD8+ T-cell responses, as well as protecting by direct cytotoxic effector functions. However potent Th1 adjuvant activity is typically associated with unacceptable toxicity, as exhibited by CFA. Thus a major challenge for adjuvant discovery is to gain Th1 stimulatory activity without exacerbating toxicity. SMAs, in particular, offer the potential to develop adjuvants with desirable, highly tailored properties.

Different adjuvants seem to behave differently for different vaccines and in different formulations. Indeed, many commercial adjuvants are combinations of molecules with different immunostimulatory properties [142]. The novel adjuvant IC31, for example, consists of an antibacterial peptide (KLKL(5)KLK) and a synthetic oligodeoxynucleotide, ODN1a, that signals through TLR9 [143]. As there is no universally effective vaccine, likewise there is no universally effective adjuvant. There are many reasons for this. In this context, a key underappreciated problem with adjuvants is that they have been and are being discovered in an unsystematic uncoordinated irrational fashion. Much as vaccines have been, and are being, discovered in an uncoordinated and haphazard fashion. Even the idiosyncratic and haphazard world of preclinical drug discovery is better organised than this.

Although as-yet-underexplored, SMAs are widely applicable and can open up a whole new area of therapeutic discovery without the pharmacodynamic, pharmacokinetic, and toxicological restrictions imposed by the once- or twice-a-day dosing of small-molecule drugs. The ADMET (Absorption Disposition Metabolism Excretion/Toxicology) properties of adjuvants (dosed at most once or twice a year) need not be identical to those of commercially marketed drugs, though they may overlap. Orally bioavailability is the prime goal, but other delivery mechanisms may be possible. Nonetheless, obtaining a range of properties and pharmacological readout will be vital to the discovery of clinically useful and deployable molecules.

Compared to proteins or synthetically obdurate natural products, SMAs have many seeming advantages. As drug-like small molecules, their properties may be precisely tailored. Their discovery is also amenable to SB-VS, and the optimisation of their specificity and properties can be undertaken using parallel synthesis, QSAR, and medicinal chemistry. It is feasible to manipulate in a rational way the structure of such compounds and thus create adjuvant compounds with enhanced in vivo characteristics. A drug dosed once or twice in a lifetime should not need all the properties we crave in the next blockbuster drug, though being as close as possible to an optimal pharmacokinetic profile would be a clear benefit.

By using the large amounts of macromolecular structure data now available for PRRs, VS should now prove the ideal starting point for the discovery of SMAs. Following the strategy outlined above will deliver this information, allowing us to understand, optimise, and ultimately fully commercialise our discoveries. If the effort invested worldwide were properly coordinated rather than directed towards short-term goals and cupidity, the whole process could be effectively systematised and the discovery of protein adjuvants, natural product-based adjuvants, and SMAs could thus be expedited.

Acknowledgements I should like to thank all my colleagues who have influenced me positively or negatively through my career, and have thus been instrumental in forming the opinions expressed above. In particular, Dr. David Tough, Dr. Jagedesch Bayry, Professor Peter Beverley, and Dr. Elma Tchillian.

References

1. Glenny AT, Pope CG, Waddington H, Wallace U (1926) The antigenic value of toxoid precipitated by potassium alum. J Pathol Bacteriol 29:38–45
2. Volk VK, Bunney WE (1942) Reimmunization against diphtheria of previously immunized children. Am J Public Health Nations Health 32(7):700–708
3. Volk VK, Bunney WE (1942) Diphtheria immunization with fluid toxoid and alum-precipitated toxoid. Am J Public Health Nations Health 32(7):690–699
4. Aguilar JC, Rodriguez EG (2007) Vaccine adjuvants revisited. Vaccine 25(19):3752–3762
5. McCluskie MJ, Weeratna RD (2001) Novel adjuvant systems. Curr Drug Targets Infect Disord 1(3):263–271
6. Spickler AR, Roth JA (2003) Adjuvants in veterinary vaccines: modes of action and adverse effects. J Vet Intern Med 17(3):273–281
7. Gupta RK et al (1993) Adjuvants—a balance between toxicity and adjuvanticity. Vaccine 11 (3):293–306
8. Gupta RK, Siber GR (1995) Adjuvants for human vaccines—current status, problems and future prospects. Vaccine 13(14):1263–1276
9. Jensen OM, Koch C (1988) On the effect of Al(Oh)3 as an immunological adjuvant. APMIS 96(3):257–264
10. Gupta RK, Siber GR (1994) Comparison of adjuvant activities of aluminium phosphate, calcium phosphate and stearyl tyrosine for tetanus toxoid. Biologicals 22(1):53–63
11. Gupta RK (1998) Aluminum compounds as vaccine adjuvants. Adv Drug Deliv Rev 32 (3):155–172
12. Marshall DJ et al (2006) Interleukin-18 enhances Th1 immunity and tumor protection of a DNA vaccine. Vaccine 24(3):244–253
13. Relyveld EH, Bizzini B, Gupta RK (1998) Rational approaches to reduce adverse reactions in man to vaccines containing tetanus and diphtheria toxoids. Vaccine 16(9–10):1016–1023
14. Anon (1963) Jules Freund, 1890–1960. J Immunol 90:331–336
15. Anon (1960) Jules Freund. Lancet 1(7132):1031–1032
16. Claassen E et al (1992) Freund's complete adjuvant: an effective but disagreeable formula. Res Immunol 143(5):478–483; discussion 572
17. Evans JT et al (2003) Enhancement of antigen-specific immunity via the TLR4 ligands MPL adjuvant and Ribi.529. Expert Rev Vaccines 2(2):219–229

18. Tejada-Simon MV, Pestka JJ (1998) Production of polyclonal antibody against ergosterol hemisuccinate using Freund's and Titermax adjuvants. J Food Prot 61(8):1060–1063
19. Allison AC, Byars NE (1992) Syntex adjuvant formulation. Res Immunol 143(5):519–525
20. Brey RN (1995) Development of vaccines based on formulations containing nonionic block copolymers. Pharm Biotechnol 6:297–311
21. O'Hagan DT, Wack A, Podda A (2007) MF59 is a safe and potent vaccine adjuvant for flu vaccines in humans: what did we learn during its development? Clin Pharmacol Ther 82 (6):740–744
22. O'Hagan DT (2007) MF59 is a safe and potent vaccine adjuvant that enhances protection against influenza virus infection. Expert Rev Vaccines 6(5):699–710
23. Walker WT, Faust SN (2010) Monovalent inactivated split-virion AS03-adjuvanted pandemic influenza A (H1N1) vaccine. Expert Rev Vaccines 9(12):1385–1398
24. Waddington C et al (2010) Open-label, randomised, parallel-group, multicentre study to evaluate the safety, tolerability and immunogenicity of an AS03(B)/oil-in-water emulsion-adjuvanted (AS03(B)) split-virion versus non-adjuvanted whole-virion H1N1 influenza vaccine in UK children 6 months to 12 years of age. Health Technol Assess 14(46):1–130
25. Wack A et al (2008) Combination adjuvants for the induction of potent, long-lasting antibody and T-cell responses to influenza vaccine in mice. Vaccine 26(4):552–561
26. Pellegrini M et al (2009) MF59-adjuvanted versus non-adjuvanted influenza vaccines: integrated analysis from a large safety database. Vaccine 27(49):6959–6965
27. Schwarz TF (2009) Clinical update of the AS04-adjuvanted human papillomavirus-16/18 cervical cancer vaccine, Cervarix. Adv Ther 26(11):983–998
28. Tritto E, Mosca F, De Gregorio E (2009) Mechanism of action of licensed vaccine adjuvants. Vaccine 27(25–26):3331–3334
29. Lambrecht BN et al (2009) Mechanism of action of clinically approved adjuvants. Curr Opin Immunol 21(1):23–29
30. Noe SM et al (2010) Mechanism of immunopotentiation by aluminum-containing adjuvants elucidated by the relationship between antigen retention at the inoculation site and the immune response. Vaccine 28(20):3588–3594
31. Zaborsky N et al (2010) Antigen aggregation decides the fate of the allergic immune response. J Immunol 184(2):725–735
32. Li H, Nookala S, Re F (2007) Aluminum hydroxide adjuvants activate caspase-1 and induce IL-1beta and IL-18 release. J Immunol 178(8):5271–5276
33. Li H et al (2008) Cutting edge: inflammasome activation by alum and alum's adjuvant effect are mediated by NLRP3. J Immunol 181(1):17–21
34. Aimanianda V et al (2009) Novel cellular and molecular mechanisms of induction of immune responses by aluminum adjuvants. Trends Pharmacol Sci 30(6):287–295
35. Eisenbarth SC et al (2008) Crucial role for the Nalp3 inflammasome in the immunostimulatory properties of aluminium adjuvants. Nature 453(7198):1122–1126
36. Bianchi ME (2007) DAMPs, PAMPs and alarmins: all we need to know about danger. J Leukoc Biol 81(1):1–5
37. Schenten D, Medzhitov R (2011) The control of adaptive immune responses by the innate immune system. Adv Immunol 109:87–124
38. Matzinger P (2002) An innate sense of danger. Ann N Y Acad Sci 961:341–342
39. Matzinger P (2002) The danger model: a renewed sense of self. Science 296(5566):301–305
40. Gasse P et al (2009) Uric acid is a danger signal activating NALP3 inflammasome in lung injury inflammation and fibrosis. Am J Respir Crit Care Med 179(10):903–913
41. Denoble AE et al (2011) Uric acid is a danger signal of increasing risk for osteoarthritis through inflammasome activation. Proc Natl Acad Sci U S A 108(5):2088–2093
42. Miyaji EN et al (2011) Trends in adjuvant development for vaccines: DAMPs and PAMPs as potential new adjuvants. Braz J Med Biol Res 44(6):500–513
43. Olive C (2012) Pattern recognition receptors: sentinels in innate immunity and targets of new vaccine adjuvants. Expert Rev Vaccines 11(2):237–256

44. Bayry J et al (2008) From 'perfect mix' to 'potion magique'—regulatory T cells and anti-inflammatory cytokines as adjuvant targets. Nat Rev Microbiol 6(1):C1; author reply C2
45. Kornbluth RS, Stone GW (2006) Immunostimulatory combinations: designing the next generation of vaccine adjuvants. J Leukoc Biol 80(5):1084–1102
46. Carlring J, Barr T, Heath AW (2005) Adjuvanticity of anti-CD40 in vaccine development. Curr Opin Mol Ther 7(1):73–77
47. Kanagavelu SK et al (2012) Soluble multi-trimeric TNF superfamily ligand adjuvants enhance immune responses to a HIV-1 Gag DNA vaccine. Vaccine 30(4):691–702
48. Higgins SC, Mills KH (2010) TLR, NLR agonists, and other immune modulators as infectious disease vaccine adjuvants. Curr Infect Dis Rep 12(1):4–12
49. Gherardi MM, Ramirez JC, Esteban M (2001) Towards a new generation of vaccines: the cytokine IL-12 as an adjuvant to enhance cellular immune responses to pathogens during prime-booster vaccination regimens. Histol Histopathol 16(2):655–667
50. Yoon HA et al (2006) Cytokine GM-CSF genetic adjuvant facilitates prophylactic DNA vaccine against pseudorabies virus through enhanced immune responses. Microbiol Immunol 50(2):83–92
51. Portielje JE et al (2003) IL-12: a promising adjuvant for cancer vaccination. Cancer Immunol Immunother 52(3):133–144
52. Metzger DW (2009) IL-12 as an adjuvant for the enhancement of protective humoral immunity. Expert Rev Vaccines 8(5):515–518
53. Wright AK et al (2011) rhIL-12 as adjuvant augments lung cell cytokine responses to pneumococcal whole cell antigen. Immunobiology 216(10):1143–1147
54. Palma C et al (2008) The LTK63 adjuvant improves protection conferred by Ag85B DNA-protein prime-boosting vaccination against Mycobacterium tuberculosis infection by dampening IFN-gamma response. Vaccine 26(33):4237–4243
55. McSorley SJ et al (2002) Bacterial flagellin is an effective adjuvant for CD4+ T cells in vivo. J Immunol 169(7):3914–3919
56. Gupta S et al (2011) EBV LMP1, a viral mimic of CD40, activates dendritic cells and functions as a molecular adjuvant when incorporated into an HIV vaccine. J Leukoc Biol 90(2):389–398
57. Rey-Ladino J et al (2011) Natural products and the search for novel vaccine adjuvants. Vaccine 29(38):6464–6471
58. Ragupathi G et al (2011) Natural and synthetic saponin adjuvant QS-21 for vaccines against cancer. Expert Rev Vaccines 10(4):463–470
59. Kensil CR, Kammer R (1998) QS-21: a water-soluble triterpene glycoside adjuvant. Expert Opin Investig Drugs 7(9):1475–1482
60. Liu G et al (2002) QS-21 structure/function studies: effect of acylation on adjuvant activity. Vaccine 20(21–22):2808–2815
61. Evans TG et al (2001) QS-21 promotes an adjuvant effect allowing for reduced antigen dose during HIV-1 envelope subunit immunization in humans. Vaccine 19(15–16):2080–2091
62. Ogawa C, Liu YJ, Kobayashi KS (2011) Muramyl dipeptide and its derivatives: peptide adjuvant in immunological disorders and cancer therapy. Curr Bioact Compd 7(3):180–197
63. Aucouturier J et al (2002) Montanide ISA 720 and 51: a new generation of water in oil emulsions as adjuvants for human vaccines. Expert Rev Vaccines 1(1):111–118
64. Enoksson M et al (2011) Human cord blood-derived mast cells are activated by the Nod1 agonist M-TriDAP to release pro-inflammatory cytokines and chemokines. J Innate Immun 3 (2):142–149
65. Mata-Haro V et al (2007) The vaccine adjuvant monophosphoryl lipid A as a TRIF-biased agonist of TLR4. Science 316(5831):1628–1632
66. Cluff CW (2010) Monophosphoryl lipid A (MPL) as an adjuvant for anti-cancer vaccines: clinical results. Adv Exp Med Biol 667:111–123
67. Schromm AB et al (2007) Physicochemical and biological analysis of synthetic bacterial lipopeptides: validity of the concept of endotoxic conformation. J Biol Chem 282 (15):11030–11037

68. Coler RN et al (2010) A synthetic adjuvant to enhance and expand immune responses to influenza vaccines. PLoS One 5(10):e13677
69. Raman VS et al (2010) Applying TLR synergy in immunotherapy: implications in cutaneous leishmaniasis. J Immunol 185(3):1701–1710
70. Buwitt-Beckmann U et al (2005) Toll-like receptor 6-independent signaling by diacylated lipopeptides. Eur J Immunol 35(1):282–289
71. Allison AC (1999) Squalene and squalane emulsions as adjuvants. Methods 19(1):87–93
72. Kalvodova L (2010) Squalene-based oil-in-water emulsion adjuvants perturb metabolism of neutral lipids and enhance lipid droplet formation. Biochem Biophys Res Commun 393 (3):350–355
73. Brito LA et al (2011) An alternative renewable source of squalene for use in emulsion adjuvants. Vaccine 29(37):6262–6268
74. Kensil CR et al (1998) QS-21 and QS-7: purified saponin adjuvants. Dev Biol Stand 92:41–47
75. Kensil CR, Wu JY, Soltysik S (1995) Structural and immunological characterization of the vaccine adjuvant QS-21. Pharm Biotechnol 6:525–541
76. Chapman PB et al (2000) Induction of antibodies against GM2 ganglioside by immunizing melanoma patients using GM2-keyhole limpet hemocyanin + QS21 vaccine: a dose–response study. Clin Cancer Res 6(3):874–879
77. Moreno CA et al (1999) Preclinical evaluation of a synthetic Plasmodium falciparum MAP malaria vaccine in Aotus monkeys and mice. Vaccine 18(1–2):89–99
78. Hancock GE et al (1995) Formulation of the purified fusion protein of respiratory syncytial virus with the saponin QS-21 induces protective immune responses in Balb/c mice that are similar to those generated by experimental infection. Vaccine 13(4):391–400
79. Oliveira-Freitas E et al (2006) Acylated and deacylated saponins of Quillaja saponaria mixture as adjuvants for the FML-vaccine against visceral leishmaniasis. Vaccine 24 (18):3909–3920
80. Soltysik S et al (1995) Structure/function studies of QS-21 adjuvant: assessment of triterpene aldehyde and glucuronic acid roles in adjuvant function. Vaccine 13(15):1403–1410
81. Yan W et al (2010) Bryostatin-I: a dendritic cell stimulator for chemokines induction and a promising adjuvant for a peptide based cancer vaccine. Cytokine 52(3):238–244
82. Clamp A, Jayson GC (2002) The clinical development of the bryostatins. Anticancer Drugs 13(7):673–683
83. Pettit GR et al (1991) Isolation and structure of the cell growth inhibitory constituents from the western Pacific marine sponge Axinella sp. J Med Chem 34(11):3339–3340
84. Do Y et al (2004) Bryostatin-1 enhances the maturation and antigen-presenting ability of murine and human dendritic cells. Cancer Res 64(18):6756–6765
85. Li H et al (2006) IFN-gamma and T-bet expression in human dendritic cells from normal donors and cancer patients is controlled through mechanisms involving ERK-1/2-dependent and IL-12-independent pathways. J Immunol 177(6):3554–3563
86. Yan H, Chen W (2010) 3′,5′-Cyclic diguanylic acid: a small nucleotide that makes big impacts. Chem Soc Rev 39(8):2914–2924
87. Chen W, Kuolee R, Yan H (2010) The potential of 3′,5′-cyclic diguanylic acid (c-di-GMP) as an effective vaccine adjuvant. Vaccine 28(18):3080–3085
88. Ebensen T et al (2011) Bis-(3′,5′)-cyclic dimeric adenosine monophosphate: strong Th1/Th2/Th17 promoting mucosal adjuvant. Vaccine 29(32):5210–5220
89. Madhun AS et al (2011) Intranasal c-di-GMP-adjuvanted plant-derived H5 influenza vaccine induces multifunctional Th1 CD4+ cells and strong mucosal and systemic antibody responses in mice. Vaccine 29(31):4973–4982
90. Bode C et al (2011) CpG DNA as a vaccine adjuvant. Expert Rev Vaccines 10(4):499–511
91. Klinman DM et al (2009) CpG oligonucleotides as adjuvants for vaccines targeting infectious diseases. Adv Drug Deliv Rev 61(3):248–255
92. Klinman D et al (2008) Synthetic oligonucleotides as modulators of inflammation. J Leukoc Biol 84(4):958–964
93. Ballas ZK et al (2001) Divergent therapeutic and immunologic effects of oligodeoxynucleotides with distinct CpG motifs. J Immunol 167(9):4878–4886

94. Stacey KJ, Blackwell JM (1999) Immunostimulatory DNA as an adjuvant in vaccination against Leishmania major. Infect Immun 67(8):3719–3726
95. Cui Z, Qiu F (2006) Synthetic double-stranded RNA poly(I:C) as a potent peptide vaccine adjuvant: therapeutic activity against human cervical cancer in a rodent model. Cancer Immunol Immunother 55(10):1267–1279
96. Luganini A et al (2008) Phosphorothioate-modified oligodeoxynucleotides inhibit human cytomegalovirus replication by blocking virus entry. Antimicrob Agents Chemother 52 (3):1111–1120
97. Sasaki S et al (1998) Adjuvant effect of Ubenimex on a DNA vaccine for HIV-1. Clin Exp Immunol 111(1):30–35
98. Peng HJ et al (2004) Comparison of different adjuvants of protein and DNA vaccination for the prophylaxis of IgE antibody formation. Vaccine 22(5–6):755–761
99. Huang CF et al (2012) Induction of specific Th1 responses and suppression of IgE antibody formation by vaccination with plasmid DNA encoding Cyn d 1. Int Arch Allergy Immunol 158(2):142–150
100. Lu H et al (2008) Enhancing effects of the chemical adjuvant levamisole on the DNA vaccine pVIR-P12A-IL18-3C. Microbiol Immunol 52(9):440–446
101. Alavian SM, Tabatabaei SV (2010) Effects of oral levamisole as an adjuvant to hepatitis B vaccine in adults with end-stage renal disease: a meta-analysis of controlled clinical trials. Clin Ther 32(1):1–10
102. Smahel M et al (2011) Systemic administration of CpG oligodeoxynucleotide and levamisole as adjuvants for gene-gun-delivered antitumor DNA vaccines. Clin Dev Immunol 2011:176759
103. Wang B et al (1993) Gene inoculation generates immune responses against human immunodeficiency virus type 1. Proc Natl Acad Sci U S A 90(9):4156–4160
104. Jin H et al (2004) Effect of chemical adjuvants on DNA vaccination. Vaccine 22 (21–22):2925–2935
105. McLachlan JB et al (2008) Mast cell activators: a new class of highly effective vaccine adjuvants. Nat Med 14(5):536–541
106. Stevenson HC et al (1991) Levamisole—known effects on the immune-system, clinical-results, and future applications to the treatment of cancer. J Clin Oncol 9(11):2052–2066
107. Suda H et al (1976) Inhibition of aminopeptidase-B and leucine aminopeptidase by bestatin and its stereoisomer. Arch Biochem Biophys 177(1):196–200
108. Umezawa H et al (1976) Bestatin, an inhibitor of aminopeptidase-B, produced by actinomycetes. J Antibiot 29(1):97–99
109. Brown TCK (2012) History of pediatric regional anesthesia. Pediatr Anaesth 22(1):3–9
110. Miller RL et al (1999) Treatment of primary herpes simplex virus infection in guinea pigs by imiquimod. Antiviral Res 44(1):31–42
111. Sauder DN (2000) Immunomodulatory and pharmacologic properties of imiquimod. J Am Acad Dermatol 43(1):S6–S11
112. Suzuki H et al (2000) Imiquimod, a topical immune response modifier, induces migration of Langerhans cells. J Invest Dermatol 114(1):135–141
113. Tomai MA et al (2007) Resiquimod and other immune response modifiers as vaccine adjuvants. Expert Rev Vaccines 6(5):835–847
114. Ma F, Zhang J, Zhang C (2010) The TLR7 agonists imiquimod and gardiquimod improve DC-based immunotherapy for melanoma in mice. Cell Mol Immunol 7(5):381–388
115. Dzopalic T et al (2010) Loxoribine, a selective Toll-like receptor 7 agonist, induces maturation of human monocyte-derived dendritic cells and stimulates their Th-1- and Th-17-polarizing capability. Int Immunopharmacol 10(11):1428–1433
116. Sharma BS et al (1991) Potentiation of the efficacy of murine L1210 leukemia vaccine by a novel immunostimulator 7-thia-8-oxoguanosine: increased survival after immunization with vaccine plus 7-thia-8-oxoguanosine. Cancer Immunol Immunother 33(2):109–114
117. McInnes C (2007) Virtual screening strategies in drug discovery. Curr Opin Chem Biol 11 (5):494–502

118. Ripphausen P et al (2010) Quo vadis, virtual screening? A comprehensive survey of prospective applications. J Med Chem 53(24):8461–8467
119. Bajorath J (2010) Computational studies, virtual screening, and theoretical molecular models. J Med Chem 53(1):1–2
120. Hattotuwagama CK, Davies MN, Flower DR (2006) Receptor-ligand binding sites and virtual screening. Curr Med Chem 13(11):1283–1304
121. Irwin JJ, Shoichet BK (2005) ZINC–a free database of commercially available compounds for virtual screening. J Chem Inf Model 45(1):177–182
122. Flower DR (1998) DISSIM: a program for the analysis of chemical diversity. J Mol Graph Model 16(4–6):239–253, 264
123. Davis AM et al (2005) Components of successful lead generation. Curr Top Med Chem 5 (4):421–439
124. Lagorce D et al (2011) The FAF-Drugs2 server: a multistep engine to prepare electronic chemical compound collections. Bioinformatics 27(14):2018–2020
125. Lagorce D et al (2008) FAF-Drugs2: free ADME/tox filtering tool to assist drug discovery and chemical biology projects. BMC Bioinformatics 9:396
126. Miteva MA et al (2006) FAF-drugs: free ADME/tox filtering of compound collections. Nucleic Acids Res 34(Web Server issue):W738–W744
127. Khan MT, Sylte I (2007) Predictive QSAR modeling for the successful predictions of the ADMET properties of candidate drug molecules. Curr Drug Discov Technol 4(3):141–149
128. Khan MT (2010) Predictions of the ADMET properties of candidate drug molecules utilizing different QSAR/QSPR modelling approaches. Curr Drug Metab 11(4):285–295
129. Moroy G et al (2012) Toward in silico structure-based ADMET prediction in drug discovery. Drug Discov Today 17(1–2):44–55
130. Charoenvit Y et al (2004) CEL-1000—a peptide with adjuvant activity for Th1 immune responses. Vaccine 22(19):2368–2373
131. Luster AD (1998) Chemokines—chemotactic cytokines that mediate inflammation. N Engl J Med 338(7):436–445
132. Rees S, Morrow D, Kenakin T (2002) GPCR drug discovery through the exploitation of allosteric drug binding sites. Receptors Channels 8(5–6):261–268
133. Gether U et al (2002) Structural basis for activation of G-protein-coupled receptors. Pharmacol Toxicol 91(6):304–312
134. Feng Y et al (1996) HIV-1 entry cofactor: functional cDNA cloning of a seven-transmembrane, G protein-coupled receptor. Science 272(5263):872–877
135. Bayry J et al (2008) In silico identified CCR4 antagonists target regulatory T cells and exert adjuvant activity in vaccination. Proc Natl Acad Sci U S A 105(29):10221–10226
136. Davies MN et al (2009) Toward the discovery of vaccine adjuvants: coupling in silico screening and in vitro analysis of antagonist binding to human and mouse CCR4 receptors. PLoS One 4(11):e8084
137. Pere H et al (2011) A CCR4 antagonist combined with vaccines induces antigen-specific CD8 + T cells and tumor immunity against self antigens. Blood 118(18):4853–4862
138. Schijns VE, Tangeras A (2005) Vaccine adjuvant technology: from theoretical mechanisms to practical approaches. Dev Biol (Basel) 121:127–134
139. Degen WG, Jansen T, Schijns VE (2003) Vaccine adjuvant technology: from mechanistic concepts to practical applications. Expert Rev Vaccines 2(2):327–335
140. Schijns VE (2003) Mechanisms of vaccine adjuvant activity: initiation and regulation of immune responses by vaccine adjuvants. Vaccine 21(9–10):829–831
141. Schijns VE (2000) Immunological concepts of vaccine adjuvant activity. Curr Opin Immunol 12(4):456–463
142. Garcon N, Van Mechelen M (2011) Recent clinical experience with vaccines using MPL- and QS-21-containing adjuvant systems. Expert Rev Vaccines 10(4):471–486
143. Schellack C et al (2006) IC31, a novel adjuvant signaling via TLR9, induces potent cellular and humoral immune responses. Vaccine 24(26):5461–5472

Chapter 10
Designing Liposomes as Vaccine Adjuvants

Malou Henriksen-Lacey and Yvonne Perrie

Abstract The most important perquisite in modern-day prophylactic vaccine development is the production of safe, nonreverting vaccines. To do this there has been a distinct move towards peptide or protein antigen-based vaccines, which are incapable of becoming virulent or mutating. However, whilst such vaccines appear desirable on paper, they are generally poorly immunogenic. Consequently, there has been intense development in the field of adjuvants and delivery systems, which are capable of fulfilling two important functions: firstly that antigen is delivered to an immunologically relevant cell, and secondly that antigen is recognised as being immunogenic and subsequently processed.

Whilst many adjuvants are successful at ticking one of these parameters, few can act as the combined immunostimulatory delivery systems. Liposomes are among some of the successful formulations, which have been pursued as clinically relevant adjuvants (equally there are many liposome formulations which have been ignored due to their inability to be both delivery vehicle and immunostimulatory). However, in this chapter we will focus on the successful design of adjuvantal liposomes, which are of interest to vaccine developers focusing on life-threatening diseases of both the developing and developed world. Particular emphasis will be given to structural considerations and how varying these have an effect on the observed immunological outcome, measured in either in vitro, in vivo or ex vivo studies.

10.1 Introduction—Basics in Liposome Geometry

Liposomes are composed of lipid monomers, which align in an energy-dependent process to form bilayered vesicles. The liposomes may be single or multilamellar in structure, and form part of a population that can be considered homo- or

Y. Perrie (✉)
School of Life and Health Sciences, Aston University, Birmingham, UK
e-mail: y.perrie@aston.ac.uk

D.R. Flower and Y. Perrie (eds.), *Immunomic Discovery of Adjuvants and Candidate Subunit Vaccines*, Immunomics Reviews: 5, DOI 10.1007/978-1-4614-5070-2_10,

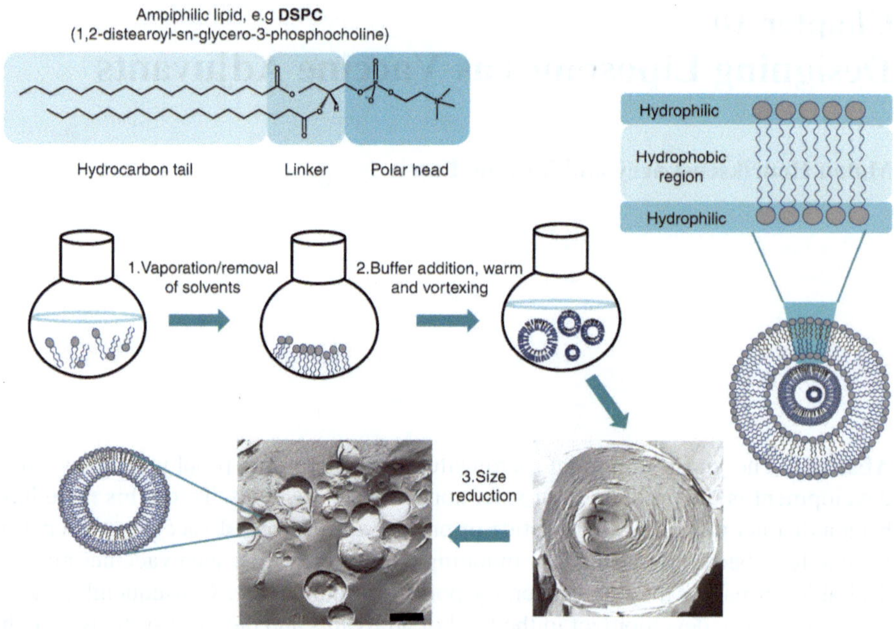

Fig. 10.1 Outline of lipid structure and the liposome formation process

heterogeneous based on the size distribution of the vesicles (Fig. 10.1). Whilst heat is often required for the lipid monomers to rearrange into a liposomal bilayer, for some liposome compositions it is not a necessity. The geometry of liposomes is therefore principally determined by their lipid, or other, constituents although post-formulation techniques can be used to promote the formation of a more "desirable" physical characteristic. Traditional examples include sonication, whereby disruptive energy causes large vesicles to rearrange into smaller ones, and size-extrusion, in which vesicles are forced through defined pore sizes. Whilst these techniques are principally used as size-reduction techniques, they can also be used as methods to promote or improve antigen and liposome association [27]. When no such technique is applied, antigen and liposome association will be dependent on electrostatic interactions. The overall charge of a peptide or protein will be dependent on its amino acids and will change according to the pH of the solution it is suspended in. Know as the pI (or isoelectric point), this is an important factor to consider when designing liposomes as adjuvants for specific disease antigens.

As shown in Fig. 10.1, lipids are composed of three sections (tail, linker and head) and due to the hydrophobic and hydrophilic natures of the tail and head, respectively, the water-loving head group is directed outwards. Liposome charge is dependent on the presence of anions or cations found on the head group of the lipid monomers. Consequently, liposomes and antigens which express opposite ionic charges will be able to interact electrostatically. It is important to remember that these interactions are not permanent and that no covalent bond is formed—this feature allows a single liposome formulation to be designed to associate with numerous antigens, assuming that their electrostatic charges are compatible.

10.1.1 Variations on a Theme

Liposomes are not the only vesicular adjuvants which are able to interact with peptide/protein antigens. Structures such as nanoparticles, microspheres, virosomes, and bilosomes have all been developed as antigen delivery systems with the ability to either encapsulate or surface-associate with antigen. There is no "best adjuvant" to choose from, rather some have properties which are more suitable for certain applications. For example, bilosomes which contain bile salts are being developed as vaccines suited to oral administration as the inclusion of bile salts in the formulation prevents natural stomach digestive enzymes from disrupting the bilayered membrane, hence improving formulation stability. Likewise, as the name suggests, virosomes are highly efficient at delivering viral antigens and have been successfully licenced as adjuvants in vaccines against Hepatitis A and influenza [9].

10.2 Liposomes as Antigen Delivery Systems

Whilst vaccines aim to stimulate the adaptive immune system, which leads to memory formation and hence the ability to respond quickly and effectively to future pathogenic exposure, by including adjuvants which are immunomodulatory to the innate immune system, the chances of resulting in successful immunisation are heightened (Fig. 10.2). In this sense, one of the stand-out points relating to liposomes is their versatile structure which allows inclusion of various lipophilic components such as bacterial derived glycolipids in the bilayered membrane, or surface-bound nucleotide-based molecules, both of which are known to stimulate the immune system. In particular, there has been much interest over the past 10 years in toll-like receptors (TLRs) and their natural and synthetic agonists, many of which can be incorporated into liposome design with the aim to produce immunostimulatory antigen delivery systems.

10.2.1 Immunomodulation

Current adjuvant design is focusing on pathogen mimicry by including synthetic ligands to cellular receptors, known to stimulate the innate responses. An example of this is the AS04 adjuvant (GlaxoSmithKline (GSK) Biologicals, Belgium) which includes synthetic monophosphoryl lipid A (MPL), a component of bacterial cell

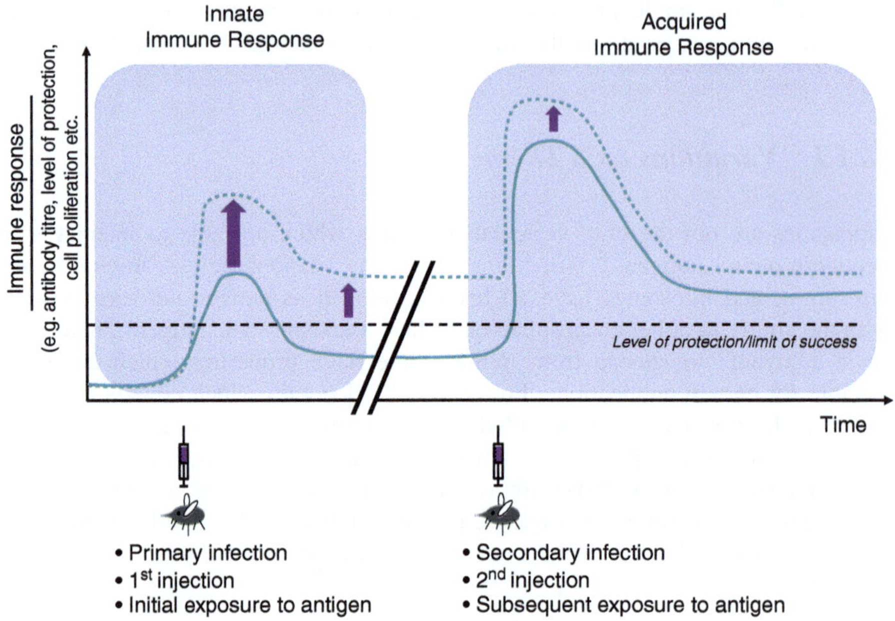

Fig. 10.2 Schematic depicting how adjuvants aim to raise the immune response in both the innate and acquired responses

walls. MPL is a ligand for TLR 4 and is discussed in more detail below. Other examples of pathogen mimicry in adjuvant formulations, although yet to be licensed, include synthetic nucleic acids, lipopeptides and lipopolysaccharide (LPS). Another method to stimulate the innate immune system is structurally, either by causing non-specific tissue damage, or due to lengthening the retention of the vaccine at the injection site. Aluminium hydroxide and other mineral salts grouped in the "Alum" category act by a combination of these mechanisms; both increased antigen retention and tissue damage is observed, the latter resulting in production of endogenous inflammatory mediators and subsequent activation of intracellular signalling cascades thereby triggering a strong immune response.

10.2.2 Formulating Liposomes to Look Like Pathogens

Liposomes bear a relationship to Gram negative bacteria in that they both share a similar [phosho] lipid bilayer. This is not the case for Gram positive bacteria whose cell wall is made of peptidoglycan rather than lipids and proteins, or for viruses which are not cellular organisms. Regardless, liposomes can be designed to mimic bacteria by encapsulation of nucleic acids or addition of amphiphilic molecules such as LPS, which are also present in Gram negative bacterial cell walls. Furthermore, liposome size correlates with that of numerous pathogens (Fig. 10.3). This is

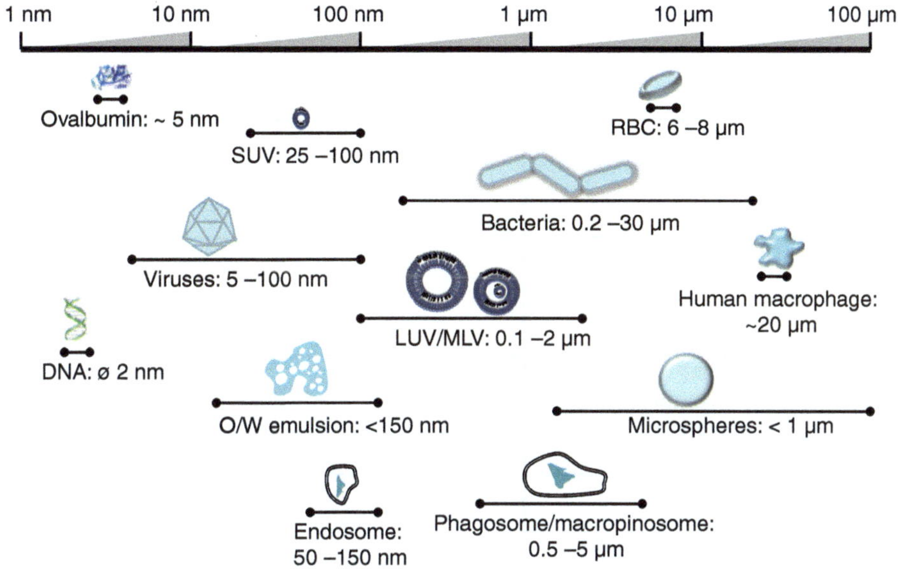

Fig. 10.3 Size comparisons of biologically relevant species with liposomes and other adjuvant systems

important because it also means that uptake of liposomes by phagocytic cells will ideally follow the same route as the pathogen against which you are vaccinating. Therefore, with careful design, liposomes can be engineered to physically look similar to a pathogen but without the pathogenic effects.

With regards to the non-structural "mechanisms" by which liposomes act, this depends on additional and generally non-lipid components. Some liposome-forming cationic lipids have been shown to be inherently immunogenic by binding to specific cellular receptors. An example is the lipid DiC14-amidine, which has been shown to activate the TLR4 pathway through binding to TLR4 or its associated molecules CD14, MD-2, and LBP [46]. DiC14-amidine and another cationic lipid DOTAP (Fig. 10.4) have also both been suggested as capable of recognising a G-protein-coupled receptor (GPCR) with activation of intracellular pathways such as MAPK, resulting in the expression of chemokines and co-stimulatory molecules [31]. However, DiC14-amidine and DOTAP share little structural similarity (Fig. 10.4), which therefore suggests involvement of either different GPCRs or additional helper molecules, such as seen with the relationship between CD14, MD-2, TRL4 and LBP.

10.2.3 PAMPS, DAMPS and MAMPS

The lipophilic nature of the liposome membrane promotes the inclusion of bacterial-modelled glycolipids such as MPL and TDB, both of which readily insert

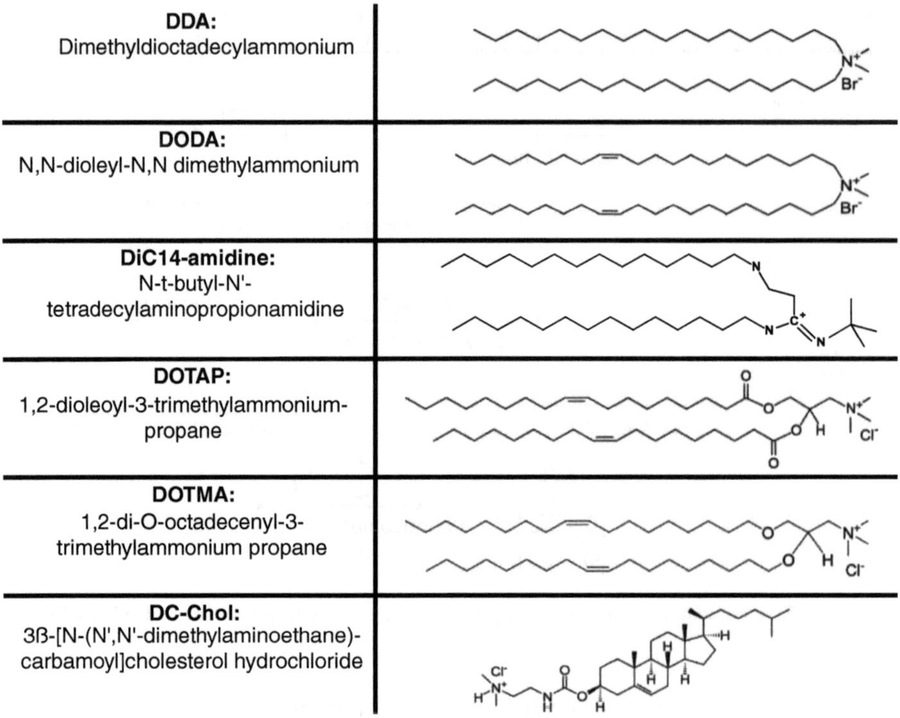

Fig. 10.4 Commonly used cationic lipids of interest in adjuvant formulation

into the bilayer and are able to bind to host pattern recognition receptors (PRRs). PRRs, which can be soluble or membrane bound, are receptors which become activated by molecules derived from either pathogens (known as pathogen-associated molecular patterns; PAMPS), cellular damage (damage-associated molecular patterns; DAMPS), or the more recently coined term MAMPS, which refers to microbe-associated molecular patterns. Whilst these subgroups sound complex, they are effectively specific terms given to molecules which are immunostimulatory and [normally] derive from an exogenous organism which can induce harm to the host. The exceptions are DAMPS, which include endogenous substances, or alarmins, which normally derive from host cells upon damage. Regardless, inclusion of such substances in adjuvant formulations, thereby designating them as "second generation" formulations [40], can improve their immunostimulatory abilities in a synergistic manner. Table 10.1 lists some PAMP-containing liposomal formulations and their respective PRRs which are currently in development. PRRs can also be divided into further subgroups. The fairly recent discovery that the inflammasome, an intracellular complex containing a PRR, is activated by Alum has reawakened interest in this group of receptors known more specifically as nucleotide-binding domain and leucine-rich repeat-containing family (NLR). These receptors and their ligands are well-known

Table 10.1 PAMP containing liposomal formulations in development

Formulation (principle lipid)	PAMP	PRR	Immune response (IR)	References
Infectious disease vaccines				
CAF01 (DDA)	TDB	Mincle	CD4 Th1/Th17 response, IgG2 humoral IR	[20] [15]
CAF05 (DDA)	TDB PolyI:C	Mincle TLR3	Strong Ag-specific CD8 T cell response with CD4, good cross-priming	[39]
CAF09 (DDA)	MMG	Non-TLR, Mincle?	CMI with mixed Th1/Th17 profile, humoral IR (IgG1, IgG2), strong cross-priming	[8] [3] [39]
CAF06 (DDA)	TDB MPL	Mincle TLR4	CD8 T cell with humoral antibody response	[39]
AS01 (proprietary formulation)	MPL	TLR4	Strong malaria antigen humoral IR with Th1 CD4 response	[17]
Cancer vaccines				
Mannosylated liposomes with ErbB2/HER2 peptide	Pam_3CAG Pam_2CAG + Pam_2CGD	TLR1/2 TLR2/6	Anti-tumour IR with < 100 % survival in primary and recall inoculations, indicative of CTL IR.	[47]
Stimuvax[a]	MPL	TLR4	Ag-specific CTL and Th1 responses	[2], www.oncothyreon.com
ONT-10[b]	PET-Lipid A	TLR4	Ag-specific CTL (90 % reduction in tumour growth) and Th1 (IgG2b, IFN-g) responses	[42]
MLB (DOTAP, DOPE)	MPL	TLR4	Inhibition of tumour metastasis High levels of IFN-γ (Th1) and IgG (humoral)	[53]

CTL cytotoxic T cell; *DDA* dimethyldioctadecylammonium bromide; *DOPE* dioleoyl phosphatidylethanolamine; *DOTAP* 1,2-dioleoyl-3-trimethylammonium-propane; *IR* immune response; *MMG* monomycoloyl glycerol; *MPL* monophosphoryl lipid A; *PET-lipid A* penta erythritol lipid A; *TDB* Trehalose 6′6-dibehenate; *TLR* Toll-like receptor

Formulation currently in Phase I trials for TB with Ag85B-ESAT-6

[a]Formulation currently in two Phase II trials for "non-small-cell" lung cancer

[a]propriety adjuvant of Oncothyreon (http://www.oncothyreon.com) currently in development as a therapeutic cancer vaccine

components in inflammation and have been linked to a wide range of autoimmune and autoinflammatory diseases [28]. Recently we and other groups detected significant amounts of the characteristic inflammasome cytokine IL-1β in the tissue of mice injected with particulate adjuvants including TDB-containing cationic liposomes and microparticles [20, 43]. Splenocytes derived from mice immunized with these formulations showed enhanced levels of IL-6 (in the case of microparticles) and IFN-γ (in the case of liposomes). Both cytokines are also pro-inflammatory and are often used as markers of inflammation or cellular activation. Whilst there are reports that non-PAMP-like substances such as HMBP can synergize with microparticles to result in IL-1β production [43], the generally accepted dogma is that for successful IL-1β production, activation of NF-κB must occur (for example due to TLR signalling), which stimulates transcription of pro-IL-1β [28]. This NF-κB link may explain the strong IL-1β production noted upon immunisation of mice with cationic liposomes containing TDB. TDB is a ligand for the plasma membrane receptor Mincle, which is assumed to signal intracellulary via the NF-κB complex. By combining both inflammatory (cationic lipid) and PRR stimulating (TDB) components in the same adjuvant formulation, a two-pronged attack is mounted. Further discussions relating to PAMPS and PRRs can be found in two in depth reviews on the subject [22, 26].

10.3 Altering In Vivo Properties Through Careful Design

There is a vast choice of lipids available for liposome production. Choices include natural or synthetic, unsaturated or saturated, long or short chain, cationic or anionic, single or double chain, in addition to whether a single lipid or a combination of lipids can or will be used. Furthermore, aspects such as the ratio of combined lipids will also have a significant effect on the characteristics of the formulation. Choosing such properties is complicated and often relies on a "trial and error" method, although the aim of many groups working with liposomes as vaccines is to determine which factors lead to the most successful formulations with regards to stability and immunogenicity.

10.3.1 Charged Vesicles

The seminal work conducted by Gall and colleagues in the 1960s lead to the discovery that a range of cationic lipids were capable of disrupting cell monolayers, causing haemolysis of sheep red blood cells and damage to tissue at the injection site [16]. In retrospect, this is probably not unusual when non-GMP grade and probably impure lipids are used. However, it did provide vital information regarding the physical properties of active lipids; a long ($>$ 12) carbon chain length and basicity are both required. In particular, lipids with a quaternary ammonium head group (see Fig. 10.4) showed particularly high levels of activity. Certainly cationic liposomes are not ideal if avoidance of the immune system is required. Their positive surface charge results in surface association with host proteins which are predominantly anionic in nature. Therefore aggregation of vesicles is commonly observed. Whilst this is a problem for formulations administered via an intravenous route whereby embolism may occur, administered via routes such as subcutaneous, intramuscular or intradermal, this does not pose such a problem. However, the aggregation of such cationic vesicles is also suggested to be part of their success as vaccine adjuvants as they result in a depot-effect whereby liposome and consequently antigen are retained in the tissue for an extended period of time.

10.3.2 Fusogenic Lipids

In addition to surface active lipids, helper lipids are frequently included in liposome formulations, either to cause vesicle formation (as not all lipids will spontaneously produce vesicles), as a "filler out" lipid, or to influence physical parameters such as liposome clearance rates or intracellular liposome stability. One such lipid is DOPE, which when exposed to a low pH environment such as found in endosomes, the lipid and therefore the liposomal bilayer break down with the subsequent release of liposomal-entrapped molecules. This characteristic is of special interest in the development of liposomal nucleic acid delivery systems whereby nuclear delivery of the genetic material is necessary for transfection to occur. Commercial products such as TransFast™ (Promega), Metafectene™ (Biontex Laboratories GmbH; Munich, Germany), ESCORT™ (Sigma, St. Louis, USA) and PerFectin™ (Genlantis, San Diego, USA) all use DOPE as a liposome–endosome fusion mediator.

10.3.3 Membrane Fluidity

Whilst fusogenic liposomes take advantage of changes in the pH, the main phase transition temperature (T_m) of a lipid will determine the fluidity of a liposomal membrane at a given temperature (Fig. 10.5). The location and degree of hydrocarbon chain saturation, in addition to hydrocarbon chain length, all affect the strength of the van der Waals forces, which hold adjacent chains together [41]. Consequently, in the in vivo environment where the temperature is 37°C, liposomes exhibiting a $T_m > 37°C$ will remain in a rigid ordered structure, however those with a $T_m < 37°C$ will become fluid and disorganized. The T_m of lipid bilayers can be calculated with the use of differential scanning calorimetry (DSC) or differential thermal analysis (DTA), both of which detect heat changes between a reference and the sample during a programmed heating or cooling programme. These techniques (also see Table 10.2) are invaluable for the detection of small structural transitions that occur in liposomal systems.

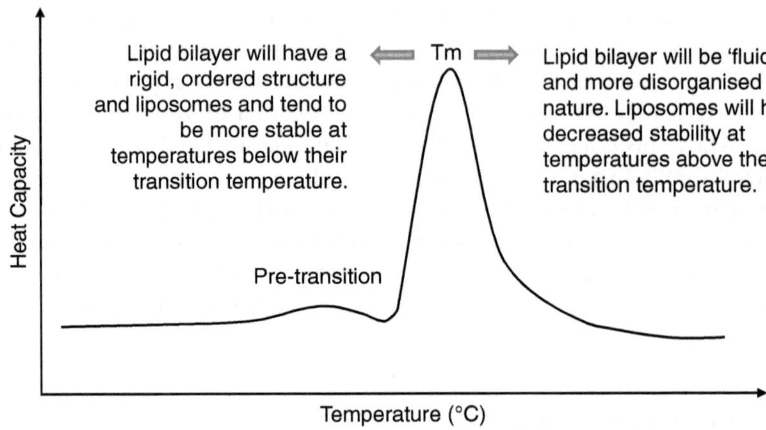

Fig. 10.5 DSC schematic showing the pretransition and main phase transition (Tm) of a lipid

The effect of changing either membrane fluidity or fusogenic ability is mainly investigated with regards to biodistribution, pharmacokinetics and stability, although these parameters also have an effect on the adjuvant activity. Cationic liposomes with a fluid bilayer have a shortened depot-effect compared to rigid-bilayered analogues (Christensen et al., paper in preparation). Furthermore, these "fluid liposomes" are poorer at inducing IFN-γ and IL-17 release, both cytokines being characteristic of a T_H1 biased immune response. Interestingly, the same study also showed an equal ability of the rigid and fluid liposomes to present antigen to T cells and cause proliferation. Therefore, whilst bilayer fluidity plays a role in the formation of memory responses, this does not appear to be due to their antigen presenting abilities.

10.3.4 Good or Bad Cholesterol?

Inclusion of cholesterol in liposomal formulations is commonly implemented to improve liposome stability although paradoxically, by inserting in the lipid bilayer, it actually disrupts the lipid monomer arrangement [32]. The immunomodulatory effect of cholesterol insertion is unclear; whilst some studies have shown improvements in the immune response [5, 49], others have noted reduced responses [35]. The contrasting results support the notion that cholesterol inclusion is one of many factors which affect the adjuvant properties of liposomes through structural changes.

Table 10.2 Liposome characterisation techniques

Technique	Detection of:	Detection range	Co-factors	Advantages	Disadvantages
DLS (also known as PCS, QELS)	Size of suspended particles, moving via Brownian motion, via the Stokes-Einstein equation	1–6 μm (typically < 1 μm though)	Temperature, viscosity, ionic strength of solution, particle shape and surface topography	Quick, ease to use, accessible with small bench top machines available, can detect molecular weight	Gives the hydrodynamic radius, only suitable for spherical particles
DSC	Heat requirement of lipid bilayers when undergoing phase transitions, cooperative unit,	−180–+2,400 °C (dependent on machine)	Sample purity	Small sample volume, sensitivity, large quantity of thermo-physical data obtained	Expensive, requires trained users, instrumentation artefacts, high sample concentration needed
Zeta potential (usually determined via LDV or PALS)	Indirect measure of the surface charge of a particle at an invisible boundary (the Stern layer) via application of a current to the dispersion	~ −200–+200 mV	Temperature, ionic strength of solution	Machines often combined with DLS, rapid, ease or use, solvent compatible,	Sample volume, contamination of probe between samples
Turbidity	Level of aggregation of a particle in suspension	Arbitary unit—dependent on a control	Particle size, concentration, temperature, viscosity	Low cost, rapid, ease of use, no sample loss	Poor precision, difficult to compare across formulations
Optical Microscopy	Size and morphology of particles in suspension	< 200 nm	Mounting method, sample purity	Low cost, rapid, qualitative data	Costain often required, low magnification, not quantitative
SEM[b]	Size and morphology of particles	5 nm–1 cm	Conductivity, state of dryness	Visually qualitative data, different shaped particles can be analysed, great depth of focus, produces 3D image	Expensive, collection of quantitative data is time-consuming and user-dependant, surface stain often required (although not necessary[a]), poor

(continued)

Table 10.2 (continued)

Technique	Detection of:	Detection range	Co-factors	Advantages	Disadvantages
					resolution (compared to TEM)
TEM	Size and morphology of particles in suspension	0.2 nm–~100 μm (dependent on grid size)	Sample thickness, ionic strength of solution or choice of solvent, particle concentration and charge	Visually qualitative data, different shaped particles can be analysed, high resolution, provides structural data	Expensive, collection of quantitative data is time-consuming and user-dependant, surface stain often required (although not necessary)

DLS dynamic light scattering; *DSC* differential scanning calorimetry; *LDV* laser Doppler velocimetry; *PALS* phase analysis light scattering; *SEM* scanning electron microscopy; *TEM* transmission electron microscopy

Technique not available in all machines

[a]For example, no stain is required for environmental SEM

[b]General overview given although variations on the technique are available (e.g., cryo-SEM)

10.4 Considerations Regarding Delivery Method and Site

Liposomes offer significantly more flexibility than other adjuvant systems with regards to their physicochemical characteristics. However do these variables also translate to different administration routes? Infectious diseases infect primarily via the mucosal route and there are a number of in-depth reviews covering this aspect of vaccine delivery [11, 36]. In fact, the liposomal formulation CAF01, which has a long history of inducing strong T_H1 biased immune responses when administered via the intramuscular (i.m) route was recently investigated as a potential mucosal adjuvant given via the intranasal (i.n) administration route for influenza vaccination [14]. Both preliminary in vitro and in vivo studies provided promising results with the immunisation study characterised by high IFN-γ and total IgG antibody levels offering significant improvements on non-adjuvanted influenza vaccination.

10.4.1 Systemic Delivery

Whilst it is recognised that i.m and subcutaneous (s.c) administration are not the most suitable of vaccine delivery routes due to the poor expression of immunocompetent cells at these sites [24], vesicular systems such as liposomes are ideally suited to this route of vaccine delivery as they are aqueous suspensions composed of vesicles, which fit the correct size range for cellular uptake either at the site of injection or the target tissue. A recent study investigating how varying the injection route of three vesicular adjuvant vaccine formulations affects immune responses (measured by IgG1/IgG2 ratios and IFN-γ and IL-4 cytokine production) showed that whilst administration route had little effect on IgG1 responses, the IgG2 response was significantly affected [33]. Intralymphatic injection, albeit an unlikely delivery method in humans, elicited strong T_H1 biased immune responses in mice. I.m and intradermal (i.d) injection of the same formulations resulted in intermediate T_H1 responses, but s.c administration failed to stimulate this arm of the immune system.

10.4.2 Novel Methods of Administration

In terms of targeting immunoprivileged sites via systemic vaccination, the epidermis is the for-runner as it has a high population of Langerhans cells, DCs and a large lymphatic network capable of transporting antigen directly to the lymph nodes [24]. However, injecting vaccines into the epidermis and not the dermis or hypodermis (both of which have a high proportion of fat and connective tissues) is a skilled technique in humans, and even more so in small rodent research models. More advanced administration tactics have therefore evolved with the development of patches and microneedles, which have shown success in both drug and vaccine delivery (reviewed in ref. [10]). One such study involving lipoplexes applied to fabric gauze and left on the skin for a 12-h period has shown promising results with T_H2 immune responses and significantly improved survival rates in a viral challenge study [13]. Patches such as these are already marketed as drug delivery systems (most famously as Nicorette®), however, their disadvantages including the time required for the drug/vaccine to traverse the stratum corneum, in addition to being highly dependent on host compliance, may indeed limit their use as vaccine delivery systems. A method of particular interest at present which can overcome these disadvantages is the microneedle array which is currently being investigated as a delivery method for a wide range of drugs and vaccines (reviewed in ref. [4]).

10.5 Analysing Liposomal Properties

One of the most important stages in the development of suitable vaccine adjuvants is their characterisation. Not only must the detailed composition of the formulation be accounted for and GMP facilities used throughout, but also the stability, pharmacokinetic, biodistribution and immunological outcome be fully analysed. A wide range of techniques are available to analyse such features and are indeed required by the World Health Organisation (WHO) for consideration as suitable formulations for vaccine adjuvants (Table 10.2).

10.5.1 Probing the Pharmacokinetics and Biodistribution of Liposomes

Liposomes can be altered to include a wide variety of tracers such as fluorescent, magnetic or radioactive molecules, which allow qualitative and quantitative measurements to be made regarding their in vitro or in vivo location. Furthermore, the gaseous or liquid component of liposomes allows these vesicles to be used as contrast agents for techniques such as magnetic resonance imaging or ultrasound. These techniques (Table 10.3) are primarily used in small animal models although some are of particular interest for clinical applications. Our own research has focused on the use of radioactive tracers to determine how changes in the liposomal physicochemical properties can alter the pharmacokinetics and biodistribution of such systems. By incorporating trace amounts of radiolabelled lipophilic compounds which have a high radioactivity:molar ratio, it is possible to keep the physicochemical characteristics of the liposomal system unaltered. Furthermore, additional components such as nucleic acids and proteins can be followed by choosing a radiolabel with a different radioactive emission (e.g., alpha/beta/

Table 10.3 Liposomal imaging and detection methods for use in vivo

Technique	Imaging agent	Example:	Pros	Cons
Scintigraphic	Radioisotopes emitting α or β particles or γ-waves	Biodistribution and pharmacokinetics	Traditional approach with wide scope of literature available, sensitive, ability to detect < 3 components simultaneously,	Strict rules and regulations with handling radiochemicals, detection can require processing techniques, cannot be used in real-time
Intravital microscopy	Fluorescence	Real-time imaging of pharmacokinetics and biodistribution	Rapid, high resolution (~1 μm), real time acquisition	Photo-bleaching, limited depth, expensive, emission in the 600–900 nm range required
Ultrasound (contrast agent)	Gas-containing liposomes	Targeted delivery and release of substances	Real time acquisition, location specific release	Expensive, liposome stability
PET	^{18}F, ^{11}C, ^{15}O, ^{64}Cu	Metabolic studies, real-time pharmacokinetics and biodistribution	Can be combined with CT to improve resolution, real-time acquisition	Strict rules and regulations with handling radiochemicals, poor resolution (1–2 mm), expensive
MRI (contrast agent)	Paramagnetic substances (Gd, Mn, ^{99m}Tc, ^{111}In)	Targeted delivery, pharmacokinetics	High soft tissue contrast, qualitative and quantitative information, 3D image, real-time acquisition	Expensive, skilled technique, signal-to-noise ratio

CT computed tomography; *MRI* magnetic resonance imagining; *PET* positron emission tomography

Table 10.4 Factors favouring the use of liposomes as drug delivery systems

Advantages of liposomes as drug delivery systems
Efficient at drug loading, either in the aqueous or lipophilic compartment
Protection of drugs from host enzymes and/or harsh production processes
Overcomes issues with drug solubility
Specific drug targeting resulting in dose sparing and reducing nonspecific toxicity
Increases drug pharmacokinetic profile
Improves intracellular delivery of drugs

gamma). The same dual-labelling strategy can also be implemented with fluorescent molecules which excite and/or emit at different wavelengths. The main advantages of many of the techniques mentioned in Table 10.3 are their non-invasive nature, in addition to the highly sensitive detection and imaging equipment readily available, therefore allowing minute quantities of the tracer molecule to be used.

The size-range of liposomes also makes them suitable for intracellular studies, although this technique may be more advantageous in a fluorescent imaging in vitro system whereby molecular processes can be studied. In combination with the wide range of inhibitory antibodies available, the specific mechanisms of liposome–cell association, uptake, activation and processing can be determined and visualised in real-time.

10.6 Clinically Relevant Liposomal Vaccines

Liposomes are successful drug delivery systems with a number of formulations being approved for clinical use (see Table 10.4 for the advantages of using liposomes for drug delivery). Examples include AmBiosome® (Astellas Pharma, Canada), Caelyx® (Scheering-Plough, Belgium) and DaunoXome® (Diatos, France). In contrast, although licensed virosomal vaccine systems exist (Epaxal® and Inflexal® V (Crucell)), there are no liposomal adjuvants or vaccines licensed for human use. Table 10.5 describes the numerous liposomal formulations currently in vaccine pre-clinical testing. These formulations include peptide, protein and nucleic acid deliverables, focused on a range of diseases including parasitic, bacterial and viral infections.

However, the question of why there are still no licensed liposomal formulations should be addressed. One issue is the diverse nature of the systems, whereby changing the ratio of two or more lipids can lead to significantly different pharmacokinetic properties, for example. Until the desirable characteristics for a liposomal vaccine adjuvant are fully determined, it is difficult to formulate good liposomes which fulfill other points such as stability, cost or antigen compatibility. With regards to the later point, this is another problem commonly faced with liposomal adjuvants, in that the same liposome but combined with two different antigens may

Table 10.5 Clinically relevant cationic liposomal formulations

Disease model/agent	Vaccine	Antigen	Relevent points	Reference
HSV	"CLDC" Liposomes composed of DOTIM lipid and cholesterol helper lipid	HSV gD2	Guinea pig model for genital herpes, s.c. injection leads to better protection than Alum/MPL adjuvant and a reduction in viral shedding. Not effective as a therapeutic vaccine	[7]
WEEV		Noncoding empty pMB75.6	Prophylactic/therapeutic challenge study via i.n/s.c and i.v routes of infection. Greatest survival rates after immunisation with CLDCs were noted after s.c viral challenge	[30]
Pneumonic infection with Francisella tularensis			i.n injection/mice; complete protection from lethal infection in challenge studies (no significant protection elicited by s.c/i.v or i.p routes). Protection dependent on NK cells and IFN-γ production	[48]
Influenza		Noncoding empty pMB75.6 and Fluzone® (split trivalent influenza vaccine)	s.c injection/mice and i.m injection/nonhuman primates; improves humoral and cell-mediated responses noted in both with improved protection in challenge studies	[29]
	"VaxiSome" Liposome composed of CSS and cholesterol helper lipid	Monovalent subunit/trivalent split virions	$>$ 41 % depending on antigen:lipid ratio, i.n or i.m administration leads to long term protective immunity characterised by high antibody titres	[25]
	Vacfectin® Liposomes composed of VC1052 lipid and DPyPE helper lipid	Trivalent split influenza vaccine	Balanced humoral and CMI noted	[45]
	"CAF01" Liposomes composed of DDA lipid and TDB immunomodulator	Vaxigrip influenza split vaccine	Antigen association N/D, i.n administration leads to significantly higher IgG and	[14]

(continued)

Table 10.5 (continued)

Disease model/agent	Vaccine	Antigen	Relevent points	Reference
			IFN-γ levels compared to nonadjuvanted controls	
Chlamydia		MOMP	Th1 response with CD4 T cell dependent protection	[18]
Malaria		Recombinant MSP-1	Antigen association N/D, strong Th1 response noted	[1]
Tuberculosis	Liposomes composed of DDA lipid and BCG derived lipid "MMG"	Recombinant subunit Ag85B-ESAT-6 protein	High level of antigen association (98 % surface adsorbed). Formulation induces mixed Th1/Th17 response with class switch to IgG2 after i.m or s.c injection.	[1, 19] [39]
	Lipofectamine™ 2000	pcDNA3.1$^+$/Ag85A	Oral delivery/mice; elevated secretory IgA and T_H1 biased immune responses	[51]
Toxoplasma gondii	"Escort™ Transreagent" Liposomes composed of DOTAP lipid and DOPE helper lipid	"pVAXGRA7" *T. Gondii* GRA7 antigen	i.m injection/sheep lead to T_H1 responses characterised by IFN-γ and IgG2 antibodies. Vaccine also contains TLR9 agonist CpG	[21]
JEV	Liposomes composed of DOTAP or DC-Chol with DOPE helper lipid	pCJ3/ME	TCI skin patch/mice; both formulations significantly improved survival rates in a challenge study with predominantly T_H2 responses	[13]
HBV, HEV	Liposomes composed of PC/DOPE/DOTAP (molar ratio 4:2:1)	Proteins: recombinant HBsAg and NEp DNA: small envelope gene of HBV and neutralizing epitope of HEV	Combination approach using DNA and/or proteins. Immunisation with liposomes +protein gave IgG1 responses whereas mixed IgG1/2 responses were noted after liposome+protein+DNA immunisation	[44]
	"JVRS-100" (cationic lipid-DNA complex)	HBs-Ag	Antigen association N/D, dual T and B cell response after i.v injection	[34]

House dust mite allergy	Liposomes composed of DiC14-amidine lipid	Recombinant proDerp1	90 % adsorption, i.p injection leads to Th1 response characterised by lack of IgE antibodies	[23, 46]
HPV type 16	"LDP" Liposomes composed of DOTAP lipid	E7 protein	95 % entrapment via freeze-drying, CTL response with tumour inhibition after s.c injection	[12, 52]

BCG Bacillus Calmette-Guérin; *CLDC* cationic liposome-DNA complex; *CMI* cell mediated immune response; *CSS* N-palmitoyl d-erythrosphingosylcarbamoylspermine; *DDA* dimethyldioctadecylammonium bromide; *DOTIM* 1-[2-(oleoyloxy)ethyl]-2-oleyl-3-(2-hydroxyethyl) imidazolinium chloride; *DC-Chol* 3β-[*N*-(*N*′,*N*′-dimethylaminoethane)-carbamoyl]cholesterol hydrochloride; *DOPE*, dioleoyl phosphatidylethanolamine; *DOTAP* 1,2-dioleoyl-3-trimethylammonium-propane; *DPyPE* 1,2-diphytanoyl-sn-glycero-3-phosphoethanolamine; *HBV* hepatitis B virus; *HEV* hepatitis E virus; *HPV* human papillomavirus; *HSV* herpes simplex virus; *i.m* intramuscular; *i.n* intranasal; *i.p* intraperitoneal; *i.v* intravenous; *JEV* Japanese encephalitis virus; *MMG* monomycoloyl glycerol; *MOMP* major outer membrane protein; *MPL* monophosphoryl lipid A; *MSP-1* merozoite surface protein-1; *NK* natural killer cells; *PC* phosphatidylcholine; *s.c* subcutaneous; *TCI* transcutaneous immunisation; *TDB* trehalose 6′6-dibehenate; *TLR* toll-like receptor; *VC1052* (±)-*N*-(3-aminopropyl)-*N*,*N*-dimethyl-2,3-bis(cis-9-tetradecenyloxy)-1-propanaminium bromide; *WEEV* western equine encephalitis virus. N/D, not determined/discussed lead to different responses. Therefore, present conditions from the WHO stipulate that liposomal adjuvants must be licensed as a vaccine formulation and not as an adjuvant which could be combined with various antigens post-licensing. The stability of liposomes is a significant concern; unlike Alum or emulsions, the pharmacokinetic properties of liposomes are affected by temperature due to the main phase transition temperature of the lipid or lipid combinations. Whilst this is frequently considered important with regards to the change in temperature between room temperature and the body, it may also be significant if liposomal vaccines are designed against diseases of hotter climates where cold-chain conditions are not always met.

As noted in Table 10.5, cationic rather than neutral or anionic liposomes appear to be more successful in clinical vaccine trials. In fact, not only cationic liposomes but various novel cationic formulations such as IC-31® (Intracell, Austria), nanoglyolipid particles [6] and micellar copolymers [50] are also proving successful as vaccine adjuvants. Whilst not liposomal, they do share various characteristics such as their charge, submicron size and ability to associate with different antigens. Therefore it seems that we are moving closer to determining the appropriate characteristics of a liposomal adjuvant.

10.7 Summary

The immunostimulatory ability of liposomes as antigen delivery systems has been documented for the past 50 years. However, still there is no truly liposomal vaccine or adjuvant licensed for human use. By gaining enhanced knowledge into the physicochemical characteristics of these systems, in addition to the receptors they bind and the intracellular signalling cascades they activate, hopefully it will soon be possible to use the immunostimulatory nature of liposomes to the full potential in the vaccine setting.

References

1. Agger EM, Rosenkrands I et al (2008) Cationic liposomes formulated with synthetic mycobacterial cordfactor (CAF01): a versatile adjuvant for vaccines with different immunological requirements. PLoS One 3(9):e3116
2. Agrawal B, Krantz MJ et al (1998) Rapid induction of primary human CD4+ and CD8+ T cell responses against cancer-associated MUC1 peptide epitopes. Int Immunol 10(12):1907–1916
3. Andersen CAS, Rosenkrands I et al (2009) Novel generation mycobacterial adjuvant based on liposome-encapsulated monomycoloyl glycerol from mycobacterium bovis bacillus calmette-guérin. J Immunol 183:2294–2302
4. Arora A, Prausnitz MR et al (2008) Micro-scale devices for transdermal drug delivery. Int J Pharm 364(2):227–236
5. Bakouche O, Gerlier D (1986) Enhancement of immunogenicity of tumour virus antigen by liposomes: the effect of lipid composition. Immunology 58:507–513

6. Ben Haij N, O Mzoughi, et al (2012) Cationic nanoglycolipidic particles as vector and adjuvant for the study of the immunogenicity of SIV Nef protein. Int J Pharm 423(1):116–123
7. Bernstein DI, Farley N et al (2010) The adjuvant CLDC increases protection of a herpes simplex type 2 glycoprotein D vaccine in guinea pigs. Vaccine 28:3748–3753
8. Bhowruth V, Minnikin DE et al (2009) Adjuvant properties of a simplified C_{32} monomycolyl glycerol analogue. Bioorg Med Chem Lett 19:2029–2032
9. Calcagnile S, Zuccotti G (2008) The virosomal adjuvanted influenza vaccine. Expert Opin Biol Ther 10(2):191–200
10. Cevc G, Vierl U (2010) Nanotechnology and the transdermal route. A state of the art review and critical appraisal. J Control Release 141:277–299
11. Chadwick S, Kriegel C et al (2010) Nanotechnology solutions for mucosal immunization. Adv Drug Deliv Rev 62(4–5):394–407
12. Chen W, Yan W et al (2008) A simple but effective cancer vaccine consisting of an antigen and a cationic lipid. Cancer Immunol Immunother 57:517–530
13. Cheng J-Y, Huang H-N et al (2009) Transcutaneous immunization by lipoplex-patch based DNA vaccines is effective vaccination against japanese encephalitis virus infection. J Control Release 135:242–249
14. Christensen D, Foged C et al (2010) CAF01 liposomes as a mucosal vaccine adjuvant: in vitro and in vivo investigations. Int J Pharm 390:19–24
15. Christensen D, Korsholm KS et al (2007) Cationic liposomes as vaccine adjuvants. Expert Rev Vaccines 6(5):785–796
16. Gall D (1966) The adjuvant activity of aliphatic nitrogenous bases. Immunology 11:369–386
17. Garçon N, Chomez P et al (2007) GlaxoSmithKline adjuvant systems in vaccines: concepts, achievements and perspectives. Expert Rev Vaccines 6(5):723–739
18. Hansen J, Jensen KT et al (2008) Liposome delivery of Chlamydia muridarum major outer membrane protein primes a Th1 response that protects against genital chlamydial infection in a mouse model. J Infect Dis 198:758–767
19. Henriksen-Lacey M, Bramwell VW et al (2009) Liposomes based on dimethyldioctadecylammonium promote a depot effect and enhance immunogenicity of soluble antigen. J Control Release 142(2):180–186
20. Henriksen-Lacey M, A Devitt, et al (2011) The vesicle size of DDA:TDB liposomal adjuvants plays a role in the cell-mediated immune response but has no significant effect on antibody production. J Control Release 154(2):131–137
21. Hiszczyńska-Sawicka E, Li H et al (2010) Comparison of immune response in sheep immunized with DNA vaccine encoding Toxoplasma gondii GRA7 antigen in different adjuvant formulations. Exp Parasitol 124:365–372
22. Ishii KJ, Koyama S et al (2008) Host innate immune receptors and beyond: making sense of microbial infections. Cell Host Microbe 3:352–363
23. Jacquet A, Vanderschrick J-F et al (2006) Vaccination with the recombinant allergen ProDer p 1 complexed with the cationic lipid DiC14-amidine prevents allergic responses to house dust mite. Mol Ther 11(6):960–968
24. Johansen P, Mohanan D et al (2010) Lympho-geographical concepts in vaccine delivery. J Control Release 148(1):56–62
25. Joseph A, Itskovitz-Cooper N et al (2006) A new intranasal influenza vaccine based on a novel polycationic lipid-ceramide carbamoyl-spermine (CCS): i. immunogenicity and efficacy studies in mice. Vaccine 24(18):3990–4006
26. Kawai T, Akira S (2010) The role of pattern-recognition receptors in innate immunity: update on Toll-like receptors. Nat Immunol 11(5):373–384
27. Kirby C, Gregoriadis G (1984) Dehydration-rehydration vesicles: a simple method for high yield drug entrapment in liposomes. Biotechnol 2:979–984
28. Kufer TA, Sansonetti PJ (2011) NLR functions beyond pathogen recognition. Nat Immunol 12 (2):121–128

29. Lay M, Callejo B et al (2009) Cationic lipid/DNA complexes (JVRS-100) combined with influenza vaccine (Fluzone®) increases antibody response, cellular immunity, and antigenically drifted protection. Vaccine 27:3811–3820
30. Logue CH, Phillips AT et al (2010) Treatment with cationic liposome-DNA complexes (CLDCs) protects mice from lethal Western equine encephalitis virus (WEEV) challenge. Antiviral Res 87:195–203
31. Lonez C, Lensink MF et al (2009) Cationic lipids activate cellular cascades. Which receptors are involved? Biochim Biophys Acta 1790(6):425–430
32. Mannock DA, Lee MYT et al (2008) Comparative calorimetric and spectroscopic studies of the effects of cholesterol and epicholesterol on the thermotropic phase behaviour of dipalmitoylphosphatidylcholine bilayer membranes. Biochim Biophys Acta 1778 (10):2191–2202
33. Mohanan D, Slütter B et al (2010) Administration routes affect the quality of immune responses: a cross-sectional evaluation of particulate antigen-delivery systems. J Control Release 147(3):342–349
34. Morrey JD, Motter NE et al (2011) Breaking B and T cell tolerance using cationic lipid-DNA complexes (CLDC) as a vaccine adjuvant with hepatitis B virus (HBV) surface antigen in transgenic mice expressing HBV. Antiviral Res 90(3):227–230
35. Nakano Y, Mori M et al (2002) Cholesterol inclusion in liposomes affects induction of antigen-specific IgG and IgE antibody production in mice by a surface-linked liposomal antigen. Bioconjug Chem 13:744–749
36. Neutra M, Kozlowski P (2006) Mucosal vaccines: the promise and the challenge. Nat Rev Immunol 6:148–158
37. Nordly P, Rose F et al (2011) Immunity by formulation design: induction of high CD8+ T-cell responses by poly(I:C) incorporated into the CAF01 adjuvant via a double emulsion method. J Control Release 150(3):307–317
38. O'Hagan DT, Gregorio ED (2009) The path to a successful vaccine adjuvant—the long and winding road. Drug Discov Today 14(11/12):541–551
39. Perrie Y, Rades T (2012) FASTtrack: pharmaceutics—drug delivery and targeting. Second Edition. London: Pharmaceutical Press
40. Pestano LA, B. Christian, et al. (2011). ONT-10, a liposomal vaccine targeting hypoglycosylated MUC1, induces a potent cellular and humoral response and suppresses the growth of MUC1 expressing tumors. Proceedings of the 102nd annual meeting of the american association for cancer research. Orlando, Florida, Philadelphia (PA): AACR
41. Sharp FA, Ruane D et al (2009) Uptake of particulate vaccine adjuvants by dendritic cells activates the NALP3 inflammasome. Proc Natl Acad Sci U S A 160(3):870–875
42. Shrivastava S, Lole KS et al (2009) Development of candidate combination vaccine for hepatitis E and hepatitis B: a liposome encapsulation approach. Vaccine 27:6582–6588
43. Sullivan SM, Doukas J et al (2010) Vaxfectin: a versatile adjuvant for plasmid DNA- and protein-based vaccines. Expert Opin Drug Deliv 7(12):1433–1446
44. Tanaka T, Legat A et al (2008) DiC14-amidine cationic liposomes stimulate myeloid dendritic cells through Toll-like receptor 4. Eur J Immunol 38:1–17
45. Thomann J-S, Heurtault B et al (2011) Antitumor activity of liposomal ErbB2/HER2 epitope peptide-based vaccine constructs incorporating TLR agonists and mannose receptor targeting. Biomaterials 32(20):4574–4583
46. Troyer RM, Propst KL et al (2009) Mucosal immunotherapy for protection from pneumonic infection with Francisella tularensis. Vaccine 27:4424–4433
47. van Houte AJ, Snippe H et al (1981) Characterization of immunogenic properties of haptenated liposomal model membranes in mice. V. Effect of membrane composition on humoral and cellular immunogenicity. Immunology 44(3):561–568
48. Voltan R, Castaldello A et al (2009) Priming with a very low dose of DNA complexed with cationic block copolymers followed by protein boost elicits broad and long-lasting antigen-specific humoral and cellular responses in mice. Vaccine 27(33):4498–4507

49. Wang D, Xu J et al (2010) Liposomal oral DNA vaccine (mycobacterium DNA) elicits immune response. Vaccine 28:3134–3142
50. Yan W, Huang L (2009) The effects of salt on the physicochemical properties and immunogenicity of protein based vaccine formulated in cationic liposome. Int J Pharm 368:56–62
51. Zhong Z, Wei X et al (2010) A novel liposomal vaccine improves humoral immunity and prevents tumor pulmonary metastasis in mice. Int J Pharm 399(1–2):156–162

Chapter 11
Designing Nonionic Surfactant Vesicles for the Delivery of Antigens for Systemic and Alternative Delivery Routes

Jitinder Wilkhu, Anil Vangala, Afzal R. Mohammed, and Yvonne Perrie

Abstract Bilayer vesicles can be prepared from a range of molecules including nonionic surfactants. Vesicles built from nonionic surfactants are known as non-ionic surfactant vesicles or niosomes. Whilst structurally similar to liposomes, the use of nonionic surfactants in a formulation may offer advantages in terms of chemical stability and reduced cost in some cases. In general, the ability of surfactant blends to form vesicles is dependent on their combined critical packing parameter, with cholesterol often being used to support the formation of vesicle constructs. To enhance the potency and delivery of antigens, niosomes can be designed to protect antigens against degradation in harsh in vivo environments, including the oral route, and enhance delivery of antigens to appropriate target sites. Key considerations in the design of niosomal adjuvants include the choice of surfactants, the surface properties of the vesicles, the method of preparation, the cholesterol content and the inclusion of immunostimulatory agents. Manipulation of these attributes allows vesicle constructs to be designed and built that can be used to deliver antigens via a range of delivery routes.

11.1 Introduction: Niosomes as Particulate Delivery Systems

There are a range of particulate constructs that are being considered for drug and vaccine delivery including solid particulate systems (which can be built from polymers, lipids, proteins, etc.) and bilayer type vesicles (which are built from molecules with surfactant type properties). Of these, liposomes are the most well-known and investigated with research stemming from their early recognition as

---

Y. Perrie (✉)
School of Life and Health Sciences, Aston University, Birmingham, UK
e-mail: y.perrie@aston.ac.uk

D.R. Flower and Y. Perrie (eds.), *Immunomic Discovery of Adjuvants and Candidate Subunit Vaccines*, Immunomics Reviews: 5, DOI 10.1007/978-1-4614-5070-2_11,

vesicles by Bangham and Horne (1964) [7] and their potential as delivery systems by Gregoriadis et al. (1971) [33]. Indeed their use as adjuvants has been discussed in the previous chapter. However, a wide number of variations, based on these initial liposome systems, have been developed including stealth liposomes to improve circulation profiles [50], vesicles built from nonionic surfactants also known as nonionic surfactant vesicles (NISVs) or niosomes (e.g. for cosmetics [36] or as drug/antigen carriers [5, 6]), surfactant polymers (e.g. polymersomes [69]), cationic systems which can electrostatically bind DNA (e.g. lipoplexes [29]), vesicles incorporating bile salts to improve stability (e.g. bilosomes [22]), or virus components (e.g. virosomes [3]) to name but a few. Many of these systems use alternatives to phospholipids to circumvent potential issues related to storage instabilities and cost (e.g. synthetic-based systems), others to improve stability within harsh biological environments (e.g. bilosomes and polymersomes), or alternatively to modulate the properties of the vesicles in terms of immunological efficacy (e.g. virosomes). Figure 11.1 gives an outline of the evolution of these various bilayer vesicles from liposomes.

Given the ability of many surfactants to form bilayer vesicles, it is no surprise that such a wide range of components have been used to construct these systems. In the case of nonionic surfactants, the ability of these molecules to act as an alternative to lipids as building blocks for bilayer vesicles (known as nonionic surfactant vesicles (NISVs) or niosomes) was first reported by Baillie et al. [6]. These niosomes offer all of the structural attributes of liposomes in terms of: their ability to entrap drugs and antigens within the bilayer and/or the aqueous phase, they can be formed in a range of sizes from small unilamellar to large multilamellar structures, and they can be surface modified in a range of ways similar to liposomes [86]. In addition to these standard attributes, niosomes have also been shown to offer additional abilities such as forming polyhedral vesicles in aqueous media [4] and have been suggested to offer greater chemical stability compared with liposomal systems and reduced special handling upon storage [6, 22], and in harsh biological environments (such as within the gastro-intestinal tract) they have been shown to offer greater stability to acidic and enzymatic degradation compared to liposomes [74, 94]. However, like liposomes, the formation of niosomes requires the input of energy in forms such as physical agitation or heat where the structure consists of an enclosed aqueous core [87].

Niosomes have been widely used in cosmetics and were first patented by L'Oreal in the 1970s with their first use being in 1979 as cosmetic products [36] and since then they have been investigated for the delivery of a wide range of drugs e.g. anticancer agents (e.g. [37, 85]), low solubility drugs (e.g. [62]), antigens (e.g. [35, 64]) and gene therapy (e.g. [39]). An early review by Gregoriadis (1990) [32] has shown that the association of antigen with liposomes improves antigen delivery to the antigen presenting cells (APCs) and this attribute is not restricted to liposomes; niosomes, have also been shown to enhance cell-mediated immunity in addition to humoural immunity [16, 17].

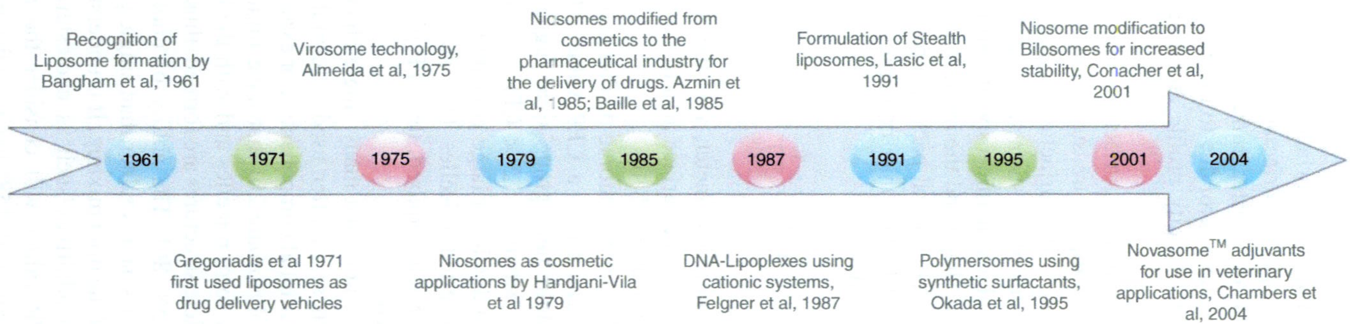

Fig. 11.1 Timeline representing use of bilayer type vesicles

11.1.1 Building Nonionic Surfactant Vesicles

There are a wide range of non-ionic surfactants that can be used to prepare niosomes and examples of the types of surfactants which can be used are given in Table 11.1. These surfactants are most commonly tested and formulated into niosomes with the presence of cholesterol due to their chemical stability, resultant sustained release of drugs, low toxicity profile and enhanced permeation when delivering via the skin [58].

In general, the formation of non-ionic surfactants into bilayer vesicles is dependent on many factors including: temperature, surfactant concentration, electrostatic and electrodynamic interactions of the surfactants within the aqueous phase. Furthermore, the molecular attributes of the surfactant is also an important parameter as the type of colloidal or vesicular structure a specific surfactant forms is to a large extent dictated by its molecular shape and the mixture of surfactant combinations used, as this will influence its geometrical packing properties in a given solution environment. The shape of a surfactant may be expressed as its critical packing parameter (CPP) which is defined as:

$$\mathrm{CPP} = \frac{v}{a_{\mathrm{o}} l_{\mathrm{c}}}$$

where CPP is the critical packing parameter, v is the molecular volume of the hydrophobic part of the lipid, a_{o} is the surface area of the hydrophilic head group, and l_{c} is the length of the hydrocarbon chain.

The CPP value can be used as an indicator to predict geometry of surfactants and the resultant structures they can form: a CPP value <0.5 (indicating a large contribution from the hydrophilic head group area) suggests the surfactant forms spherical micelles, a value between $0.5 < \mathrm{CPP} < 1$ forms bilayer vesicles (Fig. 11.2) and a $\mathrm{CPP} > 1$ (indicating a large contribution from the hydrophobic group volume) results in inverted micelles [14, 40, 41, 73, 87]. Therefore, depending upon the type of vesicle required, the CPP gives a good indication on the surfactants that can be used.

However, it is interesting to note that many single chain surfactants have CPP <0.5 and form micelles, yet these are often used to formulate niosomes, however, not without the addition of additional components. For example, soluble surfactants (such as solulan C-24 and polysorbate 20) that have high hydrophilic–lipophilic balance values (HLB) readily form micelles and with the inclusion of cholesterol into the mixture, niosome vesicle structures are formed, thus increasing the physical stability of the vesicle [20, 58, 86]. The ability of cholesterol to promote the formation of two-phase bilayer systems rather than single phase micellar solutions is related to the overall CPP of the lipid mixture. It is understood that in cases where a mixture of surfactants and additives such as cholesterol are used to prepare vesicles, the operational CPP values will consider the average of the overall components [48] and Manosroi et al. [58] have confirmed that as cholesterol is

Table 11.1 Properties of some commonly used surfactants in the preparation of niosomes

Surfactant	Structure	Molecular weight	Melting point (°C)	T_c (°C)
1-Monopalmitoyl-rac-glycerol (MPG)	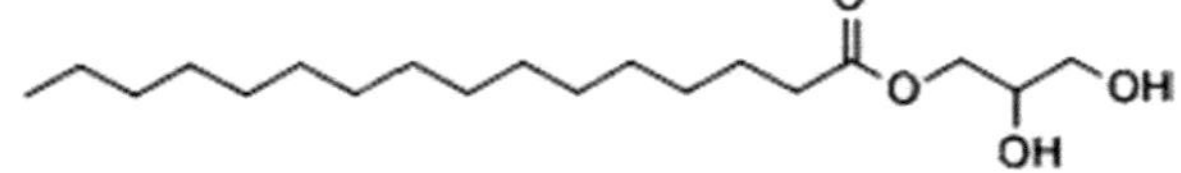	330.5	71–72	23
Dicetyl phosphate (DCP)	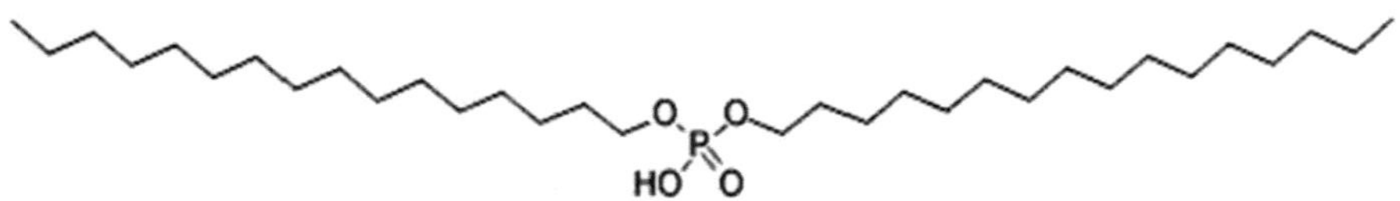	546	74–75	–
Sorbitan monostearate (span 60)	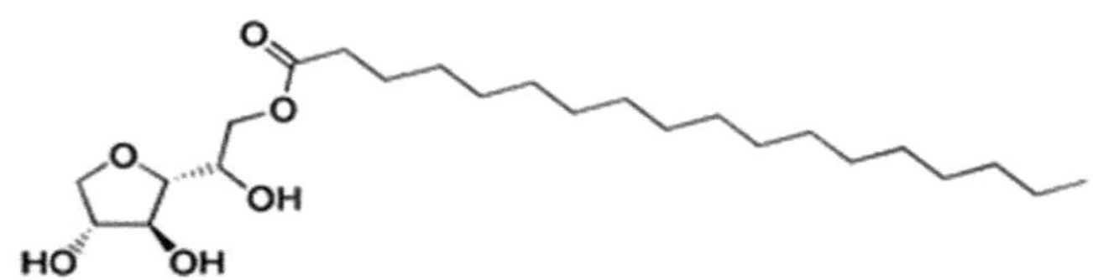	430.62	54–57	55

(continued)

Table 11.1 (continued)

Surfactant	Structure	Molecular weight	Melting point (°C)	T_c (°C)
Polyethylene glycol sorbitan monostearate (Tween 60)	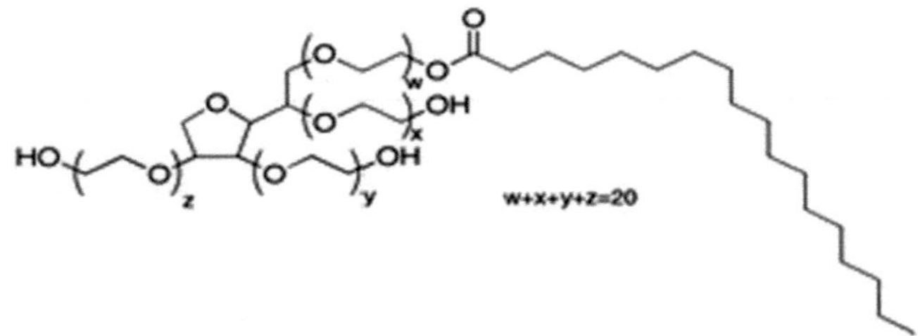	1,309	55–60	40.6
Glyceryl monostearate (GMS)	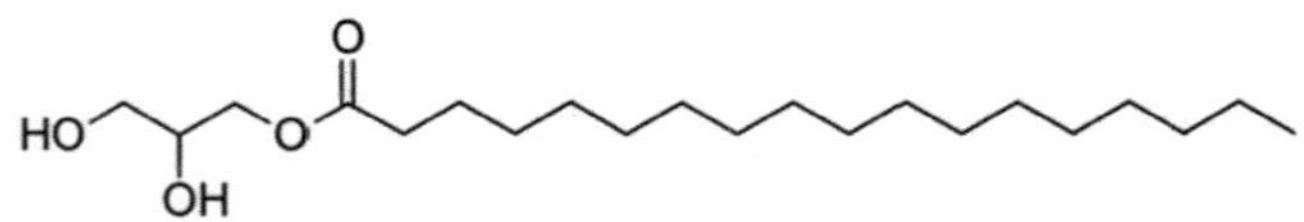	358.57	58–59	>65
Polyoxyethylene (4) lauryl ether (Brij 30)	$C_{12}H_{25}(OCH_2CH_2)_4OH$	362.5	1.67	<10
Cholesterol	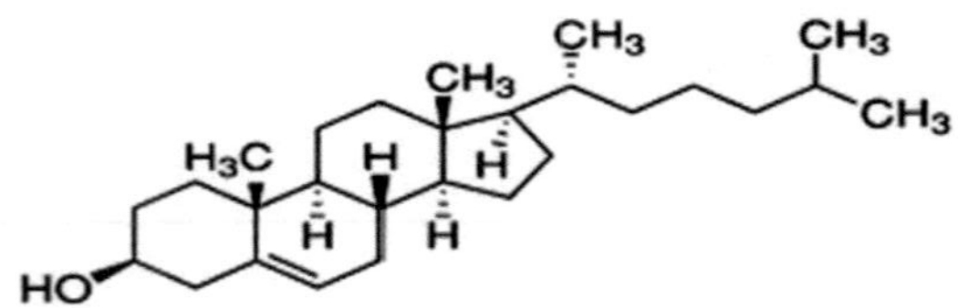	296.65	147–149	–

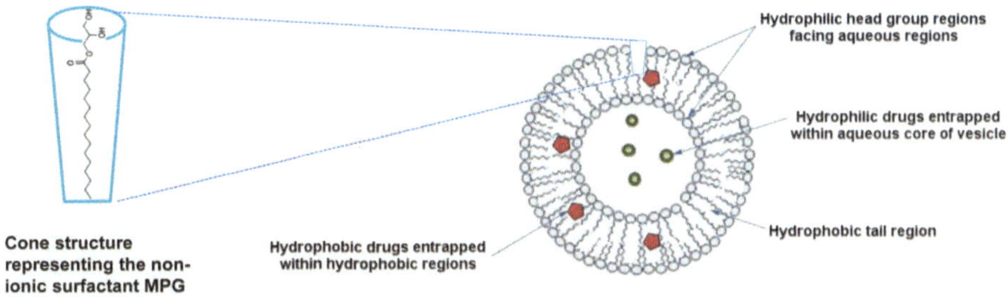

Fig. 11.2 Non-ionic surfactant MPG showing head group and tail structure and how they reside within the bilayer vesicle

incorporated within a Tween 61 surfactant mixture, an average CPP value between 0.5 and 1 was obtained, hence the formation of bilayer vesicles rather than micelles [58]. Similarly, Tween 20 has a CPP below 0.5, however, when mixed with cholesterol unilamellar vesicles were formed [20] as does with Span 60, which is widely used in the formulation of niosomes [66, 84]. This is due to the average CPP of the mixture moving into the range of 0.5–1, hence showing capabilities of forming bilayer vesicles. Due to high phase transition temperatures of Span 60 (Table 11.1), leakage of drug molecules from the bilayer has been reported [79]; the incorporation of cholesterol has also been shown to stabilise the vesicles by abolishing the phase transition temperature of the vesicles, hence avoiding leakage of drug molecules from the bilayer [79, 87]. It is clear from the thermodynamic consideration that bilayer structures do not exist as such in the absence of water because it is water that provides the driving force for surfactant molecules to assume a bilayer configuration and unlike micelles, the assembly into closed bilayers is rarely spontaneous and usually involves input of energy such as physical agitation or heat [49]. The excess free energy change between water and a hydrophobic environment explains the preference of appropriate surfactants to assemble into bilayer structures, excluding water as much as possible from their hydrophobic regions, in order to achieve the lowest free energy level and consequently the highest stability for the aggregate structure.

Another commonly used nonionic surfactant, monopalmitoyl-glycerol (MPG) used to formulate niosomes for a range of studies e.g. Brewer and Alexander [16], requires the inclusion of additional surfactants to support vesicle construction. Without the addition of cholesterol and dicetyl phosphate (DCP), MPG cannot form stable niosomes and the ratio of these combinations can dictate the physical attributes of these systems. As shown in Fig. 11.3, when the surfactant ratios of cholesterol and DCP were varied, and MPG kept constant, both the size and zeta potential of the formulation has been affected; incorporation of DCP, due to its anionic nature, provides niosomes with their net negative charge, however when high levels of DCP (25 mol%) are used a broad vesicle size range of 4.5–7 μm was noted. In contrast, when lower DCP (10 mol%) concentrations with any ratio of cholesterol produces vesicle size within the 4–4.5 μm range. This interplay between vesicle size and cholesterol content has also been noted by Van Hal et al. [88] who

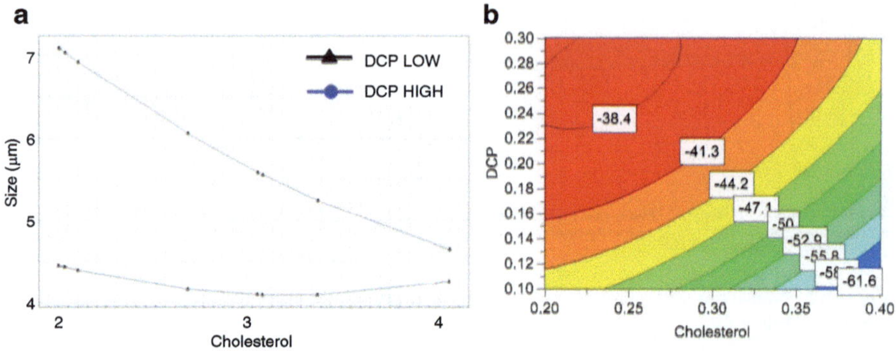

Fig. 11.3 (**a**) Vesicle size represented against specific ratios of cholesterol (Mol) with high and low DCP content, (**b**) 2D contour plot using design of experiments to determine the effect of cholesterol (Mol) and DCP (Mol) on the Zeta potential. The main surfactant used is MPG at a ratio of 5 Mol

reported a decrease in vesicle size upon increased cholesterol content. Furthermore, cholesterol has the ability to influence the packing density within the bilayer and in turn increase the planarity of the bilayer resulting in uniform bilayers [59, 88].

The Zeta potential is the simplest way to measure surface charge of vesicles and gives a representation of the stability of a formulation. A highly positive or negative zeta potential can imply that the vesicle suspension is more likely to resist aggregation [31, 34]. DCP incorporation in niosomes has been proven in several studies, including vaccine delivery to alcohol-free niosome gel formulations, to stabilise vesicles against fusion and aggregation where the vesicles obtain their net negative charge [7, 42, 86].

11.1.1.1 The Addition of Cholesterol to Niosome Formulations

Given the above outlined advantages, the addition of cholesterol can offer to a formulation, it is understandable why nearly all current studies investigating niosomes have incorporated cholesterol into the vesicle composition. Indeed when dispersed without the presence of cholesterol, whilst high solubility non-ionic surfactants form micelles, low solubility non-ionic surfactants often form a gel [95]. However, the use of cholesterol not only promotes vesicles formation from a wide range of non-ionic surfactants, its inclusion in both liposome or niosome formulations is known to remove the gel–liquid transition of the surfactant bilayer and hence influences bilayer fluidity [83]. For example, Fig. 11.4 shows a differential scanning calorimetry (DSC) scan for 1,2-distearoyl-*sn*-glycero-3-phosphocholine (DSPC) liposomes, which have a transition temperature of 54°C. The incorporation of cholesterol in a 1:1 molar ratio to this formulation results in the removal of this gel-to-liquid-crystal phase transition (Fig. 11.4). Similarly, when MPG is formulated with

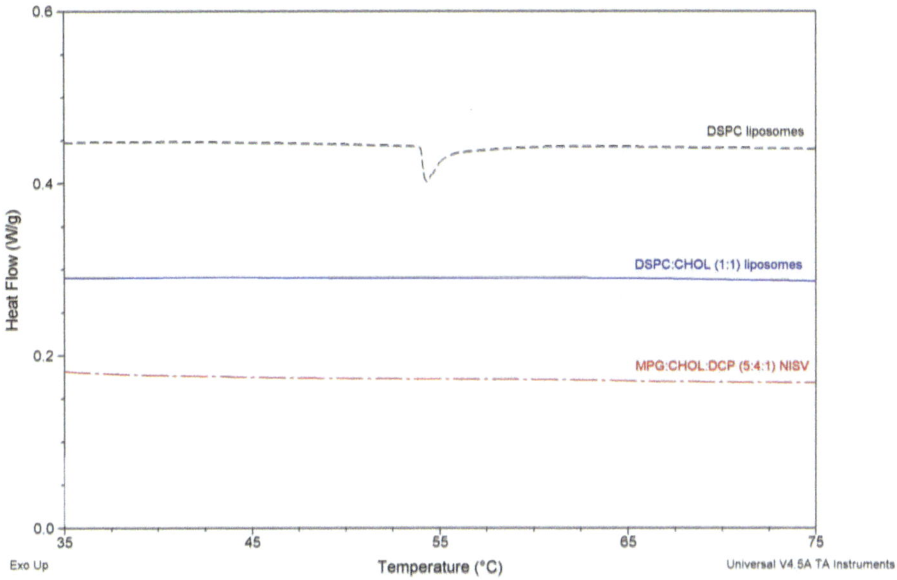

Fig. 11.4 DSC thermograms of DSPC, DSPC: CHOL and niosome formulations showing the existence or removal of the phase transition of the bilayer vesicles. Scan rate = 10 °C/min

cholesterol and DCP at 5:4:1 molar ratio as investigated by Brewer and Alexander (1992) [16] no phase transition was notable.

The preparation methods are a key parameter in the formation of structured bilayers when considering the transition temperature, e.g. the hydration temperature determines the overall size and shape of the vesicles formed. In both liposome and niosome systems the bilayer membrane is an ordered structure and may exist in the gel state, indicating a situation where the alkyl chains are tilted at a slight angle with respect to the plane of the bilayer, or the liquid crystalline state. The difference between these two phases is the degree of order, with the gel state being the most ordered structure than the liquid crystalline state. In the liquid crystalline state there is lateral diffusion of bilayer material, whereas in the gel state the alkyl chains are crystallised or otherwise less mobile. For any system, the liquid crystalline state exists at a higher temperature than the gel state. The increase in the temperature (T_c), although yielding an increase in the enthalpy term (ΔH), also results in an increase in entropy (ΔS) and thus a lowering of the free energy (ΔG) of the system occurs and it is the application of heat that is the driving force for this transition [65]. Hence the formation of niosome vesicles should occur above the T_c of the gel to liquid phase transition allowing mobility of the bilayer and hence reordering of surfactants to produce spherical uniform vesicles.

Interestingly, controlling the phase in which the bilayer is in, can influence the structure of niosomes: for example not all niosomes are spherical in nature, as is the case with polyhedral niosomes [4]. The niosomes in this study were prepared by hydrating thin films of surfactant/lipid blends where they were analysed for morphology and rheological properties. The studies showed that niosomes formed from hexadecyl diglycerol and other polyoxyethylene alkyl esters form a variety of shapes due to the differences in membrane composition. The incorporation of cholesterol results in large spherical vesicles, however the exclusion of cholesterol resulted in the formation of polyhedral niosomes [4]. These polyhedral niosomes were heated above their transition temperature, at which a reversible shape transformation into spherical niosomes occurred indicating that the niosomes go from a gel state at room temperature to a liquid-crystalline state at their T_c. As a result, the rheological properties of the polyhedral niosomes are more rigid and viscous in comparison to their spherical counterpart structures at the elevated temperatures. Therefore, when formulating niosomes for different routes of administration, characterisation should be carried out to ensure the niosomes are able to effectively perform at their intended site of action.

11.1.2 Alternatives to Cholesterol in the Formulation of Niosomes

Cholesterol is not the only component that is able to promote niosome formulation, with fatty acids also being shown to promote the formation of vesicles which can offer similar attributes to that of cholesterol-based systems. Various studies have been carried out on the replacement of cholesterol with fatty alcohols where loading efficiencies and drug release kinetics have been tested as a comparison [1, 27]. Results indicate that the replacement of cholesterol in niosome vesicles with different fatty alcohols of varying alkyl chain length exhibit a similar release profile to that of cholesterol-based niosomes. However, replacement of cholesterol with the fatty acids resulted in an overall decrease in the release rate of the drug (ketorolac tromethamine) and become even slower upon increased alkyl chain length of the fatty alcohols [27]. As a result, both studies show that fatty alcohols can replace the cholesterol when forming niosome vesicles, with release rates and entrapment being optimised by altering the ratios and contents of the surfactants [1, 27]. Furthermore, results from our lab show that attempts to formulate niosomes from MPG:DOPE: DC-Chol were unsuccessful with a precipitate forming at percentage ratios of 57:29:14%, respectively. However, the addition of 4 μmol (12.5 %) cholesterol to this composition supported the formation of vesicles [71].

11.1.3 Designing Niosomes for the Delivery of Antigens

As noted, niosome preparation can be optimised to provide a specific vesicle size, lamellarity and surface characteristics, which can then be further modified to offer enhanced antigen protection, improved delivery and controlled release [5, 6].

In drug delivery, encapsulation of drugs within niosomes can offer reduced toxicity of drugs over a broad range of therapies and delivery routes [38]. Moreover, the surfactants used are generally biodegradable and are able to improve therapeutic bioavailability by protecting drugs from the biological environment, hence increasing residence time of the vesicles. However, these comments are largely generalised and the niosome attributes are usually dictated by its composition; in the case of vaccine delivery, being non-immunogenic is not a useful attribute and therefore the bilayer composition of the niosomes can be modified by the incorporation of immunostimulatory agent [89]. The methodology of preparation must also consider the properties of the antigen to be entrapped, given that not all methods are compatible with proteins and subunit antigens. Similarly, the preparation and formulation of the niosomes can be tailored in accordance to the route of administration, i.e. oral, parenteral or topical route all require different delivery system characteristics to promote successful delivery of antigens.

11.2 Method of Preparation of Nonionic Surfactant Vesicles

Depending on the method of preparation, NISVs consist of one or more bilayer membranes (lamellae) from small unilamellar vesicles (SUV) with a diameter of about 75–100 nm, to large unilamellar vesicles (LUV) which can be several microns large, and multilamellar vesicles (MLV) which vary in size from anywhere above 100 nm to several microns. There are a wide range of methods that can be used to prepare niosomes (Fig. 11.5), and nearly all of which are adaptations from the methods used to prepare liposomes.

The method of choice, combined with the surfactant types used and drug/antigen attributes and concentration will all contribute to the vesicle size, surface characteristics, and loading efficacy and release characteristics of entrapped drug or antigen [15]. In addition to the method of preparation, the nature of the solute and hydration temperature also affects entrapment efficiency [86]. As a result, when optimising and formulating niosomes of specific characteristics the preparation method is a key consideration. For example the number of bilayers, vesicle size and distribution, and the entrapment efficiency are all influenced by the method of preparation as summarised in Table 11.2 and examples of size reduction techniques in Table 11.3.

11.2.1 Characterisation of Niosomes: Commonly Measured Parameters and Their Implication on Adjuvant Efficacy

To achieve effective subunit vaccine delivery or drug delivery via the use of niosomes, it is essential to study the physico-chemical characteristics which will

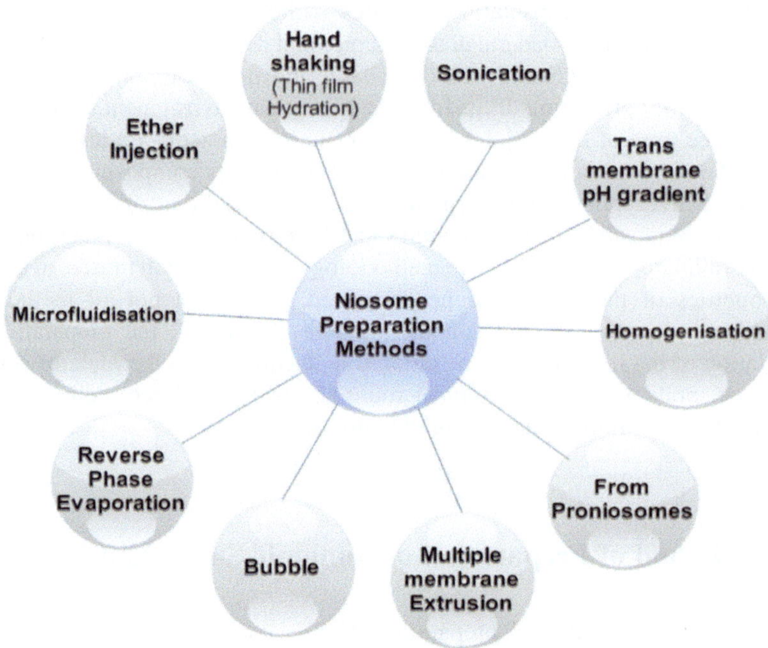

Fig. 11.5 Various methods of manufacture for niosome vesicles

determine the stability and efficacy of the delivery system. In general, there are various methods employed to characterise delivery systems which include characterisation using vesicle size, suspension pH, vesicle zeta potential, entrapment loading studies and microscopy studies such as freeze fracture, transmission electron microscopy (TEM) or basic light microscopy. It is important to ensure that the niosomes produced and tested whether in vitro or in vivo have the same characteristics in terms of charge, vesicle size, and amount of antigen or drug entrapped as differences could lead to differences in efficacy and results obtained.

Entrapment: Entrapment efficiency is obviously an important parameter as it influences surfactant/antigen ratio and total amounts of antigens needed. It can be measured using a range of techniques including: separating the unentrapped drug or antigen e.g. by centrifugation [16], dialysis [6] or gel filtration [86]. For protein and peptide-based antigen assays such as the ninhydrin assay can be used to measure entrapment of peptides and proteins within niosomes as this assay eliminates any interference of lipids or surfactants when compared to other assays such as the BCA assay [19]. In some cases the Lowry method for protein concentrations are used which works on the general principle under alkaline conditions where the divalent copper ion reacts with peptide bonds, hence forming a complex in which it is reduced to a monovalent ion. This monovalent copper ion along with the other radical groups of the reagents reacts with a Folin reagent resulting in an unstable product which is reduced to tungsten blue. The limitations of this method are that

Table 11.2 Different methods of preparation for various vesicles such as MLV, LUV and SUV

Vesicles	Method	Procedure
Multilamellar vesicles (MLV)	(a) Lipid-hydration method	Also known as thin film hydration form niosomes by the dissolution of the surfactants/cholesterol in an organic solvent such as chloroform or methanol in a round bottom flask. In this method, the organic solvent consisting a mixture of vesicle-forming ingredients, is evaporated under reduced pressure on a rotary evaporator, leaving a thin film on the wall of round bottom flask which is hydrated by shaking the film in the presence of water that contains the solute to be incorporated, above the phase-transition temperature (T_c) of the surfactant/lipid until a good dispersion of MLVs are formed [81, 89]
	(b) Dehydration-rehydration method	This method involves freeze-drying of preformed SUV mixed with the solute to be entrapped and rehydrated under controlled conditions giving MLVs with high entrapment [45]
	(c) Multiple membrane extrusion	This method is begins with the same procedure of the thin film hydration method and once formed the niosome formulation is passed through membranes of pore sizes to control the vesicle size [87]
Large unilamellar vesicles (LUV)	(a) Reverse phase evaporation method	Vesicles can be prepared when the surfactant mixture is dissolved in chloroform and to this an aqueous phase including drug is added and then sonicated to form a gel. Phosphate buffered saline (PBS) is then added and the organic phase is then removed under reduced pressure and subsequently further hydrated with PBS to form niosomes [34]
	(b) Calcium-induced fusion method	This method takes advantage of the fact that small vesicles aggregate in the presence of calcium and subsequently fuse. Large vesicles could be produced upon addition of EDTA [70]
	(c) Detergent removal method	Removal of detergent from mixed micelles formed by solubilisation of dried surfactant mixtures or preformed vesicles with a detergent containing aqueous phase, results in the formation of unilamellar vesicles. Detergents can be removed by dialysis or by gel filtration chromatography [92]
	(d) Ether injection method	Niosomes are prepared by the introduction of a surfactant/cholesterol mixture dissolved in diethyl ether and is injected into an aqueous medium such as water containing the material to be encapsulated (using a syringe-type infusion pump) at a temperature of 60°C or under reduced pressure, subsequent vaporisation of the residual ether leads to formation of unilamellar vesicles [6, 25]

(continued)

Table 11.2 (continued)

Vesicles	Method	Procedure
Small unilamellar vesicles (SUV)	(a) Sonication	Niosomes are formed by the addition of an aqueous phase in the surfactant/cholesterol mixture into a glass vial and sonicated. In addition, MLVs can also be sonicated either with a probe sonicator or a bath type sonicator leading to rapid size reduction, forming SUV [6]
	(b) French press method	A French pressure cell is used to reduce the size of MLV by extrusion under high pressure [9]. This technique yields homogenous SUV with sizes depending upon the pressure used
	(c) Ethanol injection method	This method, employs a procedure where surfactant/lipids are dissolved in ethanol and rapidly injected into a vast excess of buffer solution through a fine needle yielding a high proportion of SUVs [10]
	(d) Microfluidisation method	This method is based on submerged jet principle in which two fluidised streams interact at ultra high velocities (up to 1,700 ft/s) in precisely defined micro channels within the interaction chamber. The impingement of thin liquid sheets along a common front is arranged such that the energy applied to the system remains within the area of vesicle formation. This procedure gives SUVs with uniform size distribution of a sub 50 nm size from the energy supplied [87]
	(e) Homogenization	Homogenization of MLV by commercially available high shear homogenizers produces SUVs. The size of the vesicles depends on the speed of the probe, duration of homogenization and also on the surfactant/lipid composition. To prepare the bilayer vesicles the surfactants in the powder form are mixed at the appropriate ratio and melted in an oil bath, and while maintaining the molten mixture an emulsion is created by the addition of aqueous buffers and homogenised for 10 min. Upon cooling, the niosome formulation was incubated for 2 h with gentle shaking at 220 rpm [54]

Table 11.3 Summary of various manufacturing methods for size reduction showing resultant vesicles produced

Method	Type of vesicle
Sonication	Small unilamellar
Homogenisation	Multilamellar
Microfluidisation	Small unilamellar
Multiple membrane extrusion	Multilamellar
French press method	Small unilamellar

for the reaction to occur a pH of 9–11 needs to be maintained and that certain buffers, lipids and drugs may interfere with the assay, hence appropriate filtration and dilutions are needed before running the assay [53]. Due to the limitations of the Lowry method, a simpler and less sensitive to interference assay is the Bradford assay. The Bradford assay is analysed at a wavelength of 595 nm as this becomes the lambda max for the reagent Coomassie brilliant blue G-250 when protein binding occurs. The colour change is observed due to the stabilising effect of the anionic dye by hydrophobic and ionic interactions of the reaction [47].

Vesicle diameter size and morphology: The vesicle size and polydispersity of a niosome suspension can be determined using various techniques including: e.g. light microscopy, freeze fracture electron microscopy and laser diffraction. Laser diffraction is commonly used in the analysis of particle size for suspensions, aerosols, emulsions and other pharmaceutical products. Of the physical attributes, particle size and polydispersity are often seen as key factors that may affect product stability and in vivo efficacy. Indeed, the vesicle size range is crucial as it determines the end location of the vesicle in vivo. Studies show that when injecting liposome vesicles, the vesicle size has an important role in providing adjuvant effects. For example, a study by Desjardins et al. [26] showed that MLV preparations of DSPC and Dipalmitoylphosphatidylcholine (DPPC) liposomes resulted in a high response from the popliteal lymph nodes [26] compared to MLV formulations prepared from low T_c lipids such as egg phosphatidylcholine. The MLV preparations resulted in increased numbers of $CD4^+$, $CD8^+$, $CD69^+$, Ig^+ subsets and IL-2 receptor cells in relation to the smaller sized SUV preparations of same lipid composition which resulted in reduced immunoactivating potential at the popliteal lymph nodes [26]. Consideration of the delivery route plays an important role in the consideration of the required size range of vesicles for vaccine delivery: when orally administering vesicles where the target site for orally delivered vesicles are the immuno-competent cells within the gut which are known as Peyer's patches, studies by Eldridge et al. [28] on vesicle size uptake in the Peyer's patches show that uptake is dependent on both the vesicle size and hydrophobicity [28]. The results from their experiments indicate that a vesicle size of 10 μm or less are taken up by the Peyer's patches; however, particles with a size less than 5 μm can traffic to other tissue cells by a process of lymphoid drainage. Therefore, the vesicle size plays a crucial role when designing vaccine carrier systems to successfully allow the vaccine and the carrier to reach and retain at the target site to allow them to exert their therapeutic effect.

In addition to laser diffraction, it is important to confirm the shape and structure of the niosomes and microscopy techniques can be used to consider this. A review by Bibi et al. discusses the advantages and limitations of specific microscopy techniques to analyse vesicles [13]. Although there are several microscopy techniques available for the image analysis of vesicles, techniques such as light microscopy offers basic conformation of morphology and size of the vesicles. However, when examining vesicles in greater detail, advanced microscopy techniques are available such as the various TEM techniques which include, negative stain TEM, Cryo-TEM and freeze fracture TEM. An example of

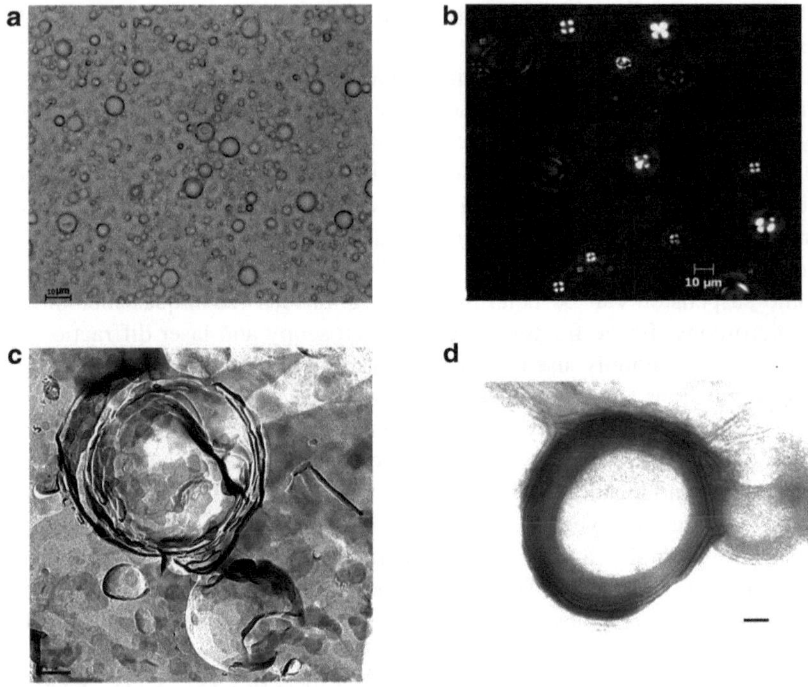

Fig. 11.6 (**a**) Light microscopy of a niosome formulation at ×40 objective showing spherical vesicles ranging from larger and smaller ones in the same formulation. (**b**) Polarised light microscopy of niosome vesicles showing the presence of a Maltese cross. (**c**) Freeze fracture image of a niosome formulation showing spherical vesicles and the multiple layers within the vesicle. (**d**) Transmission electron micrograph of surfactant vesicle composed of 1-monopalmitoyl glycerol, cholesterol, DDA, TDB (16:16:4:0.5 μmoles) showing multilamellar bilayers. Bar = 100 nm (*Reprinted from International Journal of Pharmaceutics, Microscopy imaging of liposomes: From coverslips to environmental SEM, 417/1-2, Sagida Bibi, Randip Kaur, Malou Henriksen-Lacey, Sarah E. McNeil, Jitinder Wilkhu, Eric Lattmann, Dennis Christensen, Afzal R. Mohammed, Yvonne Perrie, Copyright (2011) with permission from Elsevier.)

microscopy images of niosomes collated from a range of techniques is shown in Fig. 11.6, in particular, the use of freeze-fracture can give greater detail on both the size and number of bilayers the niosomes have; however, general light microscopy can offer a good overview of heterogenicity.

Surface charge: Zeta potential is a function of the vesicle surface charge which is calculated at the surface interface and the nature of the surrounding medium. The Zeta potential is the nearest experimental approximation of surface potential, as both the surface potential and stern potential are difficult to measure. When an electric current is passed through each particle and its ions in the region move throughout the solution. The rate and extent of movement within the layers and the surrounding medium can be used to determine the zeta potential. Hence, the Zeta potential is the potential at the surface of shear which is measured by electrophoresis and reflects the effective charge on the vesicles and the repulsion between them, in turn giving an insight into the stability and flocculation of the suspension.

Hydrophobicity: Further to surface charge of vesicles, the hydrophobicity/hydrophilicity of particles can play an important role in vesicle delivery and uptake. For example, liposome uptake within the body can be influenced by the presence of a Polyethylene glycol coating on the vesicle surface which modifies the surface hydrophilicity and in return reduces opsonisation and macrophage recognition [2]. By reducing opsonisation, the liposomes increase their circulation time within the body; however, for a vaccine delivery system this may be counter-productive. As a result the hydrophobicity of the vesicles should be taken into consideration when optimising bilayer vesicles for adjuvant activity.

11.3 Formulation Design of Niosomes Used as Vaccine Adjuvants

Niosomes have been widely studied as carrier systems over a range of administration routes which include e.g. intravenous [37], oral [43], transdermal [57, 86], peroral [74] and parenteral routes [64]. Incorporating antigens within the surfactant vesicles aid in the protection and enhanced delivery of antigens by a variety of routes provide sustained antigen release, targeting the antigen into appropriate APCs and promotes intracellular delivery of antigen contributing to cytotoxic T cell response. This way the particulate adjuvants could play a fundamental role, alone or as part of a formulation, acting as carrier to target immune cells and as depot [75].

In terms of niosomes use for antigen delivery, the niosome formulation of 1-monopalmitoyl glycerol, cholesterol and DCP is commonly adopted [15]. Given the DCP content of these systems, their highly charged surface can offer enhanced stability due to the electrostatic repulsive forces between the vesicles, hence restricts aggregation [11, 95] and has been reported to aid in uptake when delivering antigens via the oral route [28]. Indeed this formulation stems from initial investigations into the adjuvanticity of niosomes prepared from 1-monopalmitoyl glycerol, cholesterol and DCP at a 5:4:1 molar ratio. The formulation demonstrated in mice that, on subcutaneous administration of niosomes incorporating bovine serum albumin (BSA) [16], ovalbumin (OVA) [18], or a synthetic peptide containing a known T-cell epitope [18] that niosomes were generally better stimulators of IgG2a than Freud's complete adjuvant, but weak stimulators for IgG1. In addition, the adjuvant activity of niosomes was wholly dependent on the model antigen being entrapped within the vesicles while mixing free antigen with the preformed vesicles were unable to illicit a significant immune responses [16]. This was attributed to the ability of niosomes retaining the antigen for a prolonged period and promoting APC uptake through active or passive targeting to cells [16, 22]. The same niosome system has also been shown to act as a vaccine adjuvant when administered intraperitoneally to severe combined immunodeficiency mice reconstituted with peripheral blood lymphocytes (PBL-SCID mice) [93]. This mouse model was designed to mimic the human response to an antigen challenge.

The 1-monopalmitoyl glycerol-based niosomes have also been considered for the delivery of DNA vaccines. Formulated by the dehydration–rehydration method (DRV), MPG-based niosomes incorporating cationic surfactants (DC-Chol) rather than anionic surfactants have been shown to offer an increased stability and increased plasmid DNA retention in the presence of competitive anions when compared to similarly formulated PC-based liposomes [68]. This niosome formulation was able to engender transgene-specific immune responses comparable with their liposomal counterparts [68, 71, 72].

Murdan et al. [64], have worked on the use of sorbitan monostearate/polysorbate 20 organogels, which contain niosomes. The aim of the study was to establish whether vesicle-in-water-in-oil (v/w/o) gels could potentially be used as vehicles for vaccine delivery. For incorporation of BSA niosome formulations were prepared using thin film hydration method, whereas for haemagglutinin (HA), niosomes were prepared by a dehydration–rehydration method [45, 64]. The preparation of the organogels involved the addition of the aqueous niosome formulation at 60°C into an organic solution which produces an emulsion and upon cooling forms an opaque semisolid v/w/o gel. Results from the radiolabelled BSA niosomes showed a depot effect after IM administration, hence retaining the BSA at the site of injection (SOI) and then over a period of days migrates from the SOI. The hypothesis is that when in vivo, the aqueous areas penetrate into the gel thus causing the gel to break up into smaller fragments, allowing for the release of the niosomes and the antigen. These findings were confirmed by in vitro tests which were carried out, and also showed that the interstitial fluid penetrates the gel, hence resulting in disintegration of the v/w/o gel [64]. In terms of the immunogenicity studies with the HA antigen, the v/w/o gel and a control gel consisting of just radiolabelled BSA (w/o) both possessed immunoadjuvant properties enhancing the primary and secondary antibody titres to the antigen.

When considering the industrial large scale applications of niosomes, their stability should be considered. Previous stability studies on the effect of storage of niosomes on the adjuvant activity resulted in vesicles maintaining their adjuvant activity at 10 months at various storage conditions, but by 18 months the adjuvant activity diminished [22]. However, the lyophilisation of other vesicle systems has proven to increase stability of systems such as dimethyldioctadecylammonium (DDA): trehalose 6,6′-dibehenate (TDB) vesicles [60, 61]. Lyophilised niosome preparations with sucrose have prolonged the adjuvant activity hence keeping the vesicles stable for an increased period of time whilst retaining adjuvant properties [22]. As a result, depending upon the surfactants used to prepare the vesicles the niosomes can be modified to entrap antigen and prolong the release of the antigen from the vesicles which results in an increased shelf life of the formulations. To overcome the problems of leeching and instabilities of the vesicles in the liquid state, niosome formulations can be lyophilised.

11.3.1 Addition of Immunostimulatory Agents

A range of immunostimulatory agents are available such as monophosphoryl lipid A, *Quillaja saponaria* (Quil-A), CpG oligodeoxynucleotides, trehalose 6,6-dibhenate (TDB). For example, TDB has been considered into a range of liposome and niosome formulations including DDA liposome preparations where it has been shown to increase the immune response to a tuberculosis vaccine protein (Ag85B-ESAT-6) as well as providing increased stability [24]. Similarly, MPG-based vesicles incorporating both DDA and TDB were developed by Vangala et al. [90] which resulted in an increase in the vesicle size due to the hydrophilicity of the surfactants, without altering the zeta potential of the vesicles compared to DDA: TDB vesicles. The MPG-based vesicles were proven to increase overall stability of the DDA systems whilst maintaining comparable induction of antibody responses. In terms of malarial antigens (Merozoite surface protein 1 [MSP1] and glutamate-rich protein [GLURP]), the MPG-based vesicles, in comparison to DDA liposomes, showed similarly strong Th2 humoural responses when analysing IgG1 titres; however, the MPG-based vesicles also showed high IgG2b titres unlike the DDA: TDB systems [90].

Novasome™ adjuvants, also referred to as non-phospholipid liposomes [21] are multicomponent adjuvant systems made up of dioxyethylene cetyl ether, cholesterol and oleic acid have been licensed for veterinary application (for the immunisation of fowl against Newcastle virus disease and avian rheovirus). The Novasome™ technology, made with glycerol monostearate and butyl alcohol and included the potent adjuvant monophosphoryl lipid A [21], was shown to offer protection of guinea pigs against aerosol challenge with virulent *Mycobacterium bovis*.

In addition, Quil-A saponins have been used in several studies and are generally used as part of immune-stimulating complexes (ISCOMs) where the Quil-A acts as an adjuvant [44, 46]. ISCOM use as antigen delivery systems show the formation of cationic cage-like complexes when DC–cholesterol replaces cholesterol, or the substitution of PC with dioleoyl-trimethyl-ammonium-propane. The cationic complexes formed are similar to the classical anionic ISCOMs and allow a more diverse range of antigens to be used in their formulation [51, 52]. Orally, ISCOMs have shown promising systemic immune responses by eliciting Th1, Th2 and MHC-restricted cytotoxic T-cell responses in addition to local induction of IgA [60]. As a result, the introduction of immunostimulatory agents has shown to be useful to enhance immune responses to subunit vaccines and offer a promising platform for further studies. A detailed consideration of the use of ISCOMs can be found in the chapter by Hook and Rades.

11.3.2 Design Considerations for Alternative Delivery Routes

In addition to parenteral route, a range of other routes have been explored so as to potentially improve patient acceptability and convenience. Niosomal studies by

Gupta et al. [35], involved the delivery of vaccines via topical immunisation and compared the use of transfersomes with niosome and liposome systems. The niosomes and liposomes were prepared via reverse phase evaporation technique, yielding LUV and then passed through polycarbonate membranes [35]. Gupta and co-workers employed reverse phase evaporation technique as it is known to produce high encapsulation efficiency of antigens and peptides as previously reported [80]. The immune response was assessed by measuring the serum anti-TT IgG titres after intervals following topical immunisation. Results were compared against a control tetanus toxoid which was administered intramuscularly. The encapsulation efficiency of niosomes was not significantly different to liposomes (~42% for both), as might be expected given the similar physical attributes of the structures. However, the niosome and liposome formulations elicited weak immune responses via a topical route of administration compared to alum-adsorbed tetanus toxoid formulations of the same dose administered intramuscularly [35].

A similar study by Vyas et al. [91] which also comprised of using niosomes for topical immunisation against hepatitis B showed promising results in comparison to liposomes. This study incorporated DNA-encoded hepatitis B surface antigens within the vesicles that were once again prepared by reverse phase evaporation technique [91]. Again the entrapment efficiency between the liposomes and niosomes was similar (49 ± 3 % and 45 ± 3 %, respectively). Naked DNA will undergo hydrolysis by deoxyribonuclease enzymes hence, the encapsulation of the DNA within vesicles protect the DNA from degradation and are taken up by the APCs. Vyas et al. [91] found that the niosome formulations were better carriers for DNA via the topical route compared to liposomes as the surfactants in the niosome formulations can act as penetration enhancers of the skin by reducing the barrier properties [91]. Overall the study showed that the niosomes were able to induce a strong humoural and cellular immune response after the delivery of DNA via the topical route.

Peroral vaccine delivery has also been examined by Rentel et al. [74], where OVA was encapsulated in various lyophilised formulations consisting of esters, cholesterol and DCP. The niosome formulations were then tested in vivo using BALB/c mice where the serum, saliva and intestinal washings were collected and specific antibody titres were generated using ELISA on a time schedule [74]. Results have shown that the OVA formulations encapsulated within Wasag®7 (Sucrose ester surfactant, 7 representing HLB value) niosomes induced significant antibody titres, whereas, the OVA alone and niosomes alone did not exert the same effect. Further studies by Rentel et al. [74], also showed that OVA encapsulated within Wasag®15 (Sucrose ester surfactant, 15 representing HLB value) niosome preparations also did not show significant antibody titres. The differences in HLB values could explain the differences in antibody titre levels; Wasag®15 being the more hydrophilic niosome formulation compared with Wasag®7 niosomes which induced significant antibody titres.

To improve oral delivery, Jain et al. [43] formulated niosomes by reverse phase evaporation; however, coated the vesicles upon formation with *O*-palmitoyl mannan (OPM) to protect the vesicles from degradation within the GIT when

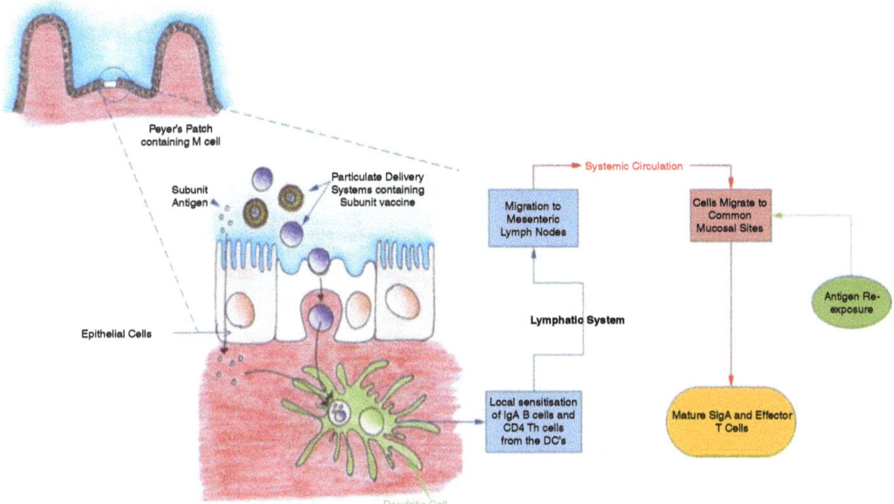

Fig. 11.7 Target site for oral delivery of vesicles and potential mechanism of action

administering orally [43]. After coating, the unbound polysaccharide was removed by one of the removal techniques mentioned previously; centrifugation through a sephadex column. The target sites of the niosomes via the oral route are the M cells within the Peyer's patches along the small intestine within the GIT (Fig. 11.7). M cells are vital in establishing mucosal immunity and allow a route for antigens to be delivered. This route delivers the antigens to underlying lymphoid tissues where a secretory immune response is initiated [23]. Although the mechanism of action upon absorption by the Peyer's patches remains unknown, M cells remain good targets for niosomes/bilosomes and other oral vaccine delivery systems, however, tolerance and mechanisms of uptake still need to be resolved and determined. The results from the Jain et al. [43] study show that the niosomes coated with OPM promoted higher mucosal IgA immune responses compared with uncoated niosomes [43]. Further the OPM-coated niosomes were able to produce both systemic and mucosal immune responses as well as a cellular immune response upon oral delivery.

11.3.3 Further Modification of Niosomes to Enhance Oral Delivery

Given the advantages the oral route offers compared to administration of vaccines via injection it is no surprise this has promoted further modifications of niosomes. The potential of vesicle lysis when administered orally has been the foundation for the development of modified lipid-based vesicles which have increased stability

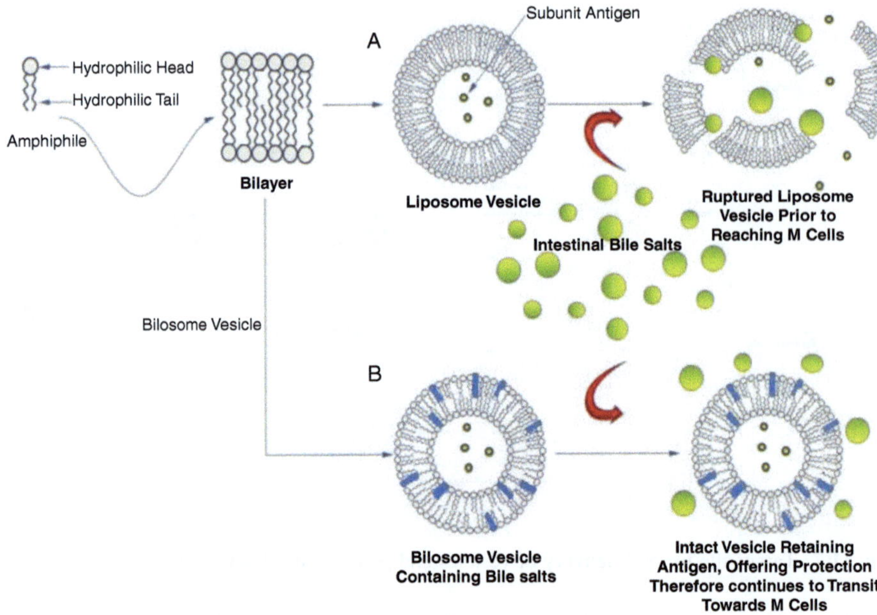

Fig. 11.8 Representation of vesicles containing bile salts showing two pathways where (**a**) is a normal lipid-based vesicle without bile salts which are disrupted by the intestinal bile salts, resulting in degradation and vesicle lysis. (**b**) Pathway represents niosome vesicles with bile salt incorporated into the bilayer structure prior to gastrointestinal exposure results in membrane stability when in the presence of intestinal bile salts

in the form of niosomes. It has been suggested that vesicles allow a greater chance for the antigen/drug to reach the site of action and to have increased absorption through the GIT compared to free antigen/drug [5, 94]. Hence, further modifications to the niosome vesicles are known as bilosomes which are a novel drug delivery system for oral vaccine delivery. Bilosomes intend to protect antigens from the enzymes present in the GIT and the rupturing from the bile acids, and can act as potent immunological adjuvants. Alexander and Brewer first developed and formulated bilosomes by exploiting NISV technology [22]. They achieve this by incorporating bile salts such as sodium deoxycholate into the formulation thereby increasing the stability of the carrier thus, preventing premature release of the protein/antigen via the oral route. Schubert et al. [76] suggest that by incorporating bile salts into the vesicles they resist degradation and disruption from the digestive enzymes (Fig. 11.8) therefore making the formulation more stable and giving the potential rise for an oral route of delivery for vaccines [76]. By preventing premature release, bilosomes deliver the vaccines to the mucosal tissue. Thus, requiring smaller concentrations of antigen to elicit an effective immune response.

Recent studies using bilosomes incorporating several antigens have proven to be successful in various animal models e.g. the A/panama [54], tetanus toxoid [55] and hepatitis B [78]. In the bilosome studies by Bennett et al. [12] and Mann et al. [54–56] the anionic surfactant DCP is again used in the formulation of bilosomes.

These studies all show that, by orally administering the bilosome vesicles with entrapped antigen, a mucosal immune response is elicited with specific IgA production increased. The production of IgA levels suggests that the oral immune response has been successfully initiated as this is one of the steps in the stimulation of a mucosal immune response. As mentioned the incorporation of the DCP lipid within the formulation results in the vesicles having a highly negative surface charge, which could potentially be the reason for such increased levels of immunity achieved from orally dosing the bilosome vesicles. These recent studies confirm previous studies by Tabata and Ikada [82] where they showed that the peak uptake of particles occurs with a zeta potential of −70 mV in the epithelial cells [82]. This is also in line with studies by Norris et al. [67] and Eldridge et al. [28] where they also found that the uptake of negatively charged particulates is favoured [28, 67]. In addition, the work carried out by Shakweh et al. [77] also suggests that negatively charged or neutral particles in mice have a greater affinity for the Peyer's patches than positively charged particles [77]. As a result, various studies carried out on mucosal particulate uptake all stem down to the presence of a negative surface charge. This will allow uptake by the M cells within the Peyer's patches and trigger the dendritic cells and initiate the immune response.

11.4 Summary

Niosomes have evolved over the years from their first appearance in cosmetics to technologies used in the pharmaceutical industry to improve delivery of antigens and drugs to the human body. The incorporation of drugs or antigens into niosomes to enhance their delivery is continually being researched and developments in the field offer promising insight into the future. With the further development of a range of synthetic lipids the ability to draw the classical distinctions between liposomes and niosomes becomes more difficult, particularly given many such niosomes incorporate charged surfactants such as DCP. Niosome studies are comparable to studies carried out with liposomes; however, niosomal formulations are proposed to be more economical and are potentially safe due to the biocompatibility of the surfactants used. The use of cost effective, highly stable surfactants within a formulation continues to offer key advantages in the development of vesicles for drug and vaccine delivery. Furthermore, the ability for these systems to be further customised for particular delivery routes, such as with the development of bilosomes gives them a wider platform of effective use. In terms of niosomes as vaccine adjuvant delivery systems, current work shows a promising future by the immune response elicited via the various routes of administration; however, further exploration is required to potentially bring a niosomal vaccine product to the commercial market.

References

1. Ali MH, Kirby DJ, Mohammed AR, Perrie Y (2010) Solubilisation of drugs within liposomal bilayers: alternatives to cholesterol as a membrane stabilising agent. J Pharm Pharmacol 62 (11):1646–1655
2. Allen TM, Hansen CB, de Menezes DEL (1995) Pharmacokinetics of long-circulating liposomes. Adv Drug Deliv Rev 16(2–3):267–284
3. Almeida J, Edwards DC, Brand C, Heath T (1975) Formation of virosomes from influenza subunits and liposomes. Lancet 306(7941):899–901
4. Arunothayanun P, Uchegbu IF, Craig DQM, Turton JA, Florence AT (1999) In vitro/in vivo characterisation of polyhedral niosomes. Int J Pharm 183(1):57–61
5. Azmin MN, Florence AT, Handjani-Vila RM, Stuart JF, Vanlerberghe G, Whittaker JS (1985) The effect of non-ionic surfactant vesicle (niosome) entrapment on the absorption and distribution of methotrexate in mice. J Pharm Pharmacol 37(4):237–242
6. Baillie AJ, Florence AT, Hume LR, Muirhead GT, Rogerson A (1985) The preparation and properties of niosomes—non-ionic surfactant vesicles. J Pharm Pharmacol 37(12):863–868
7. Bangham AD, Horne RW (1964) Negative staining of phospholipids and their structural modification by surface-active agents as observed in the electron microscope. J Mol Biol 8(5):660-668
8. Barakat HS, Darwish IA, El-Khordagui LK, Khalafallah NM (2009) Development of naftifine hydrochloride alcohol-free niosome gel. Drug Dev Ind Pharm 35(5):631–637
9. Barenholzt Y, Amselem S, Lichtenberg D (1979) A new method for preparation of phospholipid vesicles (liposomes)—French press. FEBS Lett 99(1):210–214
10. Batzri S, Korn ED (1973) Single bilayer liposomes prepared without sonication. Biochim Biophys Acta 298(4):1015–1019
11. Bayindir ZS, Yuksel N (2010) Characterization of niosomes prepared with various nonionic surfactants for paclitaxel oral delivery. J Pharm Sci 99(4):2049–2060
12. Bennett E, Mullen AB, Ferro VA (2009) Translational modifications to improve vaccine efficacy in an oral influenza vaccine. Methods 49(4):322–327
13. Bibi S, Kaur R, Henriksen-Lacey M, McNeil SE, Wilkhu J, Lattmann E, Christensen D, Mohammed AR, Perrie Y (2011) Microscopy imaging of liposomes: from coverslips to environmental SEM. Int J Pharm 417(1–2):138–150
14. Biswal S, Murthy PN, Sahu J, Sahoo P, Amir F (2008) Vesicles of non-ionic surfactants (niosomes) and drug delivery potential. Int J Pharm Sci Nanotechnol 1(1):1–8
15. Bramwell VW, Perrie Y (2005) The rational design of vaccines. Drug Discov Today 10 (22):1527–1534
16. Brewer JM, Alexander J (1992) The adjuvant activity of non-ionic surfactant vesicles (niosomes) on the BALB/c humoral response to bovine serum albumin. Immunology 75 (4):570–575
17. Brewer JM, Alexander J (1994) Studies on the adjuvant activity of non-ionic surfactant vesicles: adjuvant-driven IgG2a production independent of MHC control. Vaccine 12 (7):613–619
18. Brewer JM, Conacher M, Satoskar A, Bluethmann H, Alexander J (1996) In interleukin-4-deficient mice, alum not only generates T helper 1 responses equivalent to Freund's complete adjuvant, but continues to induce T helper 2 cytokine production. Eur J Immunol 26 (9):2062–2066
19. Brewer JM, Roberts CW, Stimson WH, Alexander J (1995) Accurate determination of adjuvant-associated protein or peptide by ninhydrin assay. Vaccine 13(15):1441–1444
20. Carafa M, Santucci E, Alhaique F, Coviello T, Murtas E, Riccieri FM, Lucania G, Torrisi MR (1998) Preparation and properties of new unilamellar non-ionic/ionic surfactant vesicles. Int J Pharm 160(1):51–59
21. Chambers MA, Wright DC, Brisker J, Williams A, Hatch G, Gavier-Widen D, Hall G, Marsh PD, Glyn Hewinson R (2004) A single dose of killed Mycobacterium bovis BCG in a novel

class of adjuvant (Novasome) protects guinea pigs from lethal tuberculosis. Vaccine 22 (8):1063–1071
22. Conacher M, Alexander J, Brewer JM (2001) Oral immunisation with peptide and protein antigens by formulation in lipid vesicles incorporating bile salts (bilosomes). Vaccine 19 (20–22):2965–2974
23. Corr SC, Gahan CCGM, Hill C (2008) M-cells: origin, morphology and role in mucosal immunity and microbial pathogenesis. FEMS Immunol Med Microbiol 52(1):2–12
24. Davidsen J, Rosenkrands I, Christensen D, Vangala A, Kirby D, Perrie Y, Agger EM, Andersen P (2005) Characterization of cationic liposomes based on dimethyldioctadecylammonium and synthetic cord factor from M. tuberculosis (trehalose 6,6′-dibehenate)—a novel adjuvant inducing both strong CMI and antibody responses. Biochim Biophys Acta 1718 (1–2):22–31
25. Deamer D, Bangham AD (1976) Large volume liposomes by an ether vaporization method. Biochim Biophys Acta 443(3):629–634
26. Desjardins R, Krzystyniak K, Thérien H-M, Banska W, Tancrede P, Fournier M (1995) Immunoactivating potential of multilamellar liposome vesicles (MLV) in murine popliteal lymph node (PLN) test. Int J Immunopharmacol 17(5):367–374
27. Devaraj GN, Parakh SR, Devraj R, Apte SS, Rao BR, Rambhau D (2002) Release studies on niosomes containing fatty alcohols as bilayer stabilizers instead of cholesterol. J Colloid Interface Sci 251(2):360–365
28. Eldridge JH, Hammond CJ, Meulbroek JA, Staas JK, Gilley RM, Tice TR (1990) Controlled vaccine release in the gut-associated lymphoid tissues. I. Orally administered biodegradable microspheres target the peyer's patches. J Control Release 11(1–3):205–214
29. Felgner PL, Gadek TR, Holm M, Roman R, Chan HW, Wenz M, Northrop JP, Ringold GM, Danielsen M (1987) Lipofection: a highly efficient, lipid-mediated DNA-transfection procedure. Proc Natl Acad Sci U S A 84(21):7413–7417
30. Freitas C, Müller RH (1998) Effect of light and temperature on zeta potential and physical stability in solid lipid nanoparticle (SLN™) dispersions. Int J Pharm 168(2):221–229
31. González-Rodríguez M, Rabasco A (2011) Charged liposomes as carriers to enhance the permeation through the skin. Expert Opin Drug Deliv 8(7):857–871
32. Gregoriadis G (1990) Immunological adjuvants: a role for liposomes. Immunology Today 11:89–97
33. Gregoriadis G, Leathwood PD, et al (1971) Enzyme entrapment in liposomes. FEBS Letters 14(2):95–99
34. Guinedi AS, Mortada ND, Mansour S, Hathout RM (2005) Preparation and evaluation of reverse-phase evaporation and multilamellar niosomes as ophthalmic carriers of acetazolamide. Int J Pharm 306(1–2):71–82
35. Gupta PN, Mishra V, Rawat A, Dubey P, Mahor S, Jain S, Chatterji DP, Vyas SP (2005) Non-invasive vaccine delivery in transfersomes, niosomes and liposomes: a comparative study. Int J Pharm 293(1–2):73–82
36. Handjani-Vila RM, Ribier A, Rondot B, Vanlerberghie G (1979) Dispersions of lamellar phases of non-ionic lipids in cosmetic products. Int J Cosmet Sci 1(5):303–314
37. Hong M, Zhu S, Jiang Y, Tang G, Pei Y (2009) Efficient tumor targeting of hydroxycamptothecin loaded PEGylated niosomes modified with transferrin. J Control Release 133 (2):96–102
38. Hood E, Gonzalez M, Plaas A, Strom J, VanAuker M (2007) Immuno-targeting of nonionic surfactant vesicles to inflammation. Int J Pharm 339(1–2):222–230
39. Huang Y-Z, Gao J-Q, Chen J-L, Liang W-Q (2006) Cationic liposomes modified with non-ionic surfactants as effective non-viral carrier for gene transfer. Colloids Surf B Biointerfaces 49(2):158–164
40. Israelachvili JN, Mitchell DJ (1975) A model for the packing of lipids in bilayer membranes. Biochim Biophys Acta 389(1):13–19

41. Israelachvili JN, Mitchell DJ, Ninham BW (1977) Theory of self-assembly of lipid bilayers and vesicles. Biochim Biophys Acta 470(2):185–201
42. Jadon P, Gajbhiye V, Jadon R, Gajbhiye K, Ganesh N (2009) Enhanced oral bioavailability of griseofulvin via niosomes. AAPS PharmSciTech 10(4):1186–1192
43. Jain S, Singh P, Mishra V, Vyas SP (2005) Mannosylated niosomes as adjuvant-carrier system for oral genetic immunization against Hepatitis B. Immunol Lett 101(1):41–49
44. Kensil CR (1996) Saponins as vaccine adjuvants. Crit Rev Ther Drug Carrier Syst 13 (1–2):1–55
45. Kirby C, Gregoriadis G (1984) Dehydration-rehydration vesicles: a simple method for high yield drug entrapment in liposomes. Nat Biotechnol 2(11):979–984
46. Konnings S, Copland MJ, Davies NM, Rades T (2002) A method for the incorporation of ovalbumin into immune stimulating complexes prepared by the hydration method. Int J Pharm 241(2):385–389
47. Kruger NJ (2002) The Bradford method for protein quantitation. In: Walker JM (ed) The protein protocols handbook. Humana Press, Totowa, pp 15–21
48. Kumar VV (1991) Complementary molecular shapes and additivity of the packing parameter of lipids. Proc Natl Acad Sci U S A 88(2):444–448
49. Lasic DD (1990) On the thermodynamic stability of liposomes. J Colloid Interface Sci 140 (1):302–304
50. Lasic DD, Martin FJ, Gabizon A, Huang SK, Papahadjopoulos D (1991) Sterically stabilized liposomes: a hypothesis on the molecular origin of the extended circulation times. Biochim Biophys Acta 1070(1):187–192
51. Lendemans DG, Egert AM, Hook S, Rades T (2007) Cage-like complexes formed by DOTAP, Quil-A and cholesterol. Int J Pharm 332(1–2):192–195
52. Lendemans DG, Myschik J, Hook S, Rades T (2005) Cationic cage-like complexes formed by DC-cholesterol, Quil-A, and phospholipid. J Pharm Sci 94(8):1794–1807
53. Lowry OH, Rosebrough NJ, Farr AL, Randall RJ (1951) Protein measurement with the folin phenol reagent. J Biol Chem 193(1):265–275
54. Mann JFS, Ferro VA, Mullen AB, Tetley L, Mullen M, Carter KC, Alexander J, Stimson WH (2004) Optimisation of a lipid based oral delivery system containing A/Panama influenza haemagglutinin. Vaccine 22(19):2425–2429
55. Mann JFS, Scales HE, Shakir E, Alexander J, Carter KC, Mullen AB, Ferro VA (2006) Oral delivery of tetanus toxoid using vesicles containing bile salts (bilosomes) induces significant systemic and mucosal immunity. Methods 38(2):90–95
56. Mann JFS, Shakir E, Carter KC, Mullen AB, Alexander J, Ferro VA (2009) Lipid vesicle size of an oral influenza vaccine delivery vehicle influences the Th1/Th2 bias in the immune response and protection against infection. Vaccine 27(27):3643–3649
57. Manosroi A, Khanrin P, Lohcharoenkal W, Werner RG, Götz F, Manosroi W, Manosroi J (2010) Transdermal absorption enhancement through rat skin of gallidermin loaded in niosomes. Int J Pharm 392(1–2):304–310
58. Manosroi A, Wongtrakul P, Manosroi J, Sakai H, Sugawara F, Yuasa M, Abe M (2003) Characterization of vesicles prepared with various non-ionic surfactants mixed with cholesterol. Colloids Surf B Biointerfaces 30(1–2):129–138
59. Moghaddam B, Ali MH, Wilkhu J, Kirby DJ, Mohammed AR, Zheng Q, Perrie Y (2011) The application of monolayer studies in the understanding of liposomal formulations. Int J Pharm 417(1–2):235–244
60. Mohammed AR, Bramwell VW, Coombes AGA, Perrie Y (2006) Lyophilisation and sterilisation of liposomal vaccines to produce stable and sterile products. Methods 40(1):30–38
61. Mohammed AR, Bramwell VW, Kirby DJ, McNeil SE, Perrie Y (2010) Increased potential of a cationic liposome-based delivery system: enhancing stability and sustained immunological activity in pre-clinical development. Eur J Pharm Biopharm 76(3):404–412

62. Mokhtar M, Sammour OA, Hammad MA, Megrab NA (2008) Effect of some formulation parameters on flurbiprofen encapsulation and release rates of niosomes prepared from proniosomes. Int J Pharm 361(1–2):104–111
63. Mowat MA (2003) Anatomical basis of tolerance and immunity to intestinal antigens. Nature 3:331–341
64. Murdan S, Gregoriadis G, Florence AT (1999) Sorbitan monostearate/polysorbate 20 organogels containing niosomes: a delivery vehicle for antigens? Eur J Pharm Sci 8 (3):177–185
65. New R (1990) Liposomes a practical approach. Oxford University Press, New York, pp 1–32
66. Ning M, Guo Y, Pan H, Yu H, Gu Z (2005) Niosomes with sorbitan monoester as a carrier for vaginal delivery of insulin: studies in rats. Drug Deliv 12(6):399–407
67. Norris DA, Puri N, Sinko PJ (1998) The effect of physical barriers and properties on the oral absorption of particulates. Adv Drug Deliv Rev 34(2–3):135–154
68. Obrenovic MM, Perrie Y, Gregoriadis G (1998) Entrapment of plasmid DNA into niosomes: characterization studies. J Pharm Pharmacol 50(S9):155
69. Okada JI, Cohen S, Langer R (1995) In vitro evaluation of polymerized liposomes as an oral drug delivery system. Pharm Res 12(4):576–582
70. Papahadjopoulos D, Vail WJ, Jacobson K, Poste G (1975) Cochleate lipid cylinders: formation by fusion of unilamellar lipid vesicles. Biochim Biophys Acta 394(3):483–491
71. Perrie Y, Barralet JE, McNeil S, Vangala A (2004) Surfactant vesicle-mediated delivery of DNA vaccines via the subcutaneous route. Int J Pharm 284(1–2):31–41
72. Perrie Y, Obrenovic M, McCarthy D, Gregoriadis G (2002) Liposome (Lipodine™)-mediated DNA vaccination by the oral route. J Liposome Res 12(1–2):185–197
73. Perrie Y, Rades T (2012) FASTtrack: pharmaceutics—drug delivery and targeting. 2nd edn. Pharmaceutical Press, London
74. Rentel CO, Bouwstra JA, Naisbett B, Junginger HE (1999) Niosomes as a novel peroral vaccine delivery system. Int J Pharm 186(2):161–167
75. Sasaki S, Takeshita F, Xin K-Q, Ishii N, Okuda K (2003) Adjuvant formulations and delivery systems for DNA vaccines. Methods 31(3):243–254
76. Schubert R, Jaroni H, Schoelmerich J, Schmidt KH (1983) Studies on the mechanism of bile salt-induced liposomal membrane damage. Digestion 28(3):181–190
77. Shakweh M, Besnard M, Nicolas V, Fattal E (2005) Poly (lactide-co-glycolide) particles of different physicochemical properties and their uptake by peyer's patches in mice. Eur J Pharm Biopharm 61:1–13
78. Shukla A, Katare OP, Singh B, Vyas SP (2010) M-cell targeted delivery of recombinant hepatitis B surface antigen using cholera toxin B subunit conjugated bilosomes. Int J Pharm 385(1–2):47–52
79. Srinivas S, Kumar YA, Hemanth A, Anitha M (2010) Preparation and evaluation of niosomes containing aceclofenac. Digest J Nanomater Biostruct 5(1):249–254
80. Szoka F, Papahadjopoulos D (1978) Procedure for preparation of liposomes with large internal aqueous space and high capture by reverse-phase evaporation. Proc Natl Acad Sci U S A 75 (9):4194–4198
81. Szoka F, Papahadjopoulos D (1980) Comparative properties and methods of preparation of lipid vesicles (liposomes). Annu Rev Biophys Bioeng 9(1):467–508
82. Tabata Y, Ikada Y (1988) Effect of the size and surface charge of polymer microspheres on their phagocytosis by macrophage. Biomaterials 9(4):356–362
83. Taylor KMG, Morris RM (1995) Thermal analysis of phase transition behaviour in liposomes. Thermochim Acta 248:289–301
84. Uchegbu IF, Double JA, Turton JA, Florence AT (1995) Distribution, metabolism and tumoricidal activity of doxorubicin administered in sorbitan monostearate (Span 60) niosomes in the mouse. Pharm Res 12(7):1019–1024

85. Uchegbu IF, Duncan R (1997) Niosomes containing N-(2-hydroxypropyl)methacrylamide copolymer-doxorubicin (PK1): effect of method of preparation and choice of surfactant on niosome characteristics and a preliminary study of body distribution. Int J Pharm 155(1):7–17
86. Uchegbu IF, Florence AT (1995) Non-ionic surfactant vesicles (niosomes): physical and pharmaceutical chemistry. Adv Colloid Interface Sci 58(1):1–55
87. Uchegbu IF, Vyas SP (1998) Non-ionic surfactant based vesicles (niosomes) in drug delivery. Int J Pharm 172(1–2):33–70
88. van Hal DA, Bouwstra JA, van Rensen A, Jeremiasse E, de Vringer T, Junginger HE (1996) Preparation and characterization of nonionic surfactant vesicles. J Colloid Interface Sci 178 (1):263–273
89. Vangala A, Bramwell VW, McNeil S, Christensen D, Agger EM, Perrie Y (2007) Comparison of vesicle based antigen delivery systems for delivery of hepatitis B surface antigen. J Control Release 119(1):102–110
90. Vangala A, Kirby D, Rosenkrands I, Agger EM, Andersen P, Perrie Y (2006) A comparative study of cationic liposome and niosome-based adjuvant systems for protein subunit vaccines: characterisation, environmental scanning electron microscopy and immunisation studies in mice. J Pharm Pharmacol 58(6):787–799
91. Vyas SP, Singh RP, Jain S, Mishra V, Mahor S, Singh P, Gupta PN, Rawat A, Dubey P (2005) Non-ionic surfactant based vesicles (niosomes) for non-invasive topical genetic immunization against hepatitis B. Int J Pharm 296(1–2):80–86
92. Wacker M, Schubert R (1998) From mixed micelles to liposomes: critical steps during detergent removal by membrane dialysis. Int J Pharm 162(1–2):171–175
93. Walker W, Brewer JM, Alexander J (1996) Lipid vesicle-entrapped influenza A antigen modulates the influenza A-specific human antibody response in immune reconstituted SCID-human mice. Eur J Immunol 26(7):1664–1667
94. Yoshida H, Lehr CM, Kok W, Junginger HE, Verhoef JC, Bouwstra JA (1992) Niosomes for oral delivery of peptide drugs. J Control Release 21(1–3):145–153
95. Yoshioka T, Sternberg B, Florence AT (1994) Preparation and properties of vesicles (niosomes) of sorbitan monoesters (Span 20, 40, 60 and 80) and a sorbitan triester (Span 85). Int J Pharm 105(1):1–6

Chapter 12
Immune Stimulating Complexes (ISCOMs) and Quil-A Containing Particulate Formulations as Vaccine Delivery Systems

S. Hook and T. Rades

Abstract Immune stimulating complexes (ISCOMs) belong to the group of particulate vaccine delivery systems. These particles have received considerable attention in the field of vaccine delivery systems, especially for subunit vaccines. ISCOMs have a spherical, open and cage-like structure and a particle size of around 40 nm. They contain an adjuvant (Quil A or QS 21) and an antigen incorporated into or associated with their colloidal structure, making ISCOMs particulate antigen delivery systems which allow co-delivery of antigen and adjuvant. In this chapter we initially describe the components, microstructures and preparation methods of ISCOMs followed by their mechanism of immune stimulation and their use as vaccines.

12.1 Introduction

Immune stimulating complexes (ISCOMs) belong to the group of particulate vaccine delivery systems. ISCOMs typically have a spherical, open and cage-like structure and a particle size of around 40 nm [5]. Figure 12.1 shows an electron micrograph of the appearance of this nanoparticulate vaccine delivery system.

ISCOMs are composed of a mixture of three types of polar lipids, namely a saponin or saponin mixture, cholesterol and phospholipid. Antigen (mostly in form of an amphipathic protein) can be either incorporated into or associated with the structure. Empty ISCOMs, i.e. ISCOMs without an antigen, are termed ISCOM matrix [64]. The saponin, usually Quil A or its purified version QS 21, have adjuvant properties and thus ISCOMs combine antigen and adjuvant in a single colloidal particle [5].

S. Hook (✉)
New Zealand's National School of Pharmacy, University of Otago, Dunedin, New Zealand
e-mail: sarah.hook@otago.ac.nz

D.R. Flower and Y. Perrie (eds.), *Immunomic Discovery of Adjuvants and Candidate Subunit Vaccines*, Immunomics Reviews: 5, DOI 10.1007/978-1-4614-5070-2_12,

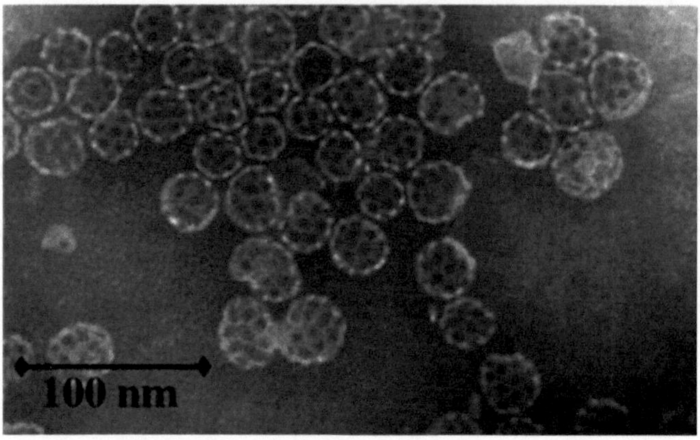

Fig. 12.1 Negative staining transmission electron micrograph of an ISCOM matrix dispersion. Bar represents 100 nm (adapted from Demana et al. [18])

In this chapter we initially discuss the components, structures and preparation methods of ISCOMs followed by their mechanism of immune stimulation and their use as vaccines.

12.2 ISCOM Components

ISCOMs typically consist of antigen and a colloidal structure formed by a combination of three types of polar lipids (saponin, cholesterol and phospholipid) in an aqueous dispersion. Whilst aqueous dispersions of phospholipid and cholesterol typically lead to the formation of liposomes, the addition of the saponin to phospholipid /cholesterol mixtures leads to structural changes on the colloidal level, resulting in a number of predominantly micellar structures, depending on the ratio of the three components and also on the preparation method used [16, 18]. Details on the colloidal structures resulting from the combination of these three polar lipid components in aqueous dispersion, as well as the various preparation methods for ISCOMs will be described in the next sections of this chapter. In this section, information is provided on the components of ISCOMs.

12.2.1 Quillaja Saponins, Quil A and QS 21

Quillaja saponins are isolated by aqueous extraction from the cortex of *Quillaja saponaria* Molina, a South America tree, also known as Soapbark tree or Panama wood [6, 39]. The extract at this stage still contains tannins and polyphenols together with a complex mixture of saponins, and can be further purified by ion-exchange chromatography and gel filtration, into a fractionated extract known as

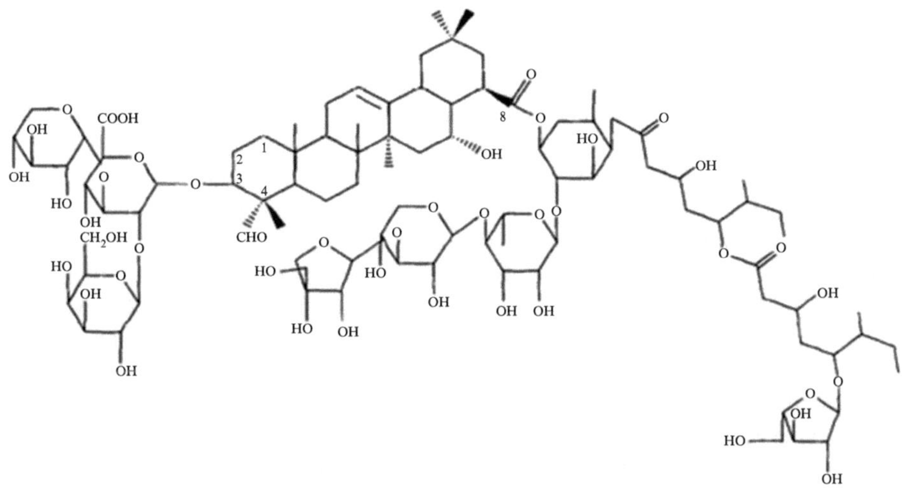

Fig. 12.2 Chemical structure of QS21 (adapted from Soltysik et al. [99])

Quil A [31]. Quil A is typically used to prepare ISCOMs, but is still a heterogeneous saponin mixture and has thus been further fractionated by reversed phase HPLC. This process leads to more than 20 sub-fractions containing more than 60 individual compounds [11, 39]. Some of the sub-fractions (termed QH-A and QH-C) retain their adjuvant activity whilst showing a lower toxicity profile than Quil A (reduced hemolytic activity) [38, 90]. Finally, purification to the level of a single saponin (termed QS21) has been performed [28, 30]. The chemical structure of QS21 is shown in Fig. 12.2 [99].

Chemically, Quillaja saponins are triterpene glycosides. Quillaic acid is the aglycon and sugar moieties are attached to C3 and C28 of the aglycon. The sugar moiety on C3 consists of two or three sugar units (in the case of QS21 these are glucoronic acid, xylose and galactose). Glucoronic acid is present in most of the Quillaja saponins and is responsible for the overall negative charge of the molecules. The sugar chain on C28 of quillaic acid is more variable but usually contains fucose bound to the aglycon (and rhamnose, xylose and apiose, in case of QS21). On C3 or C4 of fucose a further acyl chain may be attached, which in turn, in the case of QS21, is bound to arabinose.

The overall structure of the Quillaja saponins is that of a bisdesmosidic triterpene. These structures are surfactant type molecules, with a hydrophilic (sugars)-lipophilic (aglycon)-hydrophilic (sugars) structure. In fact, Quil A was found to form micelles above its critical micelle concentration (CMC) of 0.03 % [79].

12.2.2 *Cholesterol and Phospholipids*

As stated above, Quillaja saponins (for example in the fractionated form of Quil A) are surfactant type molecules (albeit with a rather unusual structure), forming micelles at concentrations above their CMC. It is thus not surprising that in order to form ISCOM matrix structures, the addition of other polar lipid components is necessary. Usually cholesterol and phospholipids are used together with Quil A to form ISCOM matrices. It has long been known that cholesterol interacts with saponins [25]. Initially, it was thought that the addition of cholesterol to Quil A was sufficient for the production of the ISCOM matrix structure, i.e. that ISCOM matrix structure formation might be possible without phospholipids, whilst phospholipids were thought to be necessary to facilitate the incorporation of antigen into the ISCOM matrix [55]. Kersten et al., however, have stated that both phospholipids and cholesterol are required, for the formation of ISCOMs and ISCOM matrices [41]. Practically all ISCOM and ISCOM matrix preparations in fact contain both cholesterol and phospholipid, albeit at different ratios, depending for example on the preparation method (see below).

As cholesterol is a neutral molecule, and phospholipids (at least the ones used in the preparation of ISCOMs) are zwitter-ionic, the overall ISCOM structure has a negative charge (which reveals itself in form of a negative zeta-potential), due to the negative charge of the carboxylic acid group of the glucoronic acid moiety of the Quillaja saponins at neutral pH conditions. As most antigens are also negatively charged, this may present a problem in loading the ISCOM matrix with the antigen. To improve loading, several attempts have been made to prepare positively charged ISCOM matrices. In principal, two strategies are possible; either to replace (or partly replace) the zwitter-ionic phospholipid with a cationic phospholipid [46], or to replace (or partly replace) cholesterol with a cationic alternative. Partial (Posintro) or complete (Pluscoms) replacement of cholesterol with DC-cholesterol, has led to ISCOM-like structures, either still being negatively charged, but containing positively charged sites (Posintro) [58] or indeed having a positive zeta potential (Pluscoms) [48]. The chemical structures of cholesterol, DC-cholesterol and phosphatidylcholine (a typically used phospholipid in the formation of ISCOMs), are shown in Fig. 12.3.

12.2.3 Antigen

In contrast to liposomes, ISCOMs and the ISCOM matrix are open structures. It is therefore generally not possible, to incorporate a hydrophilic antigen into the ISCOM matrix [65]. Similarly, if an antigen is too lipophilic, incorporation into ISCOM matrices is difficult, due to the inherent nature of these antigens to aggregate in aqueous dispersion [40]. It is thus not surprising, that the majority of antigens that have been incorporated successfully into the ISCOM structure are amphipathic in nature. These include proteins or glyco-proteins anchored in the cell or viral membrane by a hydrophobic transmembrane domain [31]. This transmembrane domain then anchors the antigen in the ISCOM structure.

Interestingly, and perhaps surprisingly, when amphipathic antigens have been incorporated into the ISCOM matrix, the resulting ISCOM is usually

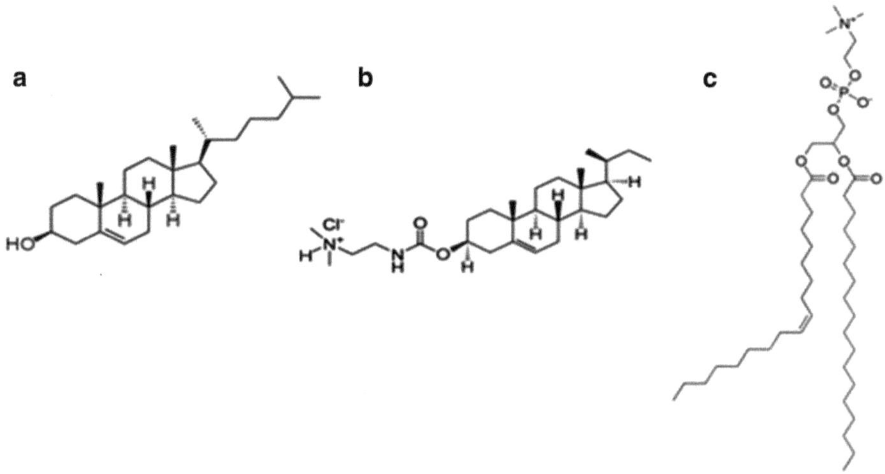

Fig. 12.3 Chemical structures of (a) cholesterol, (b) DC-cholesterol and (c) phosphatidylcholine (a typically used phospholipid in the formation of ISCOMs)

indistinguishable from the matrix, with a similar appearance in the electron microscope and similar sedimentation rates upon ultracentrifugation [4]. This may be a consequence of only a partial incorporation or a low number of antigen molecules actually being incorporated into the ISCOM structure. However, when high levels of influenza hemagglutinin were incorporated into an ISCOM matrix, typical “spikes” of the antigen could be visualised on the surface of these ISCOMs [4].

If the antigen to be incorporated into the ISCOM matrix is not amphipathic, a number of methods may be employed to either expose hydrophobic regions in the antigen or to introduce hydrophobic domains to the antigen. These hydrophobic parts of the antigen can then in turn act as anchoring regions for incorporation of the antigen into the ISCOM structure.

Methods that have been investigated to expose hydrophobic regions in the antigen include acid treatment [65], or the partial denaturation of the protein by urea or mercaptoethanol [1]. Whilst there are examples in the literature of these methods being used to incorporate hydrophilic antigens into the ISOM structure, the ultimate success of these methods will strongly depend on the nature of the antigen itself.

Another way of introducing hydrophilic antigens into an ISCOM structure is the conjugation of the antigen to a preformed ISCOM containing an amphipathic coupling protein [45, 54, 96]. For example, it has been shown that the conjugation of peptides (e.g. LHRH) to ISCOMs containing the influenza virus envelope protein (which is amphipathic and can easily be incorporated into ISCOM matrices) was possible using glutaraldehyde as a coupling agent [54].

Chemical modification of a hydrophilic antigen can also be preformed. For example, the hydrophilic model antigen ovalbumin has been successfully conjugated in a simple reaction with palmitic acid, which was used in form of an activated ester (*N*-hydroxysuccinimide ester of palmitic acid) to bind to the amino groups of the protein [8, 10, 43, 84]. Alternatively, phospholipids may be conjugated to a protein via their amino group to the carboxylic acid group of the protein [21, 36, 97].

Another method to make hydrophilic antigens "suitable" for ISCOM incorporation is the modification of the protein by genetic engineering [2, 86]. For example, the *env* gene of the feline immunodeficiency virus was modified by removing a cleavage site resulting in the expression of a 150 kDa protein, that now contained the intact transmembrane domain [86].

It should be noted that all these approaches change the antigen, and care must be taken to determine if the antigen retains its antigenicity after modification and incorporation into the ISCOM structure.

Finally, if the antigen is anionic in nature, the use of positively charged ISCOMs (Pluscoms) may lead to a high antigen load on the colloidal particles through electrostatic interactions. This has been shown for ovalbumin, in which a high antigen loading onto Pluscoms was achieved, without the need of any chemical or structural modification of the protein [48, 62].

12.3 Preparation Methods

Several methods have been described in the literature to prepare ISCOMs and ISCOM matrices. In this section a brief overview of these methods will be given, together with their advantages and disadvantages. Generally speaking, these methods have devolved from those used to prepare liposomes, with the major difference being that Quil A is added as a saponin adjuvant component to the preparation.

12.3.1 Centrifugation Method

The first method described to prepare ISCOMs is the centrifugation method [31]. In this method viral proteins (antigen) are solubilised in a surfactant together with phospholipid and cholesterol, resulting in a mixed micellar solution. This solution is then centrifuged through a thin layer of an aqueous solution of 10 % sucrose and a nonionic detergent (0.5 % Triton X-100) on top of an aqueous sucrose gradient (20–50 % w/w sucrose) containing Quil A. Upon ultracentrifugation, ISCOMs form a distinct band in the sucrose gradient and can be collected. After removal of the ISCOM band from the sucrose gradient, the collected fraction is again ultracentrifuged, this time through a 20 % sucrose solution to separate the ISCOMs from excess Quil A. The ISCOMs can then be collected as a pellet from the second ultracentrifugation step. Whilst this was the first method described to prepare ISCOMs, it is rarely used today. The method may appear simple, but it is in fact quite tedious due to the preparation of a sucrose gradient and difficulties in collecting the ISCOM band.

12.3.2 Dialysis Method

The dialysis method is the most often used method to prepare ISCOMs and ISCOM matrices [35, 84, 97]. It is essentially a variation of the detergent removal technique utilised to prepare liposomes. In this method Quil A, phospholipid and cholesterol together with the antigen are solubilised in water, with the help of a nonionic surfactant, and the resulting mixed micellar solution is then loaded into a dialysis bag and extensively dialysed against a suitable buffer. Different groups have used different surfactants (mostly octylglycoside and MEGA-10), different starting concentrations of the surfactant, and different molecular weight cut-off membranes and dialysis conditions (time and temperate) [41, 55]. The dialysate is then, as in the centrifugation method, ultracentrifuged through a 20 % sucrose solution to separate the ISCOMs, which will form a pellet, from excess Quil A.

For the formation of ISCOM matrices using the dialysis method mass ratios of Quil A:cholesterol:phospholipid of 6:1:1 may be used, whilst for the preparation of ISCOMs (i.e. antigen containing particles), a mass ratio of 5:1:1 has been reported. The ratio of the three polar lipids to the surfactant used to initially solubilise the ISCOM components has been reported to be approximately 1:7 [41]. However, it should be noted that the successful preparation of ISCOMs and ISCOM matrices depends on many factors, including type and concentration of buffer salts, equilibration time for dialysis, types of phospholipid used (e.g. phosphatidylcholine vs. phosphatidylethanolamine), type of solubilising surfactant (e.g. MEGA 10 vs. octylglycoside), and in case of ISCOMs on the nature and concentration of the antigen. It follows that for each situation the optimal dialysis conditions need to be determined experimentally.

12.3.3 Hydration Method

The hydration method is based on the classical Bangham method to prepare liposomes. In this method the phospholipid and cholesterol are initially dissolved in chloroform and then dried to a thin film in a round bottom flask using a rotary evaporator. The lipid film is then hydrated with an aqueous solution of Quil A (in case of ISCOM matrix formation) or Quil A and antigen in case of an ISCOM preparation [9, 43]. Sometimes the resulting preparation is then freeze dried and redispersed in water [18]. It is believed that the freeze drying step increases the mixing of the components and leads to a more homogenous ISCOM preparation.

The hydration method is simple and fast, with no need for extensive dialysis steps, the use of ultracentrifugation or the addition of solubilising surfactants. However, it was found that formation of ISCOMs based on this method may take considerable time due to slow equilibration of the lipid components after addition of water or buffer. For this reason the freeze drying step was introduced, as after freeze drying equilibration times to form ISCOMs were found to be shorter [18].

It is interesting to note that the formation of ISCOMs by this method was found not to be successful when similar lipid ratios as in the dialysis method were used (6:1:1 Quil A:cholesterol:phospholipid). Rather a 4:1:6 ratio led to the formation of ISCOMs using the hydration method [9, 43]. Whilst the exact reason for this finding is not well understood, it is important, as it indicates that the preparation method used has an influence on the resulting colloidal particles. This further underlines the necessity to optimise ISCOM preparations for any given case.

12.3.4 Injection Method

This method is based on the ethanol injection method to prepare liposomes. Cholesterol and phospholipid are dissolved in ethanol and the resulting solution is then rapidly injected into a stirred, aqueous Quil-A solution [49]. The ethanol injection technique leads to the formation of a high number of ISCOM matrices within 2 h of preparation. This technique appears promising, as it is rapid and requires no additional surfactants. A variation to the ethanol injection method is the ether injection method [82]. Here cholesterol and phospholipids are dissolved in ether, and injected into a Quil A aqueous solution (0.01 M phosphate buffer) at 55 °C to evaporate the ether. Homogenous ISCOM matrix dispersions were produced using a weight ratio of Quil A:cholesterol:phospholipid of 3:2:5 (w/w).

12.3.5 Freeze Drying Method

In this method, ISCOMs, containing a lipopeptide as antigen, were prepared by initially dissolving cholesterol, phospholipid and sugar (sucrose or trehalose) in aqueous *tert*-butanol (1:1 v/v) [52]. The resulting solution was frozen and freeze dried overnight. ISCOMs were then prepared by hydrating the lipid/sugar matrix with an aqueous buffer containing Quil. As with the other methods, homogeneity of the resulting ISCOM dispersions depended on the lipid ratio, but also on the ratio of lipids to sugar. It was also found that less homogenous dispersions were prepared if the Quil A was added to the lipid/sugar mixture before freeze drying.

12.4 ISCOM Structure and Properties

In Fig. 12.1 the typical transmission electron-microscopic appearance of ISCOM particles is shown. They can be described as open, cage-like structures, with a typical size of around 40 nm. We have discussed above that ISCOM matrices are formed by a combination of Quil A (or QS21), cholesterol and phospholipid. Antigen may be inserted into the ISCOM structure by hydrophobic interactions of lipophilic anchoring regions in the antigen with the ISCOM matrix. Alternately, if the antigen is negatively charged (this is true for most antigens), electrostatic binding to a (partially) positively charged ISCOM (Posintro or Pluscoms) may occur. In this section we have a closer look at the microstructure of ISCOMs and of related structures that may be formed using the above mentioned preparative techniques.

The first model proposed to describe the structure of ISCOMs was based on an assembly of spherical subunits (micelles) that come together to form a pentagonal dodecahedron arrangement, exhibiting a two-, three- and five-fold symmetry [79]. The open structure of the ISCOM in this model is therefore a result of gaps between the spherical subunits. In an alternative model, the subunits of the ISCOM structure are believed to be ring-like micelles, that again, though a combination of hydrophobic interactions, electrostatic repulsion, steric factors and hydrogen bonds form the ISCOM structure [41]. Whilst both models interpret the ISCOM structure as an assembly of smaller subunits (spherical or ring-like micelles), in the latter model the open cage-like structure is a consequence of holes in the individual ring-like micelles, rather than a result of gaps between spherical micelles.

Using the hydration method and thus excluding a possible influence of surfactants (that are used in the dialysis or centrifugation methods) that may be included into the ISCOM or in some other ways influence in the ISCOM structure, pseudo-ternary diagrams were established using Quil A, cholesterol and a phospholipid (either phosphatidylcholine or phosphatidylethanolamine) at a total lipid concentration of 6.7 mg/mL in either water or Tris buffer [16, 18]. Using a total of 66 samples per pseudo-ternary diagram, it could be shown that ISCOM matrices are not the only colloidal structure formed by the combination of the three polar lipids. This supported earlier data which reported that certain combinations of Quil A, cholesterol and phospholipid (prepared by the dialysis methods) can form ring-like micellar structures as well as the so-called lamellae structures in the absence of phospholipids, at high and low Quil A to cholesterol ratios, respectively [40, 41].

A typical pseudo-ternary diagram, established by the hydration method is shown in Fig. 12.4.

Depending on the mass ratio of the three polar lipids, a range of colloidal structures were indentified using negative staining transmission electron microscopy. If only Quil A was present (Quil A apex of the pseudo-ternary diagram), Quil A micelles were found as the only colloidal structure. It had previously been reported that Quil A behaves like a typical surfactant, with a CMC of 0.03 %, i.e. below the Quil A concentration in these samples. An electron micrograph of the typical appearance of a Quil A micellar solution is shown in Fig. 12.5.

If phosphatidylcholine was the only lipid in the formulation (phosphatidylcholine apex of the ternary diagram) as expected, lamellar, liposomal structures were found, whereas in the samples only containing cholesterol (cholesterol apex of the ternary diagram) cholesterol crystals dispersed in the aqueous phase was observed.

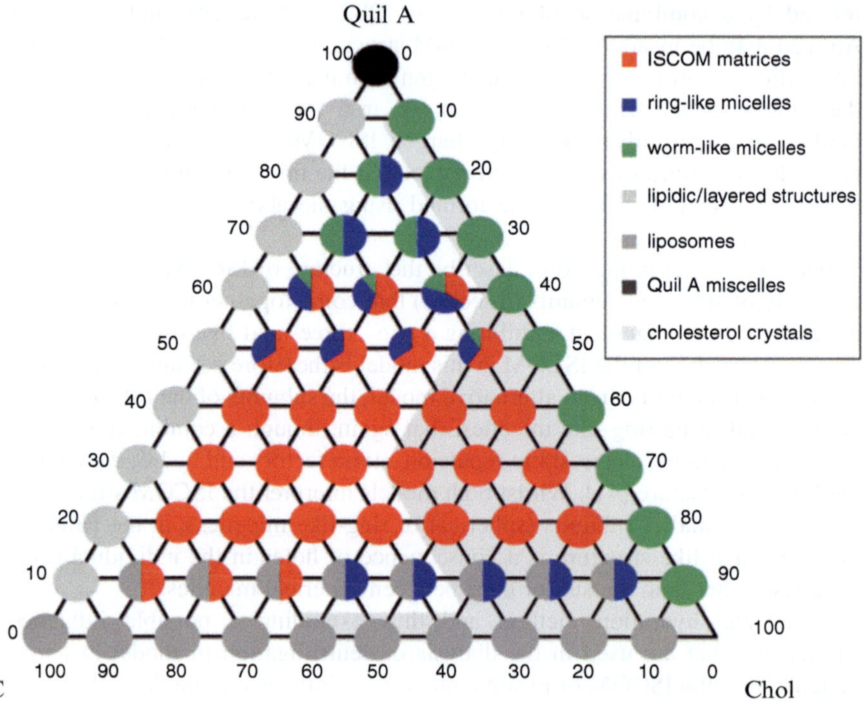

Fig. 12.4 Pseudo-ternary diagram for mixtures of Quil A, cholesterol and phosphatidylcholine hydrated in water and equilibrated for 2 months at 4 °C. Samples were prepared using the hydration method (adapted from Demana et al. [18])

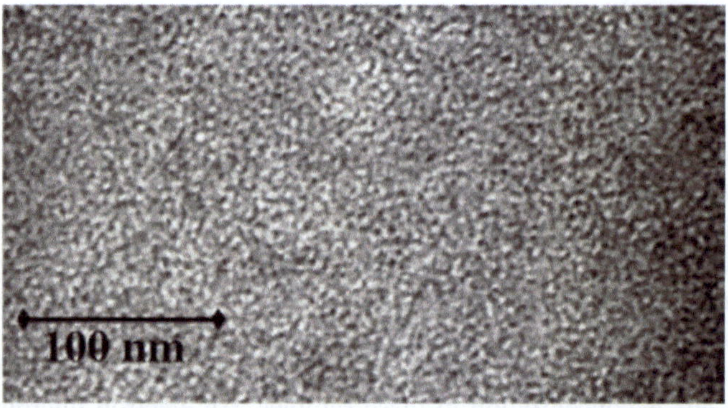

Fig. 12.5 Transmission electron micrograph of a micellar Quil A solution. Samples were prepared by negative staining. The bar represents 100 nm (adapted from Demana et al. [18])

In the pseudo-binary mixtures, liposomal structures were found for phosphatidylcholine/cholesterol systems, whereas layered lipid structures were detected for phosphatidylcholine/Quil A systems, and worm-like micelles for Quil A/cholesterol pseudo-binary mixtures. No ISCOM matrix formation was observed in any of

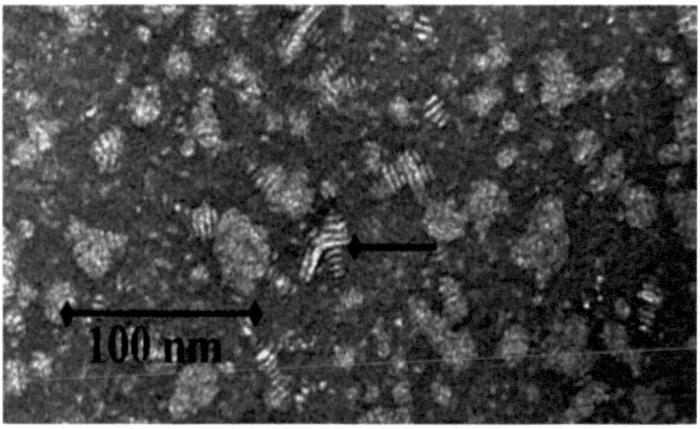

Fig. 12.6 Transmission electron micrograph of layered lipid structures formed from pseudo-binary mixture of Quil A and cholesterol. Samples were prepared by negative staining. The bar represents 100 nm (adapted from Demana et al. [18])

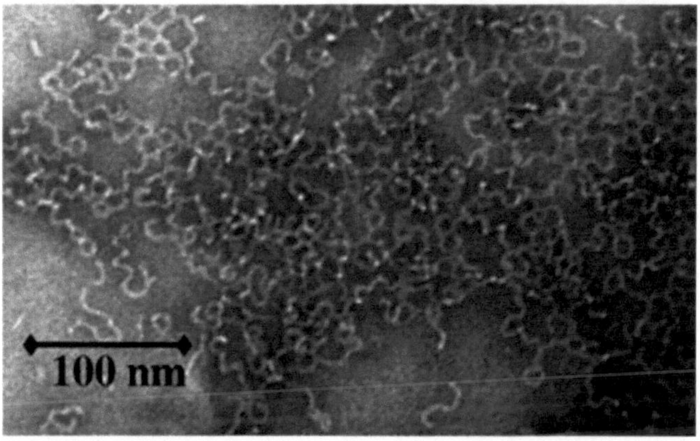

Fig. 12.7 Transmission electron micrograph of worm-like micelles formed from pseudo-binary mixture of Quil A and phospholipid. Samples were prepared by negative staining. The bar represents 100 nm (adapted from Demana et al. [18])

the binary combinations. An electron micrograph of the typical appearance of a layered lipid structures is shown in Fig. 12.6. Figure 12.7 shows the typical appearance of worm-like micelles.

The largest area in the pseudo-ternary diagram (after an equilibration time of 2 months) was indeed occupied by samples containing either exclusively or predominantly ISCOM matrix structures (see Fig. 12.1). However, immediately after preparation the ISCOM matrix area in the pseudo-ternary diagram was much smaller, and predominantly ring-like micelles were found (Fig. 12.8).

Even after prolonged equilibration times, many samples did contain several minor colloidal structures including lamellae structures (Fig. 12.9) and helical structures (Fig. 12.10) together with predominantly ISCOM matrices.

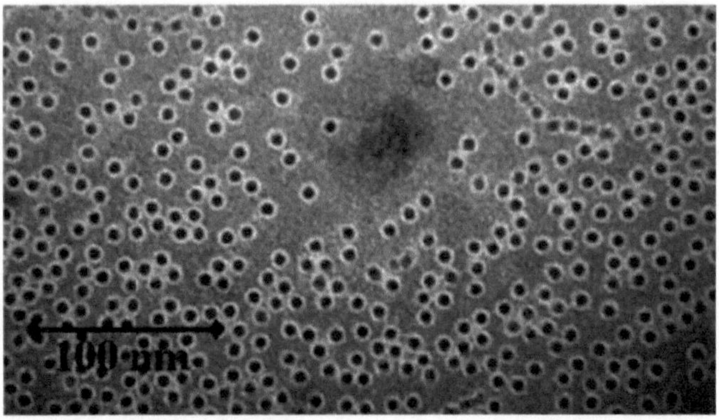

Fig. 12.8 Transmission electron micrograph of ring-like micelles formed from pseudo-ternary mixtures of Quil A, cholesterol and phospholipid. Samples were prepared by negative staining. The bar represents 100 nm (adapted from Demana et al. [18])

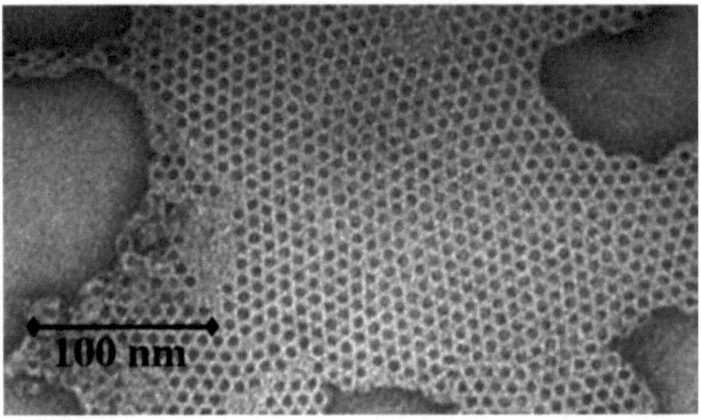

Fig. 12.9 Transmission electron micrograph of lamellae structures formed from pseudo-ternary mixtures of Quil A, cholesterol and phospholipid. These structures were present as minor structures in predominantly ISCOM containing samples. Samples were prepared by negative staining. The bar represents 100 nm (adapted from Demana et al. [18])

The above reported microscopic findings suggest that ISCOM matrices may have formed over time by the association of ring-like micelles into the typical ISCOM matrix structure but also that this process may take some time, at least if the preparation is made by the hydration method. In fact associations of ring-like micelles that may be regarded as a precursor for ISCOM matrix formation were frequently detected in the samples (Fig. 12.11).

Upon addition of Quil A to liposomal structures formed from phospholipid/cholesterol aqueous dispersions, microscopic evidence was also found for a direct conversion of lamellar vesicles to ISCOMs (Fig. 12.12).

At higher Quil A concentrations (towards the Quil A apex of the pseudo-ternary diagram), even after equilibration, predominantly ring- and worm-like micelles

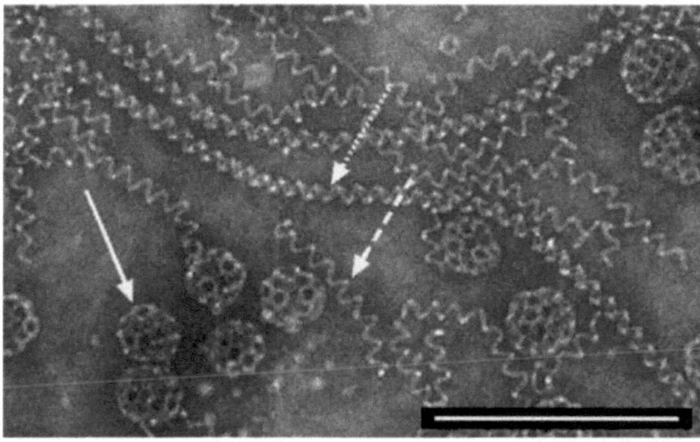

Fig. 12.10 Transmission electron micrograph of helical micelles formed from pseudo-ternary mixtures of Quil A, cholesterol and phospholipid. Samples were prepared by negative staining. These structures were present as minor structures in predominantly ISCOM containing samples. The *solid arrow* shows ISCOM particles, the *dashed arrow* shows a helical micelle and the *dotted arrow* shows helical micelles forming a double helix. The bar represents 100 nm (adapted from Myschik et al. [71])

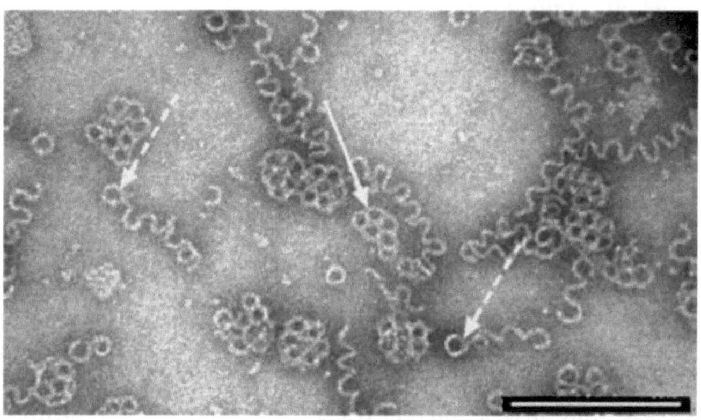

Fig. 12.11 Transmission electron micrograph of partially associated ring-like micelles formed from pseudo-ternary mixtures of Quil A, cholesterol and phospholipid (*solid arrow*). *Dashed arrows* show worm-like micelles possibly forming ring-like micelles. Samples were prepared by negative staining. The bar represents 100 nm (adapted from Myschik et al. [71])

were found. Interestingly, at low Quil A concentrations (below 5 %), many samples still showed liposomal structures, indicating that Quil A to a small extent can be incorporated into liposomes, without changing the colloidal structure of the vesicles.

All of the colloidal structures, described above were also found if similar preparations were prepared in the presence of ovalbumin, conjugated with either palmitic acid or phospholipid, which had previously been shown to be easily

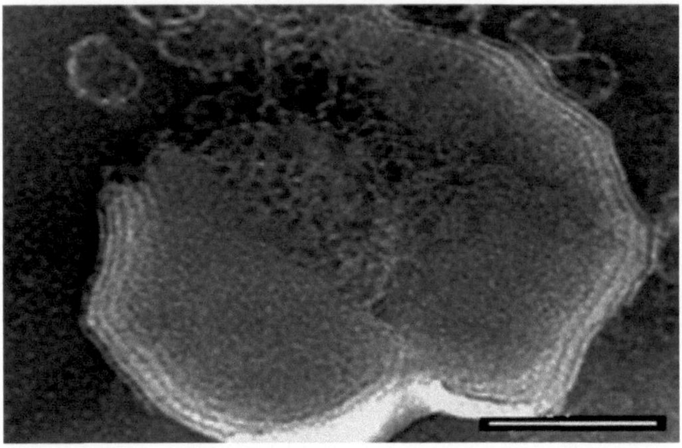

Fig. 12.12 Transmission electron micrograph of liposomal structures and micelles formed from pseudo-binary mixtures of phospholipid and cholesterol after the addition of aqueous Quil A solution. The budding off of ISCOM matrices from the vesicles is shown. Samples were prepared by negative staining. The bar represents 100 nm (adapted from Myschik et al. [71])

incorporated into the colloidal structures formed. It may therefore be concluded that these structures are present not only in ISCOM matrix but also in ISCOM preparations.

From the above findings it can be concluded that ISCOM matrix and ISCOM structures are the most stable forms of colloidal structures formed from most pseudo-ternary systems of Quil A, cholesterol and phospholipids. In fact, these systems have been found to be remarkably stable, for time periods of over a year [66]. ISCOM dispersions can also be freeze-dried and reconstituted again to form ISCOM structures [17]. Also slow release systems have been prepared, for example by freeze drying an ISCOM dispersion (containing FITC-labelled palmitified ovalbumin as a model antigen), and mixing the resulting solid with excess cholesterol. Upon rehydration, these systems slowly release ISCOMs still containing the antigen [17].

Since ISCOMs contain a surfactant (Quil A or QS21), the question arises what happens to these systems upon dilution. It could be shown that upon dilution of ISCOM matrix dispersions in vitro to concentrations below the CMC of Quil A, the ISCOM matrix structures lose the saponin, and the remaining cholesterol and phospholipid form liposomal structures instead [47]. This is perhaps not surprising, but is poses questions as to the fate of ISCOMs in vivo, where such dilution may occur or in vitro if freeze dried preparations are diluted in saline before injection. To our knowledge no in vivo studies have been carried out to examine the colloidal structures in vivo, resulting for example after the injection of ISCOM dispersions.

12.5 Mechanism of Immune Stimulation

ISCOMs act as vaccine adjuvants due both to their nature as a particulate delivery system (PDS) and also due to the presence of Quil A, which has excellent immunostimulatory properties. How PDSs and Quil A activate the immune system is reviewed in this section.

12.5.1 Particulate Delivery Systems

For many years the only vaccine delivery system available for use in humans was alum. Recently, however, a number of new delivery systems have been licensed for use in humans and many others are undergoing clinical testing [61]. Many of these new systems are particulate in nature. PDSs have numerous advantages over solution-based systems [73]. The first of these is the ability to protect vaccine antigens from degradation. The association of peptides and proteins with PDS can provide protection from enzymatic, chemical and physical degradation. It additionally raises the possibility of needle-free delivery, for example orally delivered ISCOMs have been shown to maintain immunogenicity and to be able to induce both systemic and local immune responses [24].

PDS have also been shown to enhance uptake by antigen-presenting cells (APCs). In the case of ISCOMs it has been suggested that the presence of the saponin may facilitate uptake via DEC-205 [80], however no data supporting this has been reported. Antigen uptake can also occur naturally due to the particulate nature of ISCOMs or may be further enhanced, for example through the addition of targeting ligands or by introducing a positive surface charge (Pluscoms [62], Posintro [58]).

A more recently suggested potential mechanism by which PDS can activate APC is inspiring increasing interest. The innate immune system utilises a range of conserved pattern recognition receptors (PRRs) to detect infection and cellular insult. These PRR include the toll-like receptors (TLRs), nucleotide-binding oligomerisation domain (NOD)-like receptors (NLRs) and others [108]. The NLR family pyrin domain-containing 3 (NLRP3 or NALP3) inflammasome is a cytoplasmic protein complex containing NLR3. NLRP3 can mediate inflammatory immune responses through the activation of caspase-1 and the subsequent processing and release of interleukin-1β (IL-1β) and IL-18 [60]. A number of different NLRP3 inflammasome activators have been proposed including microorganisms, endogenous danger signals and environmental irritants [101]. The activation of the inflammasome by vaccine delivery systems was first reported by Li et al. [51]. They found that PDS and adjuvants such as alum, Quil A and chitosan induced inflammasome activation in an NLRP3-dependent manner. They suggested this may be a common mechanism of action for all PDS. This hypothesis was further investigated by Demento et al. who looked at inflammasome activation by poly(lactic-co-glycolic acid) (PLGA) nanoparticles. However they found that the nanoparticles by themselves were unable to activate the inflammasome and that the presence of a TLR ligand was necessary for activation [19]. Therefore ISCOMs which comprise both a PDS and a strong adjuvant, have great potential to access this pathway and more research needs to be done to explore this definitively.

12.5.2 Quil A

Quil A can be classified as a TLR-independent adjuvant [14]. TLRs are a type of PRR expressed by APC [63] and TLR-dependent adjuvants are a diverse group of molecules, mostly isolated or based on molecules from pathogenic microorganisms. Many of these are strong adjuvants and are undergoing pre-clinical and clinical testing for inclusion into vaccines [61]. Quil A has not been shown to interact with any known TLR [20]. However APC activation by ISCOMs and Quil A has been demonstrated both in vitro [15, 87] and in vivo [98]. ISCOMs have been shown to upregulate the expression of co-stimulatory molecules [15, 87, 105] and induce the production of inflammatory cytokines [98, 105] resulting in both T cell (predominantly Th1) and B cell activation and antibody production (reviewed in Sjölander et al. [95]). Of particular interest are the strong CD8 immune responses generated following immunisation with ISCOMs or Quil A-based formulations [59, 91]. CD8 immune responses are crucial for protection against intracellular pathogens and for killing transformed cells. These responses are often difficult to generate with non-replicative vaccines as they require escape or transfer of vaccine antigens from the endosome into the cytoplasm and then presentation on MHC class I. It has been shown that for ISCOMs the transfer of antigen into the MHC class I presentation pathway is through a proteosome-independent pathway [93].

An additional mechanism by which Quil A and ISCOMs may induce immune activation is through the formation of intercellular Schiff bases. It has been proposed that the triterpene aldehyde (see Fig. 12.2) may form a Schiff base with a cellular free amino group and thereby stabilise APC-T cell interactions [85]. Indeed this aldehyde group has been shown to be necessary for the adjuvant activity of QS-21, although direct evidence for Schiff base stabilisation has not been reported [99].

Cell lysis can be considered to be both a mechanism by which saponins such as Quil A induce acute inflammation and therefore immune activation, and an unwanted toxicity. The use of Quil A and QS-21 as vaccine adjuvants has been limited due to the occurrence of, sometimes severe, injection site reactions [37]. It has been proposed that the injection site pain is likely due to cell lysis [106]. The goal therefore must to be to balance the immune activation effects with a level of acceptable toxicity.

Saponins are able to insert into and destroy the integrity of cell membranes [25]. The lytic activity of saponins has been attributed to both the affinity of the aglycon group to cell membrane cholesterol [25, 94] and to the fatty acid moiety, with deactylated saponins being reported to be less lytic and have reduced mouse lethality [76]. Modification of the glycosidic moieties has also been shown to impact on lytic activity and the influence of the size, number, location and type of sugars present in the saponin has been examined [89]. Therefore while it appears that by modifying multiple individual components of saponins the lytic activity may be ameliorated, it is likely due to an impact on how the molecule associates conformationally with the cell membrane, in particular cholesterol, and this may impact on adjuvant activity [99].

However there is evidence that formulation approaches which reduce lysis can decrease injection pain while maintaining the adjuvant activity [106]. Approaches investigated have included the addition of excipients such as benzyl alcohol, cyclodextrin and polysorbate 80 [106] or the incorporation of the saponin into colloidal structures such as ISCOMs [67] or liposomes [53, 107].

12.6 Use as a Vaccine

12.6.1 Pre-clinical Studies

There is an extensive amount of literature on pre-clinical studies investigating the use of ISCOMs and Quil A containing formulations for vaccination (reviewed in Sanders et al. [92]). A number of slightly different approaches have been utilised, generally with the aim of overcoming issues with antigen incorporation into ISCOMs and of reducing cell lysis. The lipophilic nature of ISCOMs means that antigens with lipidic moieties, such as cell membrane antigens or lipid-modified antigens [34], are readily incorporated into the ISCOM matrix. Such vaccines have been shown to be able to induce strong cellular and humoral immune responses. However as ISCOMs have an open, cage-like structure, incorporation of hydrophilic antigens can be problematic. As discussed above, a number of approaches have been investigated to deal with this issue, one being to introduce a positive charge to the particles and thereby attach antigen through charge–charge interactions. Positively charged ISCOM particles are able to be efficiently loaded with antigen and can stimulate both cellular and humoral immune responses [62].

Another approach is to not to attempt to attach or load antigen onto the ISCOM, but to simply co-administer the antigen and ISCOM matrices. This approach has been pursued by CSL Behring (ISCOMATRIX®) and also by ISCONOVA who have developed a range of ISCOM-based adjuvants, the Matrix M™ (adjuvant for human vaccines) and AbISCO® (research reagent) adjuvants. ISCOMATRIX® vaccines have been extensively investigated in preclinical studies and have now progressed into the clinic. One of the most studied vaccines is the NY-ESO-1 ISCOMATRIX® therapeutic cancer vaccine. The vaccine is prepared by mixing recombinant NY-ESO-1 protein with ISCOMATRIX® in solution. A physical association of the two components was demonstrated by flow cytometry [59]. Interestingly, the addition of the protein caused clumping of the 40 nm particles into 1–2 μm aggregates. The authors suggest this is due to cationic residues of the protein cross-linking the anionic ISCOMATRIX®. The vaccine was efficiently taken up by APC in vitro but induced only modest maturation of the cells. However in vivo both CD8 and CD4 responses were induced and mice were protected in a tumour challenge experiment. The aggregation of the vaccine into the large antigen-adjuvant complexes is noteworthy as one of the proposed advantages of ISCOMs for vaccine delivery is the presence of the 40 nm particles reminiscent of virus particles and the size and geometry of particles has been suggested to play an important role in the development of immunity [3]. It has been proposed that particles in the nanometre size range will induce more potent immune responses as they can traffic through the lymphatics to lymph nodes and then interact directly with B cells and dendritic cells (DCs) in the lymph node. The ISCONOVA adjuvants are described as saponin cage complexes formed from specific mixtures of phospholipid, cholesterol and fractionated Quillaja saponins [83]. These complexes are then mixed with vaccine antigens. Although no data has been presented on the size of any particles in the resulting formulation it is likely, that as with the ISCOMATRIX formulations, aggregation occurs to some extent. In mice the administration of Matrix-M-adjuvanted vaccines intramuscularly resulted in the induction of both cellular (CD4 and CD8) and humoral responses and the amount of antigen required to induce protective immunity could be reduced [56, 83]. The AbISCO-100 adjuvant, which is designed for use in saponin-sensitive species [33], has similarly been used in vaccines in mice and rhesus macaques to induce strong cellular and humoral immune responses [12, 100, 109]. When immune responses generated following the subcutaneous injection of a *Chlamydia trachomatis* vaccine formulated with either AbISCO-100, DDA/TDB (dimethyldioctadecylammonium bromide, D-(+)-trehalose 6,6′-dibehenate) or CpG were examined, it was found that the CpG vaccine did not provide any protection against a vaginal challenge, AbISCO-100 provided moderate protection and the DDA/TDB vaccine provided the best protection. This was correlated with strong IFN-γ, TNF-α and IL-17 responses [109].

An alternative to ISCOM-like vaccines is to incorporate Quillaja saponins or fractionate saponins (Quil A or QS 21) into other PDSs. An attractive option is to simply decrease the amount of saponin added to phospholipid (±cholesterol) such that liposomes are formed instead of ISCOMs (as described above).

Liposomes containing 1–5 % saponin are still highly immunogenic, stimulating both cellular and humoral responses, and have the advantage that they will have an intact lipid bilayer and an internal aqueous core into which hydrophilic antigens can be loaded using a lipid film hydration process [53, 107]. Including additional adjuvants such as TLR agonists may induce a synergistic effect and further boost immune responses. Inclusion of the TLR 9 agonist CpG DNA with ISCOM vaccination has been shown to boost anti-tumour immune responses [34]. GSK has developed a number of saponin-based delivery systems. AS01 and AS15 are liposome formulations containing QS-21 and the TLR 2 and TLR 9 agonists monophosphoryl lipid A (MPL, AS01 and AS15) and CpG DNA (AS15). The AS02 formulation is an oil-in-water emulsion also containing QS-21 and MPL [7]. A head-to-head comparison of AS01B- and AS02A-adjuvanted malaria vaccines (recombinant FMP011 mixed with liquid adjuvant) in three inbred strains of mice found that both vaccines stimulated protective immune responses in two of the tested mouse strains. While the antibody responses were very similar, the liposome formulation (AS01) appeared to stimulate superior IFNγ responses [7]. Unfortunately there was no characterisation carried out on the vaccine formulations so the size of the liposomes and if there was any association of vaccine antigen with the liposomes is unknown. Antigen is unlikely to have been loaded into the liposomes to any great extent as a solution of liposomes was simply mixed with an antigen solution. Researchers wishing to utilise the excellent adjuvant activity of Quil A have incorporated it into a variety of other PDS, for example silica nanoparticles [26] and cubosomes (manuscript in preparation).

There is also the potential for generating the sustained or controlled release of ISCOM-based vaccines. This approach has been investigated in an attempt to circumvent the need for booster immunisations. ISCOMs or Quil A-containing PDS has been incorporated into chitosan [27] and alginate [36] formulations, emulsified in Freund's incomplete adjuvant [36] or formulated as sustained release lipids implants [70, 72]. Immune responses generated by these sustained release formulations were found to have both similarities and differences to those generated by repeated injection of immediate release formulations. These differences were not necessarily detrimental but highlight the need for further research in this area.

While the majority of studies have investigated the ability of ISCOMs to stimulate immune responses following either subcutaneous or intramuscular injection, the potential use of this delivery system for needle-free delivery by the oral, intranasal and transcutaneous routes has also been examined. Transcutaneous delivery is an exciting option as positively charged ISCOMs were able to enhance the penetration of small lipophilic molecules through the skin [57]. Interestingly all the individual components (Quil A, phospholipid and DC-cholesterol) in isolation were able to increase penetration raising the possibility that anionic ISCOMs may also be useful for transcutaneous immunisation. Intranasal vaccination has been investigated with a Matrix-M/DNA *Haemophilus influenzae* vaccine [42], an ISCOM/Hepatitis B surface antigen vaccine [80] and an ISCOMATRIX/H1N1 (flu-ISCOM) protein influenza vaccine [91] with the aim of stimulating local protective mucosal immunity in the lungs. The Matrix-M *H. influenza* vaccine recruited and activated DC, promoted Th1 activation and sIgA production resulting in increased clearance of *H. influenza* for up to 4 months. Hepatitis B surface antigen is a good candidate for ISCOM-based immunisation as it has transmembrane domains that will facilitate incorporation into ISCOM particles during vaccine formulation. Cellular and mucosal responses (sIgA) were again stimulated, however high doses of antigen (20 μg) were required. Similar results were seen in the influenza model where intranasal immunisation with the flu-ISCOM vaccine provided full protection to a lethal challenge with the homotypic H1N1 virus and some cross protection to heterotypic H2N2 or H3N2 viruses.

The ultimate goal for many vaccine researchers would be an oral vaccine. Mowat et al. examined the potential for ISCOM-based vaccines to stimulate both local and systemic immunity in mice using palmitified ovalbumin as a model antigen [69]. They found that mice fed reasonably large quantities of ovalbumin ISCOMs (300–600 μg ovalbumin) developed antigen-specific intestinal sIgA responses as well as systemic cytotoxic CD8 immune responses with no evidence of tolerance induction. These results are very promising and the amount of antigen required could perhaps be reduced through the use of an enteric-coated formulation to provide protection during transit through the stomach. Subsequent studies have investigated the ability of orally delivered ISCOMs to stimulate immune response to a number of different antigens. A study investigating the immune response to a rotavirus VLP-ISCOM vaccine (antigen was adsorbed onto ISCOMs) in gnotobiotic pigs found that although the virus was antigenic, it did not protect against challenge. However when it was used as a boost after priming with attenuated vaccine, protection was seen [32].

12.6.2 Veterinary Use

ISCOM-based vaccines were initially used in animals because of concerns over local injection site reactions due to saponin toxicity. It is only in recent years that human vaccines have been developed. Several companies have ISCOM or Quil A-based products on the market including ISCONOVA and Pfizer. ISCONOVA has utilised its range of Matrix™ adjuvants in vaccines to protect against equine influenza (Equilis©, Prequenza and Equip©), kennel cough caused by *Bordetella bronchiseptica* (Canvac CCi©), bovine viral diarrhoea (Pestigard©) and have developed a gonadotropin releasing factor vaccine to control oestrus in horses (Equity). Pfizer has the PreZent™-A adjuvant in which Quil A/cholesterol helices are combined with antigen in an oil formulation [81]. The reason for forming Quil A/cholesterol helices was to reduce toxicity. The adjuvant is used in the CattleMaster®GOLD™ bovine viral diarrhoea vaccine.

12.6.3 Human Use

ISCOM-based vaccines have entered clinical trials for a range of indications, however much effort has been focused on therapeutic cancer vaccines and prophylactic HIV, influenza and malaria vaccines. These are diseases where the ability of Quil A-based vaccines to stimulate cytotoxic CD8 immune responses will be most beneficial. The ISCOM adjuvants predominantly being utilised are the ISCOMATRIX and AS01/AS02/AS15 adjuvants. Initial Phase I safety data has demonstrated the saponin vaccines to be safe and in general well tolerated with injection site pain being the most common adverse event reported [13, 75]. These studies also demonstrated evidence of immune stimulation leading to the establishment of several Phase II and III studies (Table 12.1). In the area of therapeutic

Table 12.1 ISCOM and Quil-A vaccine clinical trials

Vaccine	Trial sponsor	Study details	Outcome	References
Melanoma, NY-ESO-1 ISCOMATRIX ± low dose cyclophosphamide	Ludwig Institute for Cancer Research	Phase I (completed), Phase II (2003–2011)—advanced melanoma patients	Initial results of Phase II were not promising, study was amended to include low dose cyclophosphamide (results pending)	[74]
Various cancers—peptide/protein antigens + AS02B or AS15	GSK	Phase I/II/III, cancer-various	Promising results large clinical trials ongoing	[44, 104]
Malaria, various antigens + AS01 or AS02	GSK	Phase I and II	Promising results with sustained protective immune responses generated	[77]
HIV, gp120/NefTat + AS01 or AS02	GSK	Phase I	AS01 responses most promising	[50]
Influenza, Flu-ISCOM and Flu-ISCOMATRIX	University of Massachusetts Medical School	Healthy adult volunteers	More CTL responses in Flu-ISCOM and Flu-ISCOMATRIX® groups	[22]
Influenza, PANFLUVAC, H5N1 virosome ISCOM	University of Bergen	Phase I, healthy adults	Still recruiting	–
Alzheimer's disease, V950 ISCOMATRIX	Merck	Phase I, Alzheimer's patients	Ongoing, recruitment completed	–
Alzheimer's disease, AC-001 QS-21	Pfizer	Multiple trials, Phase II, Alzheimer's patients	Still recruiting	–

cancer vaccines, the Ludwig Institute for Cancer Research has been leading the way carrying out mechanistic studies in conjunction with clinical trials on an NY-ESO-1 ISCOMATRIX® vaccine for the treatment of melanoma. In the initial double-blind placebo-controlled dose escalation clinical trial, all patients receiving the ISCOMATRIX® adjuvanted vaccine (three intramuscular immunisations at 4-weekly intervals) developed immune responses including antibody, CD4 and CD8 reactivity [13]. It was also observed that patients receiving the ISCOMATRIX® vaccine appeared to relapse less frequently. In this initial study patients were not randomised and had minimal residual disease following tumour resection. In the current open label Phase II study of patients with advance metastatic disease, although antibody responses were once again generated, the cellular responses were much reduced and no clinical responses were seen [74]. Interestingly the patients with advanced disease had higher numbers of circulating regulatory T cells and the trial has now been modified to include treatment with low dose cyclophosphamide in an attempt to selectively remove these cells [74]. The GSK Quil A-containing adjuvants have been used in a number of cancer clinical trials with the AS15 adjuvant (containing QS-21, MPL and CpG) being specifically designed to stimulate anti-tumour immune responses. Treatment of cancer patients with the AS15 vaccine has resulted in the development of antigen-specific immune responses and clinical anti-tumour responses [44, 104]. Further clinical trials are now being carried out including a large Phase III non-small cell lung cancer trial—the MAGRIT study [102].

The GSK Quil A adjuvants are also being tested (Phase I and II) as prophylactic vaccines for a number of infections including malaria and HIV. One of the most promising malaria vaccines, RTS,S/AS01E, demonstrated efficacy for 15 months in children from Kenya and Tanzania in a randomised controlled trial [77]. This vaccine is now going into Phase III trials in seven African countries. A comparison of AS01 and AS02 adjuvants was carried out for an HIV gp120/NefTat vaccine with the AS01-adjuvanted vaccine inducing the most promising response [50]. A number of phase I trials have been carried out using QS-21 alone as an adjuvant for HIV vaccines and while antigen-specific immune responses were generated there were significant local toxicities and these vaccines have not progressed to larger trials [23].

Novel influenza vaccines are always of interest due to the requirement for annual immunisations to provide protection against this constantly mutating virus. ISCOM-based vaccines have been examined for their ability to stimulate long-lived and cross-reactive CD8 responses in the hope of developing vaccines that can provide protections against the different seasonal and pandemic influenza strains. A randomised double-blind controlled clinical study in which a conventional inactivated influenza vaccine was either mixed with ISCOMATRIX or formulated as ISCOMs found more CTL responses in individuals given the ISCOM-formulated vaccines as opposed to the ISCOMATRIX-mixed vaccines. Both responses were superior to those seen in volunteers given non-adjuvanted vaccines [22]. A number of clinical trials are also underway for pandemic influenza vaccines, one such study (still in the recruitment phase) initiated by the University of Bergen utilises virosomal H5N1 in combination with an ISCOM adjuvant. The ability of this vaccine to elicit long-lived and cross-reactive immunity will be assessed.

Finally, ISCOM- and QS-21-adjuvanted vaccines have been investigated in clinical trials for the treatment of Alzheimer's Disease (AD). This is an interesting application as in this situation the desired immune response is not a cellular response but an antibody response to the amyloid-β peptide which then reduces pathology by a number proposed mechanisms including clearance of the aggregates by opsonisation and phagocytosis [68]. In this situation cellular responses may induce toxicity and unfortunately a phase IIa trial using the amyloid-β peptide AN1792 plus QS-21 was halted due to the development of inflammatory reactions in the CNS [78]. It has been debated that the adverse immune reaction was more likely due to the choice of antigen as opposed to the choice of adjuvant [103] and Wyeth has initiated another clinical trial using QS-21 as the adjuvant for a short peptide which should not stimulate an unwanted cellular autoimmune response [88]. Merck is also sponsoring an AD Phase I dose escalation trial in which the safety, tolerability and immunogenicity of an N-terminal amyloid-β peptide given with or without an ISCOMATRIX adjuvant will be assessed [29].

12.7 Summary

In this chapter we have reviewed the components, structures and preparation methods of ISCOM and Quil A-containing particulate vaccines as well as their mechanism of immune stimulation and their use as vaccines. Overall, the use of ISCOMs, ISCOM matrices or Quil A type saponins as vaccine delivery systems or adjuvant appears promising. However, more work is needed to investigate the fate of the colloidal structures in vivo, as well as to elucidate whether the antigen should be a part of the ISCOM structure, if the co-administration of ISCOM matrices with the antigen is sufficient, or if indeed Quil A (or QS 21) should be incorporated into other colloidal carriers. The answer to these questions is likely to be antigen- and disease specific. The role of saponin adjuvants, such as Quil A and QS 21 in the current and future vaccine development however, cannot be underestimated.

References

1. Akerblom L, Nara P, Dunlop N, Putney S, Morein B (1993) HIV experimental vaccines based on the iscom technology using envelope and GAG gene products. Biotechnol Ther 4 (3–4):145–161
2. Andersson C, Sandberg L, Wernérus H, Johansson M, Lövgren-Bengtsson K, Ståhl S (2000) Improved systems for hydrophobic tagging of recombinant immunogens for efficient iscom incorporation. J Immunol Methods 238(1–2):181–193
3. Bachmann MF, Jennings GT (2010) Vaccine delivery: a matter of size, geometry, kinetics and molecular patterns. Nat Rev Immunol 10(11):787–796

4. Barr IG, Mitchell GF (1996) ISCOMs (immunostimulating complexes): the first decade. Immunol Cell Biol 74(1):8–25
5. Barr IG, Sjölander A, Cox JC (1998) ISCOMs and other saponin based adjuvants. Adv Drug Deliv Rev 32(3):247–271
6. Behboudi S, Morein B, Rönnberg B (1995) Isolation and quantification of Quillaja saponaria Molina saponins and lipids in iscom-matrix and iscoms. Vaccine 13(17):1690–1696
7. Brando C, Ware LA, Freyberger H, Kathcart A, Barbosa A, Cayphas S, Demoitie M-A, Mettens P, Heppner DG, Lanar DE (2007) Murine immune responses to liver-stage antigen 1 protein FMP011, a malaria vaccine candidate, delivered with adjuvant AS01B or AS02A. Infect Immun 75(2):838–845
8. Copland MJ, Baird MA, Rades T, McKenzie JL, Becker B, Reck F, Tyler PC, Davies NM (2003) Liposomal delivery of antigen to human dendritic cells. Vaccine 21(9–10):883–890
9. Copland MJ, Rades T, Davies NM (2000) Hydration of lipid films with an aqueous solution of Quil A: a simple method for the preparation of immune-stimulating complexes. Int J Pharm 196(2):135–139
10. da Fonseca DPAJ, Frerichs J, Singh M, Snippe H, Verheul AFM (2000) Induction of antibody and T-cell responses by immunization with ISCOMS containing the 38-kilodalton protein of Mycobacterium tuberculosis. Vaccine 19(1):122–131
11. Dalsgaard K (1974) Saponin adjuvants. 3. Isolation of a substance from Quillaja saponaria Molina with adjuvant activity in food-and-mouth disease vaccines. Arch Gesamte Virusforsch 44(3):243–254
12. Dasarai V, Smith C, Zhong J, Scott G, Rawlinson W, Khanna R (2011) Recombinant glycoprotein B vaccine formulation with TLR9 agonist and immune stimulating complex induces specific immunity against multiple strains of cytomegalovirus. J Gen Virol 92:1021–1031
13. Davis ID, Chen W, Jackson H, Parente P, Shackleton M, Hopkins W, Chen Q, Dimopoulos N, Luke T, Murphy R, Scott AM, Maraskovsky E, McArthur G, MacGregor D, Sturrock S, Tai TY, Green S, Cuthbertson A, Maher D, Miloradovic L, Mitchell SV, Ritter G, Jungbluth AA, Chen Y-T, Gnjatic S, Hoffman EW, Old LJ, Cebon JS (2004) Recombinant NY-ESO-1 protein with ISCOMATRIX adjuvant induces broad integrated antibody and CD4+ and CD8 + T cell responses in humans. Proc Natl Acad Sci U S A 101(29):10697–10702
14. De Gregorio E, D'Oro U, Wack A (2009) Immunology of TLR-independent vaccine adjuvants. Curr Opin Immunol 21(3):339–345
15. Demana P, Fehske C, White K, Rades T, Hook S (2004) Effect of incorporation of the adjuvant Quil A on structure and immune stimulatory capacity of liposomes. Immunol Cell Biol 82:547–554
16. Demana PH, Berger B, Vosgerau U, Rades T, Davies NM (2004) A comparison of pseudo-ternary diagrams of aqueous mixtures of Quil A, cholesterol and phospholipid prepared by lipid-film hydration and dialysis. J Pharm Pharmacol 56(5):573–580
17. Demana PH, Davies NM, Hook S, Rades T (2005) Quil A-lipid powder formulations releasing ISCOMs and related colloidal structures upon hydration. J Control Release 103 (1):45–59
18. Demana PH, Davies NM, Vosgerau U, Rades T (2004) Pseudo-ternary phase diagrams of aqueous mixtures of Quil A, cholesterol and phospholipid prepared by the lipid-film hydration method. Int J Pharm 270(1–2):229–239
19. Demento SL, Eisenbarth SC, Foellmer HG, Platt C, Caplan MJ, Mark Saltzman W, Mellman I, Ledizet M, Fikrig E, Flavell RA, Fahmy TM (2009) Inflammasome-activating nanoparticles as modular systems for optimizing vaccine efficacy. Vaccine 27 (23):3013–3021
20. Duthie MS, Windish HP, Fox CB, Reed SG (2010) Use of defined TLR ligands as adjuvants within human vaccines. Immunol Rev 239(1):178–196
21. Ekström J, Hu K-F, Bengtsson KL, Morein B (1999) Iscom and iscom-matrix enhance by intranasal route the IgA responses to OVA and rCTB in local and remote mucosal secretions. Vaccine 17(20–21):2690–2701

22. Ennis FA, Cruz J, Jameson J, Klein M, Burt D, Thipphawong J (1999) Augmentation of human influenza A virus-specific cytotoxic T lymphocyte memory by influenza vaccine and adjuvanted carriers (ISCOMs). Virology 259(2):256–261
23. Evans TG, McElrath MJ, Matthews T, Montefiori D, Weinhold K, Wolff M, Keefer MC, Kallas EG, Corey L, Gorse GJ, Belshe R, Graham BS, Spearman PW, Schwartz D, Mulligan MJ, Goepfert P, Fast P, Berman P, Powell M, Francis D (2001) QS-21 promotes an adjuvant effect allowing for reduced antigen dose during HIV-1 envelope subunit immunization in humans. Vaccine 19(15–16):2080–2091
24. Furrie E, Smith RE, Turner MW, Strobel S, Mowat AM (2002) Induction of local innate immune responses and modulation of antigen uptake as mechanisms underlying the mucosal adjuvant properties of immune stimulating complexes (ISCOMS). Vaccine 20 (17–18):2254–2262
25. Glauert AM, Dingle JT, Lucy JA (1962) Action of saponin on biological cell membranes. Nature 196(4858):953–955
26. Gordon S, Teichmann E, Young K, Finnie K, Rades T, Hook S (2010) In vitro and in vivo investigation of thermosensitive chitosan hydrogels containing silica nanoparticles for vaccine delivery. Eur J Pharm Sci 41(2):360–368
27. Gordon S, Young K, Wilson R, Rizwan S, Kemp R, Rades T, Hook S (2010) In vitro and in vivo investigation of thermosensitive chitosan hydrogels containing silica nanoparticles for vaccine delivery. European Journal of Pharmaceutical Sciences 41(2):360–368
28. Guo S, Kenne L, Lundgren LN, Rönnberg B, Sundquist BG (1998) Triterpenoid saponins from Quillaja saponaria. Phytochemistry 48(1):175–180
29. Hawkes CA, McLaurin J (2008) Clinical immunotherapy trials in Alzheimer's disease. Drug Discov Today 5(3):177–183
30. Higuchi R, Tokimitsu Y, Komori T (1988) An acylated triterpenoid saponin from Quillaja saponaria. Phytochemistry 27(4):1165–1168
31. Hoglund S, Dalsgaard K, Lovgren K, Sundquist B, Osterhaus A, Morein B (1989) ISCOMs and immunostimulation with viral antigens. Sub-cellular biochemistry, 1st edn. Plenum Press, New York
32. Iosef C, Van Nguyen T, K-I J, Bengtsson K, Morein B, Kim Y, Chang K-O, Azevedo MSP, Yuan L, Nielsen P, Saif LJ (2002) Systemic and intestinal antibody secreting cell responses and protection in gnotobiotic pigs immunized orally with attenuated Wa human rotavirus and Wa 2/6-rotavirus-like-particles associated with immunostimulating complexes. Vaccine 20 (13–14):1741–1753
33. ISCONOVA A (2011) AbISCO® adjuvant user guide. http://www.isconova.com. Accessed 23 March 2011
34. Jacobs C, Duewell P, Heckelsmiller K, Wei J, Bauernfeind F, Ellermeier J, Kisser U, Bauer CA, Dauer M, Eigler A, Maraskovsky E, Endres S, Schnurr M (2010) An ISCOM vaccine combined with a TLR9 agonist breaks immune evasion mediated by regulatory T cells in an orthotopic model of pancreatic carcinoma. Int J Cancer 128(4):897–907
35. Johansson M, Lövgren-Bengtsson K (1999) Iscoms with different quillaja saponin components differ in their immunomodulating activities. Vaccine 17(22):2894–2900
36. Johansson M, Ranlund K, Lovgren-Bengtsson K (2000) Impaired immunogenicity of immunostimulating complexes (iscoms) by administration in slow-release formulations. Microbes Infect 2(9):1003–1010
37. Keefer M, Wolff M, Gorse G, Graham B, Corey L, Clements-Mann M, Verani-Ketter N, Erb S, Smith C, Belshe R, Wagner L, McElrath M, Schwartz D, Fast P (1997) Safety profile of phase I and II preventive HIV type 1 envelope vaccination: experience of the NIAID AIDS Vaccine Evaluation Group. AIDS Res Hum Retroviruses 13(14):1163–1177
38. Kensil C, Patel U, Lennick M, Marciani D (1991) Separation and characterization of saponins with adjuvant activity from Quillaja saponaria Molina cortex. J Immunol 146(2):431–437
39. Kensil CR (1996) Saponins as vaccine adjuvants. Crit Rev Ther Drug Carrier Syst 13 (1–2):1–55

40. Kersten GFA, Crommelin DJA (1995) Liposomes and ISCOMS as vaccine formulations. Biochim Biophys Acta 1241(2):117–138
41. Kersten GFA, Spiekstra A, Beuvery EC, Crommelin DJA (1991) On the structure of immune-stimulating saponin-lipid complexes (ISCOMs). Biochim Biophys Acta 1062(2):165–171
42. Kodama S, Hirano T, Noda K, Umemoto S, Suzuki M (2011) Nasal immunization with plasmid DNA encoding P6 protein and immunostimulatory complexes elicits nontypeable Haemophilus influenzae-specific long-term mucosal immune responses in the nasopharynx. Vaccine 29(10):1881–1890
43. Könnings S, Copland MJ, Davies NM, Rades T (2002) A method for the incorporation of ovalbumin into immune stimulating complexes prepared by the hydration method. Int J Pharm 241(2):385–389
44. Kruit W, Suciu S, Dreno B, Chiarion-Sileni V, Mortier L, Robert C, Maio M, Brichard V, Lehmann F, Keilholz U (2008) Immunization with recombinant MAGE-A3 protein combined with adjuvant systems AS15 or AS02B in patients with unresectable and progressive metastatic cutaneous melanoma: A randomized open-label phase II study of the EORTC Melanoma Group. J Clin Oncol 26(suppl 15):A9065
45. Larsson M, Lövgren K, Morein B (1993) Immunopotentiation of synthetic oligopeptides by chemical conjugation to iscoms. J Immunol Methods 162(2):257–260
46. Lendemans DG, Egert AM, Hook S, Rades T (2007) Cage-like complexes formed by DOTAP, Quil-A and cholesterol. Int J Pharm 332(1–2):192–195
47. Lendemans DG, Egert AM, Myschik J, Hook S, Rades T (2006) On the dilution behaviour of immuno-stimulating complexes (ISCOMs). Pharmazie 61(8):689–695
48. Lendemans DG, Myschik J, Hook S, Rades T (2005) Cationic cage-like complexes formed by DC-cholesterol, Quil-A, and phospholipid. J Pharm Sci 94(8):1794–1807
49. Lendemans DG, Myschik J, Hook S, Rades T (2005) Immuno-stimulating complexes prepared by ethanol injection. J Pharm Pharmacol 57(6):729–733
50. Leroux-Roels I, Koutsoukos M, Clement F, Steyaert S, Janssens M, Bourguignon P, Cohen K, Altfeld M, VandepapeliËre P, Pedneault L, McNally L, Leroux-Roels G, Voss G (2010) Strong and persistent CD4+ T-cell response in healthy adults immunized with a candidate HIV-1 vaccine containing gp120, Nef and Tat antigens formulated in three adjuvant systems. Vaccine 28(43):7016–7024
51. Li H, Willingham SB, Ting JP-Y, Re F (2008) Cutting edge: inflammasome activation by alum and alum's adjuvant effect are mediated by NLRP3. J Immunol 181(1):17–21
52. Liang M, Toth I, Davies NM (2008) A novel method for preparing immune stimulating complexes (ISCOMs) by hydration of freeze-dried lipid matrix. Eur J Pharm Biopharm 68 (3):840–845
53. Lipford GB, Wagner H, Heeg K (1994) Vaccination with immunodominant peptides encapsulated in Quil A-containing liposomes induces peptide-specific primary CD8+ cytotoxic T cells. Vaccine 12(1):73–80
54. Lövgren K, Lindmark J, Pipkorn R, Morein B (1987) Antigenic presentation of small molecules and peptides conjugated to a preformed iscom as carrier. J Immunol Methods 98 (1):137–143
55. Lövgren K, Morein B (1988) The requirement of lipids for the formation of immunostimulating complexes (ISCOMs). Biotechnol Appl Biochem 10(2):161–172
56. Madhun AS, Haaheim LR, Nilsen MV, Cox RJ (2009) Intramuscular matrix-M-adjuvanted virosomal H5N1 vaccine induces high frequencies of multifunctional Th1 CD4+ cells and strong antibody responses in mice. Vaccine 27(52):7367–7376
57. Madsen H, Ifversen P, Madsen F, Brodin B, Hausser I, Nielsen H (2009) *In vitro* cutaneous application of ISCOMs on human skin enhances delivery of hydrophobic model compounds through the stratum corneum. AAPS J 11(4):728–739
58. Madsen HB, Arboe-Andersen HM, Rozlosnik N, Madsen F, Ifversen P, Kasimova MR, Nielsen HM (2010) Investigation of the interaction between modified ISCOMs and stratum corneum lipid model systems. Biochim Biophys Acta 1798(9):1779–1789

59. Maraskovsky E, Sjölander S, Drane DP, Schnurr M, Le TTT, Mateo L, Luft T, Masterman K-A, Tai T-Y, Chen Q, Green S, Sjolander A, Pearse MJ, Lemonnier FA, Chen W, Cebon J, Suhrbier A (2004) NY-ESO-1 protein formulated in ISCOMATRIX adjuvant is a potent anticancer vaccine inducing both humoral and CD8+ T-cell-mediated immunity and protection against NY-ESO-1+ tumors. Clin Cancer Res 10(8):2879–2890
60. Martinon F, Burns K, Tschopp J (2002) The inflammasome: a molecular platform triggering activation of inflammatory caspases and processing of proIL-β. Mol Cell 10(2):417–426
61. Mbow ML, De Gregorio E, Valiante NM, Rappuoli R (2010) New adjuvants for human vaccines. Curr Opin Immunol 22(3):411–416
62. McBurney WT, Lendemans DG, Myschik J, Hennessy T, Rades T, Hook S (2008) In vivo activity of cationic immune stimulating complexes (PLUSCOMs). Vaccine 26 (35):4549–4556
63. Medzhitov R, Janeway CA (2002) Decoding the patterns of self and nonself by the innate immune system. Science 296(5566):298–300
64. Morein B, Bengtsson KL (1999) Immunomodulation by Iscoms, immune stimulating complexes. Methods 19(1):94–102
65. Morein B, Ekström J, Lövgren K (1990) Increased immunogenicity of a non-amphipathic protein (BSA) after inclusion into iscoms. J Immunol Methods 128(2):177–181
66. Morein B, Lovgren K, Ronnberg B, Sjolander A, Villacres-Eriksson M (1995) Immunostimulating complexes. Clinical potential in vaccine development. Clin Immunother 3 (6):461–475
67. Morein B, Sundquist B, Hoglund S, Dalsgaard K, Osterhaus A (1984) Iscom, a novel structure for antigenic presentation of membrane proteins from enveloped viruses. Nature 308(5958):457–460
68. Morgan D (2006) Immunotherapy for Alzheimer's disease. J Intern Med 269(1):54–63
69. Mowat A, Maloy K, Donachie AM (1993) Immune-stimulating complexes as adjuvants for inducing local and systemic immunity after oral immunization with protein antigens. Immunology 80(4):527–534
70. Myschik J, Eberhardt F, Rades T, Hook S (2008) Immunostimulatory biodegradable implants containing the adjuvant Quil-A. Part I: physicochemical characterisation. J Drug Target 16 (3):213–223
71. Myschik J, Lendemans DG, McBurney WT, Demana PH, Hook S, Rades T (2006) On the preparation, microscopic investigation and application of ISCOMs. Micron 37(8):724–734
72. Myschik J, Mcburney WT, Hennessy T, Phipps-Green A, Rades T, Hook S (2008) Immunostimulatory biodegradable implants containing the adjuvant Quil-A. Part II: in vivo evaluation. J Drug Target 16(3):224–232
73. Myschik J, Rades T, Hook S (2009) Advances in lipid-based subunit vaccine formulations. Curr Immunol Rev 5:42–48
74. Nicholaou T, Ebert LM, Davis ID, McArthur GA, Jackson H, Dimopoulos N, Tan B, Maraskovsky E, Miloradovic L, Hopkins W, Pan L, Venhaus R, Hoffman EW, Chen W, Cebon J (2009) Regulatory T-cell-mediated attenuation of T-cell responses to the NY-ESO-1 ISCOMATRIX vaccine in patients with advanced malignant melanoma. Clin Cancer Res 15 (6):2166–2173
75. Ockenhouse CF, Angov E, Kester KE, Diggs C, Soisson L, Cummings JF, Stewart AV, Palmer DR, Mahajan B, Krzych U, Tornieporth N, Delchambre M, Vanhandenhove M, Ofori-Anyinam O, Cohen J, Lyon JA, Heppner DG (2006) Phase I safety and immunogenicity trial of FMP1/AS02A, a Plasmodium falciparum MSP-1 asexual blood stage vaccine. Vaccine 24(15):3009–3017
76. Oliveira-Freitas E, Casas CP, Borja-Cabrera GP, Santos FN, Nico D, Souza LOP, Tinoco LW, da Silva BP, Palatnik M, Parente JP, Palatnik-de-Sousa CB (2006) Acylated and deacylated saponins of Quillaja saponaria mixture as adjuvants for the FML-vaccine against visceral leishmaniasis. Vaccine 24(18):3909–3920

77. Olotu A, Lusingu J, Leach A, Lievens M, Vekemans J, Msham S, Lang T, Gould J, Dubois M-C, Jongert E, Vansadia P, Carter T, Njuguna P, Awuondo KO, Malabeja A, Abdul O, Gesase S, Mturi N, Drakeley CJ, Savarese B, Villafana T, Lapierre D, Ballou WR, Cohen J, Lemnge MM, Peshu N, Marsh K, Riley EM, von Seidlein L, Bejon P (2011) Efficacy of RTS, S/AS01E malaria vaccine and exploratory analysis on anti-circumsporozoite antibody titres and protection in children aged 5–17 months in Kenya and Tanzania: a randomised controlled trial. Lancet Infect Dis 11(2):102–109
78. Orgogozo JM, Gilman S, Dartigues JF, Laurent B, Puel M, Kirby LC, Jouanny P, Dubois B, Eisner L, Flitman S, Michel BF, Boada M, Frank A, Hock C (2003) Subacute meningoencephalitis in a subset of patients with AD after ςβ42 immunization. Neurology 61(1):46–54
79. Özel M, Hlund S, Gelderblom HR, Morein B (1989) Quaternary structure of the immunostimulating complex (Iscom). J Ultrastruct Mol Struct Res 102(3):240–248
80. Pandey RS, Dixit VK (2009) Evaluation of ISCOM vaccines for mucosal immunization against hepatitis B. J Drug Target 18(4):282–291
81. Pfizer Animal Health (2004) Next generation adjuvant system: Key to enhanced protection conferred by BVDV (Types 1 and 2) components of CattleMaster ®GOLD™. Pfizer Animal Health Technical Bulletin, New York
82. Pham HL, Shaw PN, Davies NM (2006) Preparation of immuno-stimulating complexes (ISCOMs) by ether injection. Int J Pharm 310(1–2):196–202
83. Radosevic K, Rodriguez A, Mintardjo R, Tax D, Bengtsson KL, Thompson C, Zambon M, Weverling GJ, UytdeHaag F, Goudsmit J (2008) Antibody and T-cell responses to a virosomal adjuvanted H9N2 avian influenza vaccine: Impact of distinct additional adjuvants. Vaccine 26(29–30):3640–3646
84. Reid G (1992) Soluble proteins incorporate into ISCOMs after covalent attachment of fatty acid. Vaccine 10(9):597–602
85. Rhodes J (1996) Covalent chemical events in immune induction: fundamental and therapeutic effects. Immunol Today 17(7):436–441
86. Rimmelzwaan GF, Siebelink KHJ, Huisman RC, Moss B, Francis MJ, Osterhaus ADME (1994) Removal of the cleavage site of recombinant feline immunodeficiency virus envelope protein facilitates incorporation of the surface glycoprotein in immune-stimulating complexes. J Gen Virol 75(8):2097–2102
87. Robson NC, Beacock-Sharp H, Donachie AM, Mowat AM (2003) The role of antigen-presenting cells and interleukin-12 in the priming of antigen-specific CD4+ T cells by immune stimulating complexes. Immunology 110:95–104
88. Rohn TA, Bachmann MF (2010) Vaccines against non-communicable diseases. Curr Opin Immunol 22(3):391–396
89. Rönnberg B, Fekadu M, Behboudi S, Kenne L, Morein B (1997) Effects of carbohydrate modification of Quillaja saponaria Molina QH-B fraction on adjuvant activity, cholesterol-binding capacity and toxicity. Vaccine 15(17–18):1820–1826
90. Rönnberg B, Fekadu M, Morein B (1995) Adjuvant activity of non-toxic Quillaja saponaria Molina components for use in ISCOM matrix. Vaccine 13(14):1375–1382
91. Sambhara S, Kurichh A, Miranda R, Tumpey T, Rowe T, Renshaw M, Arpino R, Tamane A, Kandil A, James O, Underdown B, Klein M, Katz J, Burt D (2001) Heterosubtypic immunity against human influenza A viruses, including recently emerged avian H5 and H9 viruses, induced by FLU-ISCOM vaccine in mice requires both cytotoxic T-lymphocyte and macrophage function. Cell Immunol 211(2):143–153
92. Sanders MT, Brown LE, Deliyannis G, Pearse MJ (2005) ISCOM™-based vaccines: the second decade. Immunol Cell Biol 83(2):119–128
93. Schnurr M, Orban M, Robson NC, Shin A, Braley H, Airey D, Cebon J, Maraskovsky E, Endres S (2009) ISCOMATRIX adjuvant induces efficient cross-presentation of tumor antigen by dendritic cells via rapid cytosolic antigen delivery and processing via tripeptidyl peptidase II. J Immunol 182(3):1253–1259

94. Segal R, Shatkovsky P, Milo-Goldzweig I (1974) On the mechanism of saponin hemolysis—I: hydrolysis of the glycosidic bond. Biochem Pharmacol 23(5):973–981
95. Sjölander A, Cox J, Barr I (1998) ISCOMs: an adjuvant with multiple functions. J Leukoc Biol 64(6):713–723
96. Sjölander A, Lovgren K, Stahl S, Aslund L, Hansson M, Nygren PA, Larsson M, Hagstedt M, Wahlin B, Berzins K, Uhlen M, Morein B, Perlmann P (1991) High antibody-responses in rabbits immunized with influenza-virus iscoms containing a repeated sequence of the plasmodium-falciparum antigen pf155/resa. Vaccine 9(6):443–450
97. Sjölander A, van't Land B, Bengtsson KL (1997) Iscoms containing purified Quillaja saponins upregulate both Th1-like and Th2-like immune responses. Cell Immunol 177 (1):69–76
98. Smith RE, Donachie AM, Grdic D, Lycke N, Mowat AM (1999) Immune-stimulating complexes induce an IL-12-dependent cascade of innate immune responses. J Immunol 162(9):5536–5546
99. Soltysik S, Wu J-Y, Recchia J, Wheeler DA, Newman MJ, Coughlin RT, Kensil CR (1995) Structure/function studies of QS-21 adjuvant: assessment of triterpene aldehyde and glucuronic acid roles in adjuvant function. Vaccine 13(15):1403–1410
100. Sundling C, O'Dell S, Douagi I, Forsell MN, Morner A, Lore K, Mascola JR, Wyatt RT, Karlsson Hedestam GB (2010) Immunization with wild-type or CD4-binding-defective HIV-1 Env trimers reduces viremia equivalently following heterologous challenge with simian-human immunodeficiency virus. J Virol 84(18):9086–9095
101. Tschopp J, Schroder K (2010) NLRP3 inflammasome activation: the convergence of multiple signalling pathways on ROS production? Nat Rev Immunol 10(3):210–215
102. Tyagi P, Mirakhur B (2009) MAGRIT: the largest-ever phase III lung cancer trial aims to establish a novel tumor-specific approach to therapy. Clin Lung Cancer 10(5):371–374
103. Ubhi K, Masliah E (2011) Recent advances in the development of immunotherapies for tauopathies. Exp Neurol 230(2):157–161. doi:10.1016/j.expneurol.2010.10.007
104. Vansteenkiste J, Zielinski M, Linder A, Dahabre J, Esteban E, Malinowski W, Jassem J, Passlick B, Lehmann F, Brichard V (2007) Final results of a multi-center, double-blind, randomized, placebo-controlled phase II study to assess the efficacy of MAGE-A3 immunotherapeutic as adjuvant therapy in stage IB/II non-small cell lung cancer (NSCLC). J Clin Oncol 25(18S):7554
105. Villacres-Eriksson M, Bergström-Mollaoglu M, Kåberg H, Lövgren K, Morein B (1993) The induction of cell-associated and secreted IL-1 by iscoms, matrix or micelles in murine splenic cells. Clin Exp Immunol 93(1):120–125
106. Waite DC, Jacobson EW, Ennis FA, Edelman R, White B, Kammer R, Anderson C, Kensil CR (2001) Three double-blind, randomized trials evaluating the safety and tolerance of different formulations of the saponin adjuvant QS-21. Vaccine 19(28–29):3957–3967
107. White K, Rades T, Furneaux R, Kearns P, Toth I, Hook S (2006) Immunogenicity of liposomes containing lipid core peptides and the adjuvant Quil A. Pharm Res 23 (7):1473–1481
108. Williams A, Flavell RA, Eisenbarth SC (2010) The role of NOD-like receptors in shaping adaptive immunity. Curr Opin Immunol 22(1):34–40
109. Yu H, Jiang X, Shen C, Karunakaran KP, Jiang J, Rosin NL, Brunham RC (2010) Chlamydia muridarum T-cell antigens formulated with the adjuvant DDA/TDB induce immunity against infection that correlates with a high frequency of gamma interferon (IFN-γ)/tumor necrosis factor alpha and IFN-γ/interleukin-17 double-positive CD4+ T cells. Infect Immun 78 (5):2272–2282

Chapter 13
Formulation and Characterisation of PLGA Microspheres as Vaccine Adjuvants

Daniel J. Kirby, Randip Kaur, and Yvonne Perrie

Abstract There appear to be several factors that confirm the viability of polymeric microspheres as vaccine delivery vehicles, including the ability to enhance targeting of antigen-presenting cells, the potential for controlled, sustained release of antigen-thereby potentially eliminating the need for multiple vaccination doses-as well as the ability of the polymer matrix to not only facilitate more efficient delivery by acting as a shield from the hostile external environment, but also the potential to reduce adverse reactions and abrogate problems caused by the vaccine strain in immunocompromised individuals. In addition, microspheres offer great variability in terms of manufacturing processes, constituents (including additional adjuvants), physico-chemical properties and immunological efficacy.

This chapter investigates the advantageous properties of microspheres—and more specifically, those composed primarily of polylactide-co-glycolide—for the delivery of vaccine adjuvants by outlining the various preparation techniques and the effect of the related processing parameters, the subsequent *in vivo* efficacy, and, finally, the potential for a desirable product with an extended shelf-life.

13.1 Introduction

The use of polymeric microparticles for the delivery of vaccines has been the subject of much research in recent years [130, 137], thanks in part to the wide range of synthetic (e.g. polymethyl methacrylate, polyesters, polyanhydrides, polyamides) and natural (e.g. albumin, collagen, starch, chitosan, dextran) polymers available for their production. Of these polymers, the polyesters—and in particular the polylactides (PLAs), polyglycolides (PLGs) and their copolymers (polylactide-co-glycolide [PLGA])—have been the most widely used, since these

D.J. Kirby (✉)
School of Life and Health Sciences, Aston University, Birmingham, UK
e-mail: d.j.kirby1@aston.ac.uk

D.R. Flower and Y. Perrie (eds.), *Immunomic Discovery of Adjuvants and Candidate Subunit Vaccines*, Immunomics Reviews: 5, DOI 10.1007/978-1-4614-5070-2_13,

polymers have been tested for toxicity and safety in extensive animal studies, and are currently used to prepare controlled release delivery systems, e.g. Zoladex® (I.C.I), Decapeptyl® (Debiopharm), Prostap® (Lederle) Lupron Depot®, Nutropin Depot® and Sandostatin LAR®, which are licensed for use in humans in Europe and the USA [16, 47]. Moreover, they have also found use in humans for resorbable sutures, bone implants and screws [48, 53], graft materials for artificial organs and as supporting scaffolds in tissue engineering research [78].

13.1.1 Physico-Chemical and Biological Properties of PLGA

PLG is a crystalline, biodegradable polymer having a melting point (T_m) of 225 °C and a glass transition temperature (T_g) of 36 °C. PLG, when compared to other biodegradable polymers, is highly crystalline, with a reported crystallinity within the range of 35–75 % [109]. Jamshidi et al. [64] have reported that with a decrease of the lactide content in the copolymer composition, and with a decrease in their molecular weight, the transition temperature of PLGAs decrease [62]. The polymer PLA can exist in an optically active stereo-regular form, L-polylactide (L-PLA) and in an optically inactive racemic form D, L-PLA [63, 81]. L-PLA is biodegradable and is crystalline with a 175 °C melting point and a 65 °C glass transition temperature. Compared to PLG, L-PLA is in general less crystalline and it has been reported its crystallinity is within the range of 35 % [109]. D, L-PLA is a polymer that is entirely amorphous having a transition temperature of 57 °C. The use of D, L-PLA is preferred over L-PLA as it allows more uniform dispersion of the drug in the polymer matrix [62, 138]. The carbonyl of the ester linkage is protected from hydrolytic attack through the methyl group attached in the PLA. The PLAs, despite being related to the PLGs have chemical, physical and mechanical properties that differ, as a consequence of a pendent methyl group attached on the alpha carbon [62]. Due to its additional methyl group, PLA is more hydrophobic than PGA. Both PLA and PGA are soluble in organic solvents, such as chloroform, dichloromethane (DCM), acetone and ethylacetone to a variable extent, having dependence on copolymer composition and molecular weight [75].

13.1.2 PLGA Synthesis

The synthesis of the homo- and copolymers of lactic and glycolic acids is achieved through the ring-opening melt condensation of cyclic dimers, lactide and glycolide. Direct condensation of alpha-hydroxy acids yields low molecular weight polymers that range in size from 10 to 15 kDa [24]. Melt or bulk polymerisation is used to perform the reaction in emulsion or solution [9]. Over a period of 2–6 h the polymerisations are performed at around 175 °C. Organotin catalysts are normally utilised with stannous chloride, with stannous octoate being the most common, as it has FDA approval as a food stabiliser [37].

13.1.3 Degradation and Erosion of PLGA

PLGA can be formulated into microspheres from the nanometre to several microns in size and can encapsulate a very wide range of molecules. Following introduction of the PLGA microspheres into the body, PLGA hydrolysis produces lactic and glycolic acids, which are metabolised in the Krebs cycle to CO_2 and water. This degradation process occurs in two stages—first hydrolytic scission of the ester bonds generates oligomers and monomers and a general decrease in the polymer molecular weight. Secondly, the microspheres lose mass, and the rate of polymer chain scission may increase due to autocatalysis in the presence of acidic degradation products [51].

Molecular weight and comonomer ratio are the two factors of PLGA that determine the rate of hydrolysis [75]. As shown in Table 13.1, D, L-PLGA has a polymer mass loss half-life of 14 days when it has a 50 % molecular lactic acid and 50 % glycolic acid PLGA (50:50) comonomer composition, resulting in a 50–60 day complete resorption of the microspheres. When the comonomer ratio is shifted towards either component, this leads to a significant decrease in biodegradation [75].

13.2 PLGA Microsphere for the Delivery of Vaccines

Given the biodegradable nature and sustained release properties that PLGA can offer, microspheres formulated from these polymers appear to be an ideal candidate for the delivery of subunit vaccines, due to their relative biocompatibility, adjuvanticity and prolonged drug release profile. Given their particulate nature, such delivery systems can promote uptake, transport or presentation of the antigen to antigen-presenting cells (APCs). In addition, it has been reported that PLGA microparticles exhibit an adjuvant effect for both humoural [39, 102] and cell-mediated immunity [8]. Indeed, sub-10 μm PLGA microspheres are readily recognised and ingested by macrophages and dendritic cells, an important property for stimulating the immune response [132].

A key advantage of microspheres as vaccine adjuvants is based on their controlled release capacity to potentially allow for single-dose vaccination, thereby circumventing the need for a booster immunisation. For example, Jung et al. [69] looked at the microencapsulation of tetanus toxoid (TT) into PLGA microspheres and triblock-copolymers (PLGA-PEG-PLGA) and considered the immune responses in mice. TT was encapsulated using the double emulsion method and, whilst the copolymer system avoided the deleterious microenvironmental

Table 13.1 In vivo biodegradation times of PLGA [75]

Polymer	Approximate time for biodegradation (months)
Poly (L-lactide)	18–24
Poly (glycolide)	12–16
Poly (lactide-co-glycolide) 85:15	5
Poly (lactide-co-glycolide) 50:50	2

conditions in the degrading microspheres, both the PLGA and triblock polymer gave immune responses in line with aluminium-adsorbed TT, and also offered protection in challenge studies [69]. The authors suggest that such systems could be considered for single shot vaccine delivery systems, given their ability to elicit a long lasting and protective immune response [69]. Work by Johansen et al. [68] also proposed the use of PLGA microspheres as single-shot vaccines; in immunisation studies conducted in guinea pigs, they were able to show that PLGA 50:50 exhibited specific and sustained antibody responses over 40 weeks, comparable to the responses to alum-adjuvanted toxoid (in this study diphtheria toxoid) [68]. Investigating the feasibility of PLGA microspheres as an adjuvant for a single-dose hepatitis B vaccine, Feng et al. [43] were able to develop immune responses after a single subcutaneous injection of HBsAg-loaded PLGA microspheres. Their PLGA microspheres were able to continuously release antigen in simulated in vivo conditions for up to 63 days, with PLGA 50:50 microspheres giving slightly higher release rates than PLGA 75:25 counterparts but notable difference in immunogenicity profiles, which remained high up to 125 days after injection [43].

The ability of single-dose immunisation using microspheres has also been demonstrated in monkeys as well as mice using the SPf66 malaria vaccine [120]. Within these studies, particles with a mean particle size of 1.3 μm were prepared from either PLGA 50:50 or 75:25. Notable differences in release profiles were measured, with 50:50 formulations showing a 20 % burst release throughout the first day, followed by a lag phase for several days, followed by a second burst release occurring at day 30 and thereafter a continuous release over 8 weeks [120]. In contrast, microspheres formulated using 75:25 PLGA gave an initial 40 % burst release on the first day, followed by a low but constant SPf66 release up to day 130, without a second burst release [120]. When tested for immunogenicity in mice, both microsphere formulations gave significantly higher antibody responses after subcutaneous administration than SPf66-adsorbed alum, but comparable responses to animals receiving the antigen emulsified in Freud's Adjuvant. Over the period of the study, the authors noted no significant difference between the two microsphere formulations [120]. These systems were further tested in Aotus monkeys, and again responses from the microspheres were higher in monkeys immunised with PLGA microspheres compared to those which received SPf66-alum. However, in model protection studies, only 2 out of the 7 monkeys that received the microsphere-based vaccine were fully protected [120], demonstrating the need for the evaluation of microspheres in a range of animal models.

The use of PLGA microspheres is not limited to the parenteral route. After oral administration, PLGA microspheres have been shown to elicit immune responses in some cases comparable to parenteral routes; for example, Igartua et al. [59] compared subcutaneous and oral immunisation using PLGA microspheres. They showed that, whilst a single oral administration of microspheres was not able to induce appropriate responses, dosing on 3 consecutive days was able to induce IgG responses similar to those induced by subcutaneous immunisation, and a later booster dose provided no further advantage [59]. The success of the PLGA systems as oral delivery systems was attributed to their ability to promote an initial burst release (~20 %) followed by a sustained release (~50 % by day 35 [59]). Sartia et al. [125] were also able to stimulate immune responses to OVA delivered orally in PLGA-based particulates, with both IgG and IgA responses being measured and shown to be higher than those of OVA given orally in PBS. There have also been reports of the possibility of using PLGA microspheres to induce oral tolerance to their entrapped antigen [41]. Yet, whilst PLGA-based systems have demonstrated their ability give protection to animals in challenge studies [25, 41], like other oral particulates, studies have not yet reported a protective immunity induced in humans.

The above gives a short overview of a few examples of work undertaken to investigate PLGA vaccine adjuvants, and in addition to these, there is a substantial body of published research into the use of PLGA microspheres as vaccine adjuvants. Despite this, PLGA microspheres have yet to progress into human clinical trials [66]. Initially, their development into clinical products has been hindered by problems including degradation of antigens, either during production or whilst incorporated within the polymer matrix, leading to a range of methods being considered.

13.2.1 Preparation Methods

Numerous methods have been developed for the production of microparticles, including double emulsion—solvent evaporation [100], nano-precipitation [118], cross-flow filtration [44], salting-out techniques [3], emulsion-diffusion methods [20], jet milling [99] and spray drying [115]. However, the most common method of preparation is the double emulsion process (w/o/w), whereby an initial primary w_1/o emulsion is formed by dispersion of an aqueous antigen solution (w_1) into an organic polymer solution (Fig. 13.1). This primary emulsion is then mixed by high-speed homogenisation into a secondary water phase (w_2), often containing an emulsion stabiliser or surfactant such as poly(vinyl alcohol) (PVA), in order to form a secondary w_1/o/w_2 emulsion. The organic solvent is then allowed to evaporate to facilitate the formation and hardening of the microparticles. This formulation technique, originally developed by Vrancken and Claeys [141] and modified by Ogawa et al. [100], prevents the partition of hydrophilic drugs/antigens into the aqueous phase, thereby achieving efficient and reproducible entrapment. Other advantages include the fact that the protein is encapsulated as an aqueous solution, scaling down is possible, and high yields and encapsulation efficiencies are obtained. Nonetheless, arguments pertaining to shelf life of antigens and stability of microspheres also apply to this process [130]. Using this technique,

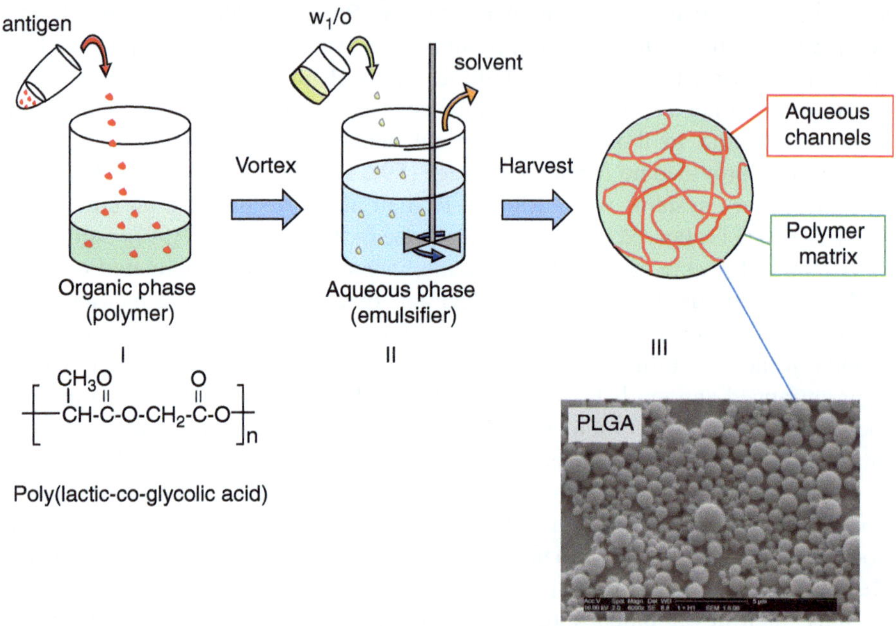

Fig. 13.1 Schematic representation of microsphere formulation by the water-in-oil-in-water double emulsion solvent evaporation process ($w_1/o/w_2$)

antigen may be entrapped within the carrier, thus acting as a shield from the hostile external environment [67], potentially reducing adverse reactions caused by the vaccine strain in immunocompromised individuals [13], whilst also exhibiting controlled release of antigen, thereby possibly eliminating the need for multiple vaccination doses [66, 78, 114].

Conversely, a variation of w/o/w process is the single oil-in-water process (o/w), whereby the initial formation of the w_1/o emulsion is omitted, with antigen being adsorbed to the surface of the microspheres following harvesting [42, 61, 86] (Fig. 13.2). This alternative process eliminates exposure of antigen to organic solvents during the formulation process, enabling delivery of several antigens simultaneously on the same formulation, at a range of different loading levels, and offering the ability to deliver either anionic or cationic moieties through the appropriate choice of polymer and/or surfactant/emulsifier. In addition, the surface characteristics and the internal morphology/porosity may be modified to yield the desired release profiles [71].

13.3 Microspheres as Adjuvants as Well as Delivery Systems

Whilst microspheres have the ability to deliver a range of moieties, including drugs and proteins, their ability to stimulate appropriate immune responses requires more than effective delivery. Therefore, to potentiate immune responses,

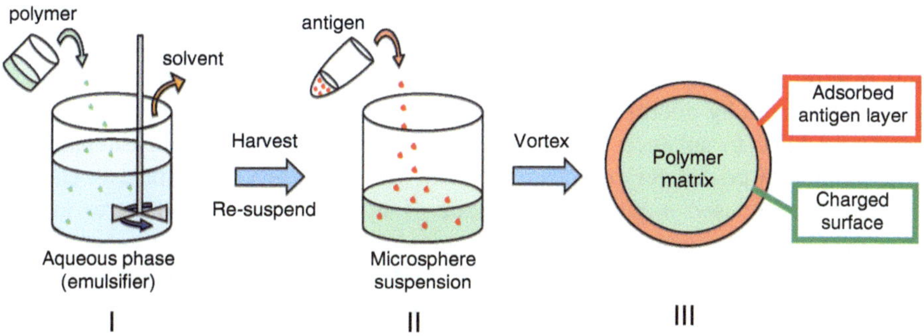

Fig. 13.2 Schematic representation of microsphere formulation by the oil-in-water single emulsion solvent evaporation process (o/w)

immunostimulatory agents are often employed within the formulations (e.g. [73, 74]). Since the structural requirements and immunological mechanisms of action of immunomodulatory adjuvants are poorly understood, they have thus been referred to as "the immunologist's dirty little secret" [65, 132]. Nevertheless, a plethora of vaccine adjuvants exists, including directly purified or synthetic derivatives of cell wall components, bacterial DNA extracts (CpG motifs) and cytokines.

Currently, the most commonly used vaccine adjuvants are aluminium based (Alum) due to their demonstrated safety profile and role in successful vaccine programmes [13]. Yet, there are concerns over severe local reactions and stability issues of such adjuvants, as well as the fact that the immune responses generated with sub-unit antigens are generally weak humoural responses, with a bias towards Th2 immunity, which is not desirable for diseases such as TB where a cell-mediated response is required [13, 97, 101, 108].

A more recently approved adjuvant is monophosphoryl lipid A (MPL), a chemically modified derivative of the lipopolysaccharide (LPS) of *Salmonella minnesota* and retains much of the immunostimulatory properties of the parent LPS without the inherent toxicity [46]. MPL acts on the TLR2 and TLR4 receptors on APC [146] and is a potent Th1 stimulator, inducing enhanced secretion of IFN-γ and IL-2, whilst also increasing migration and maturation of DCs [158], and to a lesser extent also the Th2 cytokines IL-4 and IL-5 and antibody classes IgE and IgG1 in mice [15]. As a consequence, MPL has been extensively investigated for its role in vaccine adjuvanticity [101, 147, 151] and is used as an adjuvant in the HPV vaccine Cerverix® [110].

The ability of LPS and its analogues to act as immunomodulators within particulates has also been attributed to its ability to promote preferential internalisation of particulates by dendritic cells compared to uncoated particles, and that such particles are able to rupture lysosomal compartments and destabilise inflammasomes, therefore behaving as danger signals [57], thus stimulating two innate immune response pathways [33]. For example, Sarti et al. [124] investigated PLGA microspheres for the use of oral vaccination, and in order to enhance the efficacy of their system, MPL was incorporated into the microparticles. Whilst the addition of MPL made no major difference to the microparticle physico-chemical characteristics, the authors were able to stimulate a time-dependent systemic and mucosal immune response towards the encapsulated OVA, which was higher than those stimulated by microparticles formulated from PLGA alone. Chong et al. [21] also used MPL to enhance T helper type 1 immune responses against hepatitis B core antigen by co-delivery of the antigen and MPL in PLGA microspheres. Hamdy et al. [52] also used a synthetic analogue of lipid A, 7-acyl lipid A, to induce therapeutic anti-tumour effect [150].

The immunostimulatory effects of CpG motifs, derived from bacterial DNA or synthetic oligodeoxynucleotides (ODN), have also attracted much interest, and include activation and maturation of DCs, induction of Th1 response through stimulation of cytokines and co-stimulatory molecules, and enhancement of mucosal immune responses [101, 149, 155]. McCluskie et al. [88] evaluated the combination of CpG with HBsAg or Tetanus toxoid and found that the presence of CpG augmented both systemic and mucosal immune responses against both antigens after oral delivery [88]. In terms of their use in microspheres, the co-delivery of CpG and antigen allows for enhanced immune responses; for example, Diwan et al. [35] synthesised PLGA particles co-delivering CpG and TT, and these formulations were able to induce both Th1 and Th2 immune responses but with a bias towards Th1 type, and responses were higher in mice that received the co-delivery system compared to microspheres containing TT alone [35]. However, in more recent studies, the co-encapsulation of CpG with OVA antigen within PLGA microspheres was shown to have a detrimental effect depending on the PLGA polymer used, suggesting the critical role of the polymer used in the formulation [119]. Human specific CpG motifs are available and have been shown to be potent adjuvants to pseudorabies live attenuated virus vaccine in piglet models when administered orally or subcutaneously, with both Th1 and Th2 responses being stimulated when delivered orally [83].

A surfactant commonly used within our group, and others, is dimethyldioctadecyl ammonium bromide (DDA); discovered as an adjuvant by Gall in the mid 1960s [49]. DDA is a synthetic amphiphilic lipid, comprising a hydrophilic positively charged dimethylammonium headgroup attached to two hydrophobic 18-carbon alkyl chains. DDA is known to induce cell-mediated immunity and delayed-type hypersensitivity [157], and along with its cationic nature and surfactant properties, has been shown to be an effective adjuvant in numerous applications, including mucosal immunisation [153], gene delivery [40] and subunit vaccine delivery [121, 147, 151, 154].

A second commonly investigated adjuvant within our group is trehalose 6,6′-dibehenate (TDB). Being a synthetic derivative of the mycobacterial cell wall component trehalose dimycolate (TDM), TDB has been shown to retain much of the bioactivity of the native form, whilst showing less toxicity as a result of the shorter fatty acid chains [104, 112]. Indeed, the combination of the DDA with TDB has been previously shown to be an efficient adjuvant for TB subunit vaccines (Holten-Andersen et al. 2004), inducing a strong gamma interferon (IFN-γ) response, considered to be the key cytokine for induction of a Th1 immune response, essential for effective anti-mycobacterial immunity [26, 45]. TDB is thought to act through the C-type lectin Mincle receptor [60], thereby activating NFκB via the syk-CARD9/Bcl10/Malt-1 intracellular pathway, leading to initiation of co-stimulatory and pro-inflammatory molecule transcription [126, 142].

13.3.1 Physico-Chemical Characteristics of Microspheres as Vaccine Adjuvants: The Effect of Formulation

In the formulation of particulate delivery systems, the physico-chemical properties can be a key attribute in their efficacy [13]. Therefore, it is important to understand the effect of formulation parameters in terms of both the choice of components used in the preparation of microspheres and the manufacture method adopted, as each can impact on the characteristics of the system both in terms of their physical attributes and the measured biological outputs.

13.3.2 Optimisation of Process Parameters in the Preparation of PLGA-Based Microspheres

Given the various stages involved in the preparation of microspheres formulated by the commonly used double emulsion method, we have undertaken a systematic investigation of the relationship between particle size and formulation parameters. Looking at each of the three stages in the double emulsion method, i.e. the initial polymer concentration, the homogenisation time and the emulsifier concentration, the effect of each of these parameters have been mapped onto their effect on microparticle size and heterogeneity [73, 74] (Fig. 13.3).

Considering polymer concentrations (from 0.5 to 6 %, w/v) in the organic phase, no significant change in mean particle size was observed with an increase in PLGA content from 0.5 to 3 % (w/v), but there was a significant increase in uniformity (based on the span as measured using laser diffraction; $p < 0.05$, ANOVA followed by Tukey test). The increasing polymer concentration results in an increase in viscosity, and hence stability, of the emulsion produced during the initial primary emulsification [73]. However, as polymer concentration exceeded 3 % (w/v), an overall increase in particle size can be seen; possibly due to an increased frequency in polymer globule collisions resulting in fusion of semi-formed particles [10]. Furthermore, high viscosity solutions, such as the 5 % and 6 % (w/v) polymer solution, may reduce the efficiency of homogenisation, resulting in larger microspheres (Fig. 13.3).

Following through the process, the next stage for consideration is the time of homogenisation of the secondary w/o/w emulsion. Whilst maintaining a constant speed of 6,000 rpm (with an aim of minimising antigen damage), increasing

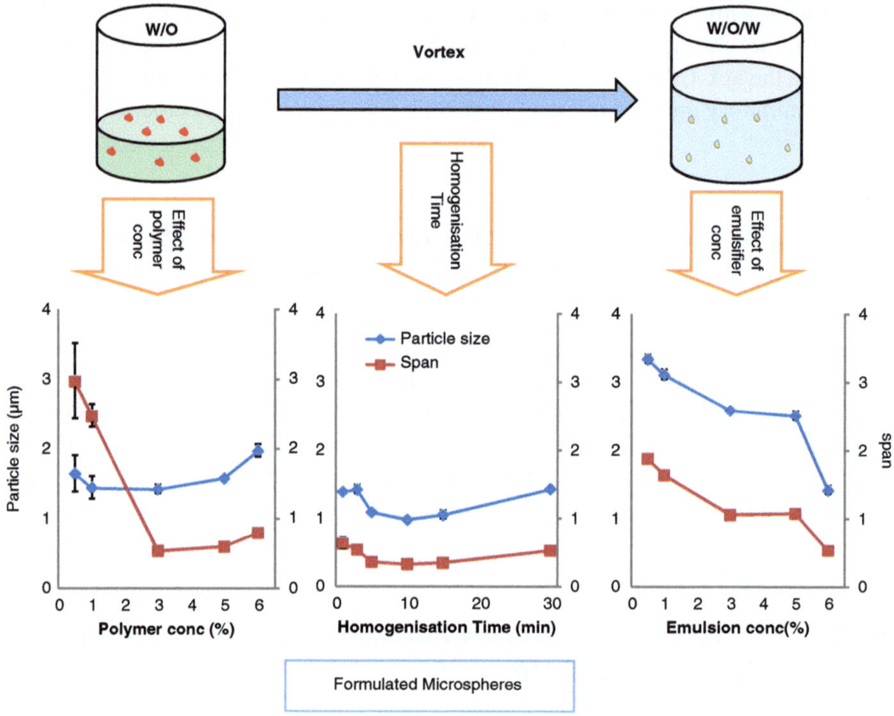

Fig. 13.3 Effect of formulation parameters on the physico-chemical characteristics of the resulting microspheres

homogenisation times from 1 to 10 min led to a general decrease in particle size (Fig. 13.3). However, homogenisation beyond this time then pushed the mean particle size up again, suggesting either fusion of semi-formed particles and/or possible instability in the emulsion due to prolonged shear forces, which also increases the possibility of antigen degradation [73].

In accordance with the empirical relationship between particle size and stabiliser concentration/viscosity [7], our results [73] also showed an increase in PVA concentration in the external aqueous phase resulted in a decrease of mean particle size and size distribution (Fig. 13.3). Indeed, this relationship appears to be relatively linear, corresponding well with similar trends reported elsewhere [17, 116].

13.3.3 Choice of Formulation Components: The Role of Emulsifier

When considering the choice of emulsifiers there are a large range of options, and this choice can have an impact on the physico-chemical characteristics, with the

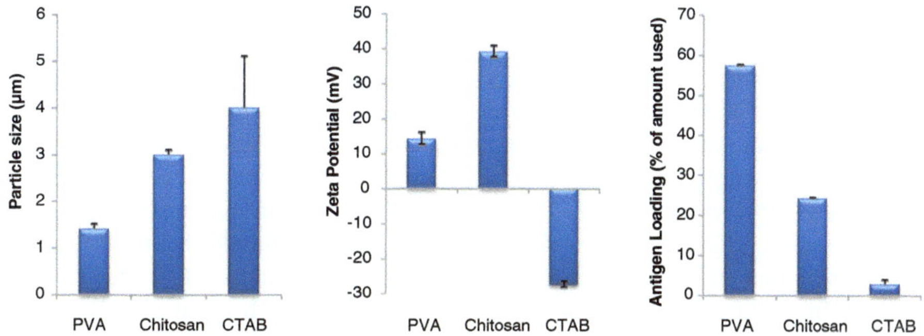

Fig. 13.4 Effect of choice of emulsifier on the physico-chemical characteristics of the resulting microspheres

ability of such formulated microspheres to carry antigen being the most notable (Fig. 13.4). This ability is directly related to the surface charge of the particulates, which can be manipulated through formulation choices. For example, PLGA (3 % w/v) microspheres containing DDA (0.6 % w/v) were prepared using the w/o/w double emulsion solvent evaporation process (Fig. 13.1) and the choice of emulsifier used to prepare the w/o/w emulsion was varied between either PVA (10 %, w/v), chitosan (0.75 %, w/v in 3 %, w/v acetic acid) or cetyl trimethyl ammonium bromide (CTAB; 0.5 %, w/v). Major differences in the formulated microspheres can be noted in size, surface charge and antigen loading (Fig. 13.4) [74].

CTAB is a cationic surfactant similar in structure to DDA, in that it possesses a quaternary ammonium head-group, although the single hydrophobic chain differs from the double hydrophobic chain present in DDA. Moreover, CTAB has previously been used to effectively prepare cationic microspheres for DNA vaccine delivery [14, 34, 103, 156], therefore making it an ideal candidate to compare with PVA.

Chitosan is a deacetylated derivative of chitin, the second most abundant polysaccharide found in nature after cellulose [106]. Derived from crustacean shell waste, once the edible parts have been removed for the food industry, chitin is available to the extent of 10 gigatons a year. Furthermore, the biocompatibility, biodegradability and low toxicity of chitosan have lent its use to a wide variety of applications in a diversity of industries, including agriculture, cosmetics, water treatment, food/nutrition, materials science [36, 54], and of course the medical sciences [70].

In terms of vaccine formulations, chitosan has been shown to stimulate macrophage function [98, 107] and cytokine production [93], possess mucoadhesive properties [145, 152] and facilitate adjuvant activity [95]. Moreover, chitosan has previously been employed in the formulation of particulate delivery vehicles [85, 117, 140], initiating enhanced Th1 immune responses [133], and therefore appears to be a viable alternative to PVA in the formulation of PLGA-based microspheres.

The PVA-stabilised microspheres exhibited relatively small, uniform particles, and it has previously been shown that PVA forms a stable layer around the microspheres, which is not fully removed on washing [11]. The relatively high antigen entrapment efficiency of the PVA-stabilised systems further supports this theory, whereas the positive charge associated with the particles is an indication of the presence of the immunomodulatory DDA (Fig. 13.4). Compared with PVA, neither Chitosan nor CTAB were as effective as emulsifiers based on the larger size of microspheres formed (Fig. 13.4a). Also, contrary to results elsewhere [40, 92], our studies [74] demonstrated that the CTAB-stabilised microspheres had an anionic surface charge, presumably due to the CTAB molecules being lost during washing of the microspheres following solvent evaporation [143]. Indeed, it is evident from the antigen entrapment efficiency (Fig. 13.4c) that CTAB, whilst producing the largest particles, is the least effective of the emulsifying agents studied in terms of stabilising the particles, since the antigen is evidently allowed to migrate to the external aqueous phase rather than remaining entrapped as an internal phase. In addition, this apparent loss of stabilising moieties did result in some aggregation of the particles following lyophilisation, as suggested by the relatively large particle size [74]. Interestingly, of the three, the Chitosan-stabilised particles exhibited a relatively high surface charge, which has been reported to enhance cellular uptake by greater interaction with the negative surface of the APC [18, 23, 34, 131]. Yet, when compared in vaccine studies, the microspheres prepared with PVA were shown to be the most effective in terms of both humoural and cellular immune responses [74].

13.3.4 The Addition of Immunomodulators

As noted, TDB is an acknowledged immunomodulator, particularly in liposomal formulations when in combination with DDA (e.g. [30]; Henriksen-Lacey et al. 2010). Such immunomodulators can also be included within microsphere formulations either with or without DDA. In recent studies from our group, we investigated using the combination of DDA and TDB within microsphere formulations, given that this combination has been shown to be highly effective when adopted in liposome formulations [56]. We are able to formulate PLGA microspheres with a combination of DDA and/or TDB; interestingly, whilst the formulations had a small effect on particle size (Fig. 13.5), loading efficiency of the Ag85B-ESAT-6 TB antigen varied significantly ($p < 0.05$) depending on the microsphere components, with antigen loading reducing from 95 to 57 % with the addition of DDA and to 80 % with the addition of TDB (Fig. 13.5). The antigen loading of microspheres prepared with the combination of DDA and TDB was not significantly different from PLGA:DDA microspheres (55 %; Fig. 13.5). These differences may be due to the choice of components within the microspheres influencing the formation of the particles both in terms of size and porosity, particularly when considering the cationic nature of DDA, which could lead to reduced antigen incorporation, yet this difference in loading capacity was not shown to influence antigen retention over a 2-month study where the microspheres were stored at 4 °C and 25 °C in sterile PBS, pH 7.4.

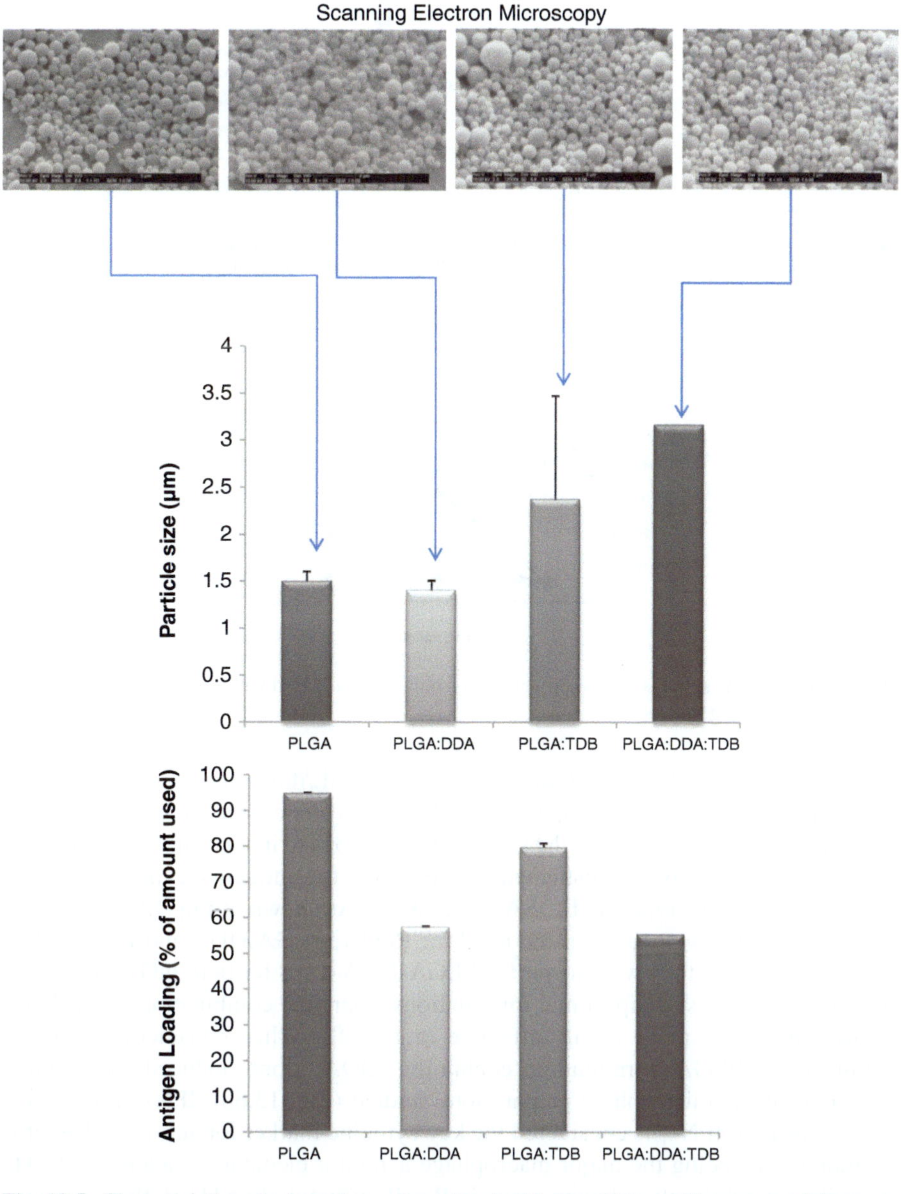

Fig. 13.5 Characteristics of microspheres formulated with the addition of immunomodulators

13.4 Adjuvant Efficacy of PLGA Microspheres for TB Vaccines: A Case Study

In our development studies of PLGA microspheres for TB vaccines, we also considered the efficacy of our systems through *in vivo* studies in mice [73, 74] (Fig. 13.6). C57BL/6 mice were subcutaneously immunised three times at 2 week

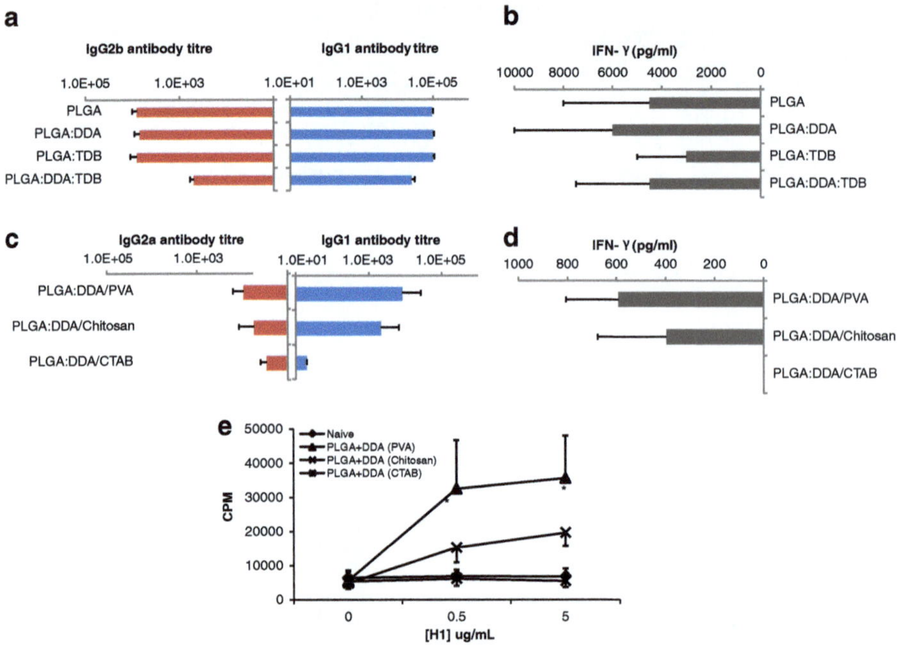

Fig. 13.6 Immune responses of microsphere formulations prepared with various adjuvants and/or various emulsifying agents

intervals with Ag85B-ESAT-6 fusion protein (0.2 mL/dose) encapsulated in PLGA microspheres containing no adjuvant, DDA or TDB alone, or a combination of both DDA and TDB. The ability of the various preparations to induce antibody responses after immunisation was investigated by measuring the antigen-specific titres of the IgG1 and IgG2b isotypes by ELISA (Fig. 13.6a). As shown in Fig. 13.6a, the IgG1 and IgG2b titres were at the same level for PLGA, PLGA:DDA and PLGA:TDB, but, interestingly, they were lower for PLGA-DDA-TDB for both IgG1 and IgG2b, which is in contrast to liposomal formulations where the combination of DDA and TDB was shown to be highly effective (e.g. [30]). When considering cytokine stimulation, PLGA formulation containing DDA alone induced the highest response of the microsphere preparations studied (Fig. 13.6b). IFN-γ levels were also measured; IFN-γ is considered the key cytokine marker for anti-mycobacterial immunity [1], being the major macrophage activator element, indicative of CD4+ recruitment, whilst also playing a role in B cell differentiation [113], therefore vital for cell-mediated immunity [96]. The levels of IFN-γ from spleen lymphocytes showed no significant difference between the four microsphere formulations (Fig. 13.6b).

When DDA, and a combination if DDA:TDB have been mixed into other delivery systems such as niosomes [139], with the addition of other surfactants in the formulation (monopalmitoyl glycerol and cholesterol) it was shown that DDA-based systems were able to effectively enhance cell-mediated Th1 immune responses against Ag85B-ESAT-6, with high IFN-γ levels compared with their niosome-based counterparts while induction of antibody responses, especially IgG1 titres, were comparable between both the systems [139]. However, a strong Th2 humoural response in terms of IgG1 titres was obtained for malarial antigens, which were comparable between the preparations, while niosome-based vesicles showed high IgG2b titres. This was attributed to the ability of vesicles to not only protect their protein content from protease attack *in vivo*, but also deliver it to APCs infiltrating the site of injection or in the lymphatics [139]. This ability to tune the immune response through formulation options offers the potential to tailor the system for the desired outcome, e.g. with malarial antigens where induction of antibody titres is vital in combating the invading parasites [139].

Using similar *in vivo* protocols, however this time in BALB/c mice, we also considered the effect of emulsifier on the immunological properties of PLGA:DDA (based on this system giving the strongest responses in Fig. 13.6a, b). The difference in the absolute readings between the experiments may be due to a number of factors including the antigen dose and the choice of mouse strain (BALB/c vs. the more traditionally used C57Bl/6).

Our results [74] show that the type of emulsifier used has a notable effect on the generation of antibodies, with PVA > Chitosan > CTAB in terms of both IgG1 and 2a (Fig. 13.6c). Indeed, the CTAB-stabilised formulation appears to offer very little immunological effect, possibly due to low antigen to polymer ratio (due to the low entrapment efficiency) and aggregation of the particles, which in turn can lead to ineffective release of antigen (Fig. 13.4) [74]. Additionally, the negative charge associated with the microspheres suggests a lack of surface modification, whilst also indicating the absence of the immunostimulatory DDA, which may potentially impair the interaction with APCs [131, 136]. Indeed, although anionic particulate carriers have been effectively employed in targeting APCs [4, 27, 55, 97, 144], other factors, such as size and protein loading, are likely to have an impact on effective presentation.

With regard to the PVA and Chitosan-stabilised PLGA:DDA particles, both formulations gave comparable IgG2a antibody responses, but the chitosan formulations achieved slightly lower IgG1 responses, which could be a consequence of the relative rigidity of the particles affecting the effective presentation of the antigen to the cells of the immune system. In addition, factors such as size and surface will also influence immune response [23, 111, 135]. As with antibody production, the type of emulsifier employed influenced IFN-γ responses, again with the trend of PVA > Chitosan > CTAB, with both the PVA and the Chitosan-stabilised formulation showed significantly increased levels of IFN-γ (Fig. 13.6d) when compared to CTAB-stabilised formulation, which showed no positive results for any cytokine assayed [74].

Once more, the physico-chemical characteristics of the microsphere formulations (Fig. 13.4) are likely to be the most influential factors in terms of efficacy in initiating an effective immune response. It has already been noted that the lack of surface modification and aggregation of the CTAB-stabilised particles will profoundly affect their interaction with APCs [23, 136]. Moreover, the positively charged systems, i.e. the PVA- and Chitosan-stabilised microspheres, will have a greater tendency to interact with the negative surfaces of the cells of the immune system (e.g. macrophages) [23, 34, 58, 129], allowing more effective presentation and processing of the antigen, as well as a greater likelihood of uptake by such cells. Indeed, it has been reported that an important mechanism of the ability of DDA (present in all formulations) to act as an adjuvant in the delivery of antigen is the immediate electrostatic interaction with the cell surface, followed by induction of active uptake [131]. This observation again implicates the loss of DDA molecules from the CTAB-stabilised formulation, thus leading to inefficient antigen uptake and lack of immunological effect.

Overall, from these studies into the development of PLGA microspheres for the delivery of a TB antigen, Ag85B-ESAT-6, it can be seen that the physico-chemical parameters of the system (which are often seen as basic and rudimentary scientific outputs) can have a significant impact on the immune response generated by the particulate systems, and there is still a need to gain more detailed appreciations of the effect of formulation parameters both on physical as well as biological outcomes in the development of vaccine adjuvants.

13.5 Enhancing the Shelf-Life of Microsphere Formulations

Whilst developing these particulate systems, a key feature of an effective formulation is the development of a stable product that offers sufficient stability on storage. With regard to vaccine products, freeze-drying is often considered as an option to improve stability. Freeze-drying, also referred to as lyophilisation, is used extensively in biological applications, particularly in the manufacture of vaccines, including BCG [50], proteins [87], blood products, antibiotics and enzymes. The process involves freezing a liquid product, and then removing the water by sublimation under reduced pressure. Under such conditions, a liquid-to-solid-to-vapour transition occurs at low temperatures and reduced pressures, resulting in a dry product with low molecular mobility, thereby suppressing potential instabilities arising from physical or chemical interactions [90].

Besides offering enhanced long-term stability, the production of a stable, dry powder product can eliminate the need for a "cold chain", which accounts for millions of wasted doses of vaccines each year [22, 127], and is of particular value in developing regions where TB is a problem (i.e. sub-Saharan Africa and South East Asia), whilst also facilitating transport as compared to bulky products such as solutions. Indeed, it has been estimated that precluding the need for a cold chain for vaccine distribution through development of thermo-stable formulations could save around $200 million annually [84], due to the costs incurred implementing necessary infrastructure, reliable transport, functioning freezers and refrigerators and effective monitoring in order to maintain the cold chain [22]. Moreover, freeze-drying has been shown to be a suitable method for improving the long-term stability of a wide variety of particulate formulations, including microspheres [19, 38], nanoparticles [12, 31, 79], liposomes [28, 90, 134] and non-viral gene delivery vectors [82, 128].

However, it is generally recognised that cryoprotectants are necessary to retain initial formulation characteristics [6, 28, 91, 122], since freeze-drying can promote aggregation or fusion of particles, a phenomenon exploited elsewhere for the production of dehydration-rehydration liposomes [72] and ISCOMs [27, 32]. Having been found to play an important role in organisms capable of withstanding dehydration [29, 77, 84], the most commonly used cryoprotectants are sugars, and more specifically the disaccharides sucrose and trehalose, which have received much attention for their role as cryoprotectants in the freeze-drying of particulate formulations [19, 89, 90, 123, 134, 148]. Various theories concerning the method of action have been proposed: the water replacement hypothesis has been postulated [28], whereby hydrogen bonding forms stable boundaries between particles; alternatively, others [77, 80] have intimated that a glassy layer, formed via vitrification of the sugars, forms a viscous matrix whereby interaction and aggregation of particles is reduced; further, Allison et al. [5] propose that particle isolation, caused by the concentration of solutes in the unfrozen fraction of the solution, is the most likely requirement for effective cryoprotection.

To investigate the potential of freeze-drying microspheres, we have undertaken studies concentrated on the use of the disaccharide sugars, sucrose and trehalose. The results (Fig. 13.7) reveal that cryoprotectants are necessary to maintain microsphere characteristics following lyophilisation. Indeed, freeze-drying of PLGA microspheres prepared by the w/o/w process, both in the presence and absence of DDA, without the use of cryoprotectants (no cryo, Fig. 13.7) leads to significant aggregation and, hence, significantly increased volume mean diameters ($p < 0.01$) as compared to before freeze-drying (bfd, Fig. 13.7). In terms of the efficiency of the disaccharides to act as cryoprotectants, sucrose, at the concentrations tested, was consistently effective in maintaining particle size, both in the presence and absence of DDA within the microparticles, with microparticles retaining a size of around 2 μm post-lyophilisation (Fig. 13.7). Trehalose, on the other hand, is only effective at preventing significant aggregation when DDA is present in the formulation.

These results suggest that the main function of the cryoprotective ability of sucrose appears to be vitrification and particle isolation [5, 76], whereas trehalose requires additional interaction with the particles, as suggested previously [105, 148]. The cationic nature of the DDA headgroup will potentially allow for ion-dipole or electrostatic interactions to be formed with the sugar, thus leading to water replacement, and hence cryoprotection. Indeed, zeta potential analysis of the formulations reveals that, although there is no evidence of an altering of the surface charge when DDA is not present in the formulation (results not shown), freeze-drying of the PLGA + DDA formulation in the presence of trehalose leads to a significant reduction in zeta potential, from 15.7 ± 0.9 mV to -15.1 ± 0.2 mV, whereas employing sucrose as cryoprotectant maintains zeta potential (16.3 ± 6.8 mV). Furthermore, although sucrose prevents significant aggregation in the PLGA formulation (i.e. without DDA), there is still an increase in mean diameter

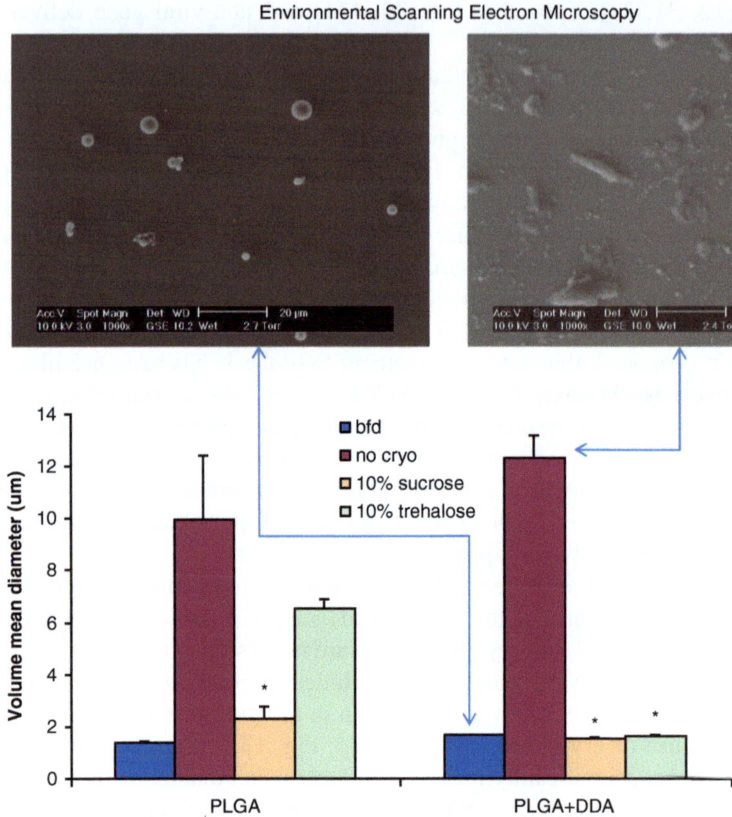

Fig. 13.7 Volume mean diameter of microspheres before and after freeze-drying in the presence of various cryoprotectants. * denotes no significant increase in mean diameter in comparison to before freeze drying (bfd) ($p>0.05$)

following lyophilisation, from 1.39 ± 0.02 μm to 2.30 ± 0.43 μm (Fig. 13.7), as well as an increase in the distribution of sizes, with an increase in span from 1.54 to 2.50 (results not shown). In contrast, the formulation containing DDA shows no significant change in mean diameter (Fig. 13.7) or span (results not shown) when freeze-dried in the presence of either cryoprotectants, suggesting interaction of both the disaccharides with the cationic DDA headgroup, leading to more efficient cryoprotection. This further supports the hypothesis that vitrification alone, although necessary, may not be sufficient for stabilisation of particulate formulations [148].

The apparent difference between the two sugars, in terms of altering the zeta potential of the formulation incorporating DDA, may be explained by the relative stability of the sugar glasses. It has previously been reported that trehalose retains a high T_g upon rehydration and thus remains in the glassy state [2, 29], whereas the lower T_g of sucrose enables the sugar glass to become more readily mobile [29].

Therefore, trehalose may be masking the charge of the microsphere surface by maintaining the glassy state around the particles, whereas the sucrose is more readily hydrated, which again implicates vitrification as a necessary function of cryoprotection in the case of the disaccharides and, subsequently, sucrose should be considered for the production of freeze-drying of microsphere formulations.

13.6 Conclusions

The development of PLGA microspheres as vaccine adjuvants remains slower than would be expected, given the supporting evidence for their efficacy. Issues that have hindered their development include potential instabilities of PLGA-encapsulated antigens, difficulties in large-scale manufacture, and lack of translation of results through various animal models. Yet, much progress has been made in terms of the formulatory considerations, although appropriate and translational pre-clinical models for testing of vaccines remains limited, with the lack of correlation between small animal models and humans continuing to be a major blockage to further development of not only PLGA systems, but many other vaccine formulations. Nevertheless, the continued unravelling of the biological mechanisms required for effective immunisation looks to address this issue, with new methods now being adopted for the detailed evaluation of vaccines. Therefore, whilst the formulation characteristics of PLGA-based microspheres have been extensively evaluated, the correlation with detailed biological outputs in appropriate models remains the key to determining if these delivery systems can be employed as vaccine adjuvants.

References

1. Agger E, Andersen P (2001) Tuberculosis subunit vaccine development: on the role of interferon-gamma. Vaccine 19:2298–2302
2. Aldous B, Auffret A, Franks F (1995) The crystallisation of hydrates from amorphous carbohydrates. Cryo Letters 16:181–186
3. Allemann E, Gurny R, Doelker E (1992) Preparation of aqueous polymeric nanodispersions by a reversible salting-out process: influence of process parameters on particle size. Int J Pharm 87:247–253
4. Allison A, Gregoriadis G (1974) Liposomes as immunological adjuvants. Nature 252:252
5. Allison S, Molina M, Anchordoquy T (2000) Stabilisation of lipid DNA complexes during the freezing step of the lyophilization process: the particle isolation hypothesis. Biochim Biophys Acta 1468:127–138
6. Anchordoquy T, Allison S, Molina M, Girouard L, Carson T (2001) Physical stabilization of DNA-based therapeutics. Drug Discov Today 6:463–470
7. Arshady R (1991) Preparation of biodegradable microspheres and microcapsules: 2. Polyactides and related polyesters. J Control Release 17:1–21

8. Audran R, Peter K, Dannull J, Men Y, Scandella E, Groettrup M, Gander B, Corradin G (2003) Encapsulation of peptides in biodegradable microspheres prolongs their MHC class-I presentation by dendritic cells and macrophages in vitro. Vaccine 21:1250–1255
9. Bendix D (1998) Chemical synthesis of polylactide and its copolymers for medical applications. Polym Degrad Stabil 59:125–135
10. Benoit M, Baras B, Gillard J (1999) Preparation and characterization of protein-loaded poly (epsilon-caprolactone) microparticles for oral vaccine delivery. Int J Pharm 184:73–84
11. Boury F, Ivanova T, Panaiotov I, Proust J, Bois A, Richou J (1995) Dynamic properties of poly(DL-lactide) and polyvinyl alcohol monolayers at the air/water and dichloromethane/water interfaces. J Colloid Interface Sci 169:380–392
12. Bozdag S, Dillen K, Vandervoort J, Ludwig A (2005) The effect of freeze-drying with different cryoprotectants and gamma-irradiation sterilization on the characteristics of ciprofloxacin HCl-loaded poly(D, L-lactide-glycolide) nanoparticles. J Pharm Pharmacol 57:699–707
13. Bramwell V, Perrie Y (2005) Particulate delivery systems for vaccines. Crit Rev Ther Drug Carrier Syst 22:151–214
14. Briones M, Singh M, Ugozzoli M, Kazzaz J, Klakamp S, Ott G, O'Hagan D (2001) The preparation, characterization, and evaluation of cationic microparticles for DNA vaccine delivery. Pharm Res 18:709–712
15. Brunner R, Wallmann J, Szalai K, Karagiannis P, Kopp T, Scheiner O, Jensen-Jarolim E, Pali-Scholl I (2007) The impact of aluminium in acid-suppressing drugs on the immune response of BALB/c mice. Clin Exp Allergy 37:1566–1573
16. Burns RJ, Vitale K, Sanders L (1990) Nafarelin controlled release injectable: theoretical clinical plasma profiles from multiple dosing and from mixtures of microspheres containing 2 per cent, 4 per cent and 7 per cent nafarelin. J Microencapsul 7:397–413
17. Capan Y, Woo B, Gebrekidan S, Ahmed S, DeLuca P (1999) Influence of formulation parameters on the characteristics of poly(D, L-lactide-co-glycolide) microspheres containing poly(L-lysine) complexed plasmid DNA. J Control Release 60:279–286
18. Carmona-Ribeiro A, Ortis F, Schumacher R, Armelin M (1997) Interactions between cationic vesicles and cultured mammalian cells. Langmuir 13:2215–2218
19. Chacon M, Molpeceres J, Berges L, Guzman M, Aberturas M (1999) Stability and freeze-drying of cyclosporine loaded poly(D, L lactide-glycolide) carriers. Eur J Pharm Sci 8:99–107
20. Choi S, Kwon H, Kim W, Kim J (2002) Thermodynamic parameters on poly(d, l-lactide-co-glycolide) particle size in emulsification-diffusion process. Colloids Surf A Physicochem Eng Asp 201:283–289
21. Chong C, Cao M, Wong W, Fischer K, Addison W, Kwon G, Tyrrell D, Samuel J (2005) Enhancement of T helper type 1 immune responses against hepatitis B virus core antigen by PLGA nanoparticle vaccine delivery. J Control Release 102:85–99
22. Christensen D, Foged C, Rosenkrands I, Nielsen H, Andersen P, Agger E (2007) Trehalose preserves DDA/TDB liposomes and their adjuvant effect during freeze-drying. Biochim Biophys Acta 1768:2120–2129
23. Chung T, Wu S, Yao M, Lu C, Lin Y, Hung Y, Mou C, Chen Y, Huang D (2007) The effect of surface charge on the uptake and biological function of mesoporous silica nanoparticles in 3T3-L1 cells and human mesenchymal stem cells. Biomaterials 28:2959–2966
24. Cohen S, Chen L, Apte R (1995) Controlled release of peptides and proteins from biodegradable polyester microspheres: an approach for treating infectious diseases and malignancies. React Polym 25:177–187
25. Conway A, Madrigal-Estebas L, McClean S, Brayden D, Mills K (2001) Protection against Bordetella pertussis infection following parenteral or oral immunization with antigens entrapped in biodegradable particles: effect of formulation and route of immunization on induction of Th1 and Th2 cells. Vaccine 19:1940–1950
26. Cooper A, Dalton D, Stewart T, Griffin J, Russell D, Orme I (1993) Disseminated tuberculosis in interferon gamma gene-disrupted mice. J Exp Med 178:2243–2247

27. Copland M, Rades T, Davies N (2000) Hydration of lipid films with an aqueous solution of Quil A: a simple method for the preparation of immune-stimulating complexes. Int J Pharm 196:135–139
28. Crowe J, Crowe L (1988) Factors affecting the stability of dry liposomes. Biochim Biophys Acta 939:327–334
29. Crowe L, Reid D, Crowe J (1996) Is trehalose special for preserving dry biomaterials? Biophys J 71:2087–2093
30. Davidsen J, Rosenkrands I, Christensen D, Vangala A, Kirby D, Perrie Y, Agger E, Andersen P (2005) Characterization of cationic liposomes based on dimethyldioctadecylammonium and synthetic cord factor from M. tuberculosis (trehalose 6,6′-dibehenate)-a novel adjuvant inducing both strong CMI and antibody responses. Biochim Biophys Acta 1718:22–31
31. de Chasteigner S, Cavé G, Fessi H, Devissaguet J-P, Puisieux F (1998) Freeze-drying of itraconazole-loaded nanosphere suspension: a feasibility study. Drug Dev Res 38:116–124
32. Demana P, Davies N, Hook S, Rades T (2005) Quil A-lipid powder formulations releasing ISCOMs and related colloidal structures upon hydration. J Control Release 103:45–59
33. Demento S, Eisenbarth S, Foellmer H, Platt C, Caplan M, Saltzman M, Mellman I, Ledizet M, Fikrig E, Flavell R, Fahmy T (2009) Inflammasome-activating nanoparticles as modular systems for optimizing vaccine efficacy. Vaccine 27:3013–3021
34. Denis-Mize K, Dupuis M, Singh M, Woo C, Ugozzoli M, O'Hagan D, Donnelly JI, Ott G, McDonald D (2003) Mechanisms of increased immunogenicity for DNA-based vaccines adsorbed onto cationic microparticles. Cell Immunol 225:12–20
35. Diwan M, Tafaghodi M, Samuel J (2002) Enhancement of immune responses by co-delivery of a CpG oligodeoxynucleotide and tetanus toxoid in biodegradable nanospheres. J Control Release 85:247–262
36. Dodane V, Vilivalam V (1998) Pharmaceutical applications of chitosan. Pharm Sci Technol Today 1:246–253
37. Domb A, Kumar N, Sheskin T, Bentolila A, Slager J, Teomim D (2002) Biodegradable polymers as drug carrier systems. In: Dumitriu S (ed) Polymeric biomaterials. Marcel Dekker, New York, pp 91–122
38. Duncan G, Jess T, Mohamed F, Price N, Kelly S, van der Walle C (2005) The influence of protein solubilisation, conformation and size on the burst release from poly(lactide-co-glycolide) microspheres. J Control Release 110:34–48
39. Eldridge J, Staas J, Meulbroek J, Tice T, Gilley R (1991) Biodegradable and biocompatible poly(DL-lactide-co-glycolide) microspheres as an adjuvant for staphylococcal enterotoxin B toxoid which enhances the level of toxin-neutralizing antibodies. Infect Immun 59: 2978–2986
40. Esposito E, Sebben S, Cortesi R, Menegatti E, Nastruzzi C (1999) Preparation and characterization of cationic microspheres for gene delivery. Int J Pharm 189:29–41
41. Fattal E, Pecquet S, Couvreur P, Andremont A (2002) Biodegradable microparticles for the mucosal delivery of antibacterial and dietary antigens. Int J Pharm 242:15–24
42. Fearon K, Marshall JD, Abbate C, Subramanian S, Yee P, Gregorio J, Teshima G, Ott G, Tuck S, Van Nest G (2003) A minimal human immunostimulatory CpG motif that potently induces IFN-gamma and IFN-alpha production. Eur J Immunol 33:2114–2159
43. Feng L, Rong X, Xing Q, Zhou J, Maitani Y, Wang S, Jiang Y, Nagai T (2006) Pharmaceutical and immunological evaluation of a single-dose hepatitis B vaccine using PLGA microspheres. J Control Release 112:35–42
44. Fessi H, Puisieux F, Devissaguet J, Ammoury N, Benita S (1989) Nanocapsule formation by interfacial polymer deposition following solvent displacement. Int J Pharm 55:1–4
45. Flynn J, Chan J, Triebold K, Dalton D, Stewart T, Bloom B (1993) An essential role for interferon gamma in resistance to Mycobacterium tuberculosis infection. J Exp Med 178:2249–2254
46. Freytag L, Clements J (2005) Mucosal adjuvants. Vaccine 23:1804–1813
47. Furr B, Hutchinson F (1985) Biodegradable sustained release formulation of the LH-RH analogue 'Zoladex' for the treatment of hormone-responsive tumours. Prog Clin Biol Res 185:143–153

48. Furukawa T, Matsusue Y, Yasunaga T, Shikinami Y, Okuno M, Nakamura T (2000) Biodegradation behavior of ultra-high-strength hydroxyapatite/poly (-lactide) composite rods for internal fixation of bone fractures. Biomaterials 21:889–898
49. Gall D (1966) The adjuvant activity of aliphatic nitrogenous bases. Immunology 11:369–386
50. Gheorghiu M, Lagranderie M, Balazuc A (1996) Stabilisation of BCG vaccines. Dev Biol Stand 87:251–261
51. Gopferich A (1996) Mechanisms of polymer degradation and erosion. Biomaterials 17:103–114
52. Hamdy S, Molavi O, Ma Z, Haddadi A, Alshamsan A, Gobti Z, Elhasi S, Samuel J, Lavasanifar A (2008) Co-delivery of cancer-associated antigen and Toll-like receptor 4 ligand in PLGA nanoparticles induces potent CD8+ T cell-mediated anti-tumor immunity. Vaccine 26:5046–5047
53. Hanafusa S, Matsusue Y, Yasunaga T, Yamamuro T, Oka M, Shikinami Y, Ikada Y (1995) Biodegradable plate fixation of rabbit femoral shaft osteotomies. A comparative study. Clin Orthop Relat Res 315:262–271
54. Harish Prashanth K, Tharanathan R (2007) Chitin/chitosan: modifications and their unlimited application potential an overview. Trends Food Sci Technol 18:117–131
55. Heath T, Lopez N, Papahadjopoulos D (1985) The effects of liposome size and surface charge on liposome-mediated delivery of methotrexate-[gamma]-aspartate to cells in vitro. Biochim Biophys Acta 820:74–84
56. Henriksen-Lacey M, Bramwell V, Christensen D, Agger E, Andersen P, Perrie Y (2010) Liposomes based on dimethyldioctadecylammonium promote a depot effect and enhance immunogenicity of soluble antigen. J Control Release 142:180–186
57. Hornung V, Bauernfeind F, Halle A, Samstad E, Kono H, Rock K, Fitzgerald K, Latz E (2008) Silica crystals and aluminum salts activate the NALP3 inflammasome through phagosomal destabilization. Nat Immunol 9:847–856
58. Huang M, Khor E, Lim L (2004) Uptake and cytotoxicity of chitosan molecules and nanoparticles: effects of molecular weight and degree of deacetylation. Pharm Res 21:344–353
59. Igartua M, Hernandez R, Esquisabel A, Gascon A, Calvo M, Pedraz J (1998) Enhanced immune response after subcutaneous and oral immunization with biodegradable PLGA microspheres. J Control Release 56:63–73
60. Ishikawa E, Ishikawa T, Morita Y, Toyonaga K, Yamada H, Takeuchi O, Kinoshita T, Akira S, Yoshikai Y, Yamasaki S (2009) Direct recognition of the mycobacterial glycolipid, trehalose dimycolate, by C-type lectin Mincle. J Exp Med 206:2879–2888
61. Jabbal-Gill I, Lin W, Jenkins P, Watts P, Jimenez M, Illum L, Davis S, Wood J, Major D, Minor P (1999) Potential of polymeric lamellar substrate particles (PLSP) as adjuvants for vaccines. Vaccine 18:238–250
62. Jain R (2000) The manufacturing techniques of various drug loaded biodegradable poly (lactide-co-glycolide) (PLGA) devices. Biomaterials 21:2475–2490
63. Jalil R, Nixon J (1990) Biodegradable poly (lactic acid) and poly (lactide-coglycolide) microcapsules: problems associated with preparative techniques and release properties. J Microencapsul 7:297–325
64. Jamshidi K, Hyon S, Ikada Y (1988) Thermal characterization of polylactides. Polymer 29:2229–2234
65. Janeway CJ (1989) Approaching the asymptote? Evolution and revolution in immunology. Cold Spring Harb Symp Quant Biol 54:1–13
66. Jiang W, Gupta R, Deshpande M, Schwendeman S (2005) Biodegradable poly(lactic-co-glycolic acid) microparticles for injectable delivery of vaccine antigens. Adv Drug Deliv Rev 57:391–410
67. Jilek S, Merkle H, Walter E (2005) DNA-loaded biodegradable microparticles as vaccine delivery systems and their interaction with dendritic cells. Adv Drug Deliv Rev 57:377–390
68. Johansen P, Moon L, Tamber H, Merkle H, Gander B, Sesardic D (1999) Immunogenicity of single-dose diphtheria vaccines based on PLA/PLGA microspheres in guinea pigs. Vaccine 18:209–215

69. Jung T, Koneberg R, Hungerer K, Kissel T (2002) Tetanus toxoid microspheres consisting of biodegradable poly(lactide-co-glycolide)- and ABA-triblock-copolymers: immune response in mice. Int J Pharm 234:75–90
70. Khor E, Lim L (2003) Implantable applications of chitin and chitosan. Biomaterials 24:2339–2349
71. Kim H, Chung H, Park T (2006) Biodegradable polymeric microspheres with open/closed pores for sustained release of human growth hormone. J Control Release 112:167–174
72. Kirby C, Gregoriadis G (1984) Preparation of liposomes containing factor VIII for oral treatment of haemophilia. J Microencapsul 1:33–45
73. Kirby D, Rosenkrands I, Agger E, Andersen P, Coombes A, Perrie Y (2008) PLGA microspheres for the delivery of a novel subunit TB vaccine. J Drug Target 16:282–293
74. Kirby D, Rosenkrands I, Agger E, Andersen P, Coombes A, Perrie Y (2008) Liposomes act as stronger subunit vaccine adjuvants when compared to microspheres. J Drug Target 16:543–554
75. Kissel T, Koneberg R (1996) Injectable biodegradable microspheres for vaccine delivery. In: Cohen S, Bernstein H (eds) Microparticulate systems for the delivery of proteins and vaccines. Marcel Dekker, New York, pp 51–88
76. Konan Y, Gurny R, Allemann E (2002) Preparation and characterization of sterile and freeze-dried sub-200 nm nanoparticles. Int J Pharm 233:239–252
77. Koster K, Leopold A (1988) Sugars and desiccation tolerance in seeds. Plant Physiol 88:829–832
78. Langer R, Folkman J (1976) Polymers for the sustained release of proteins and other macromolecules. Nature 263:797–800
79. Lemoine D, Francois C, Kedzierewicz F, Preat V, Hoffman M, Maincent P (1996) Stability study of nanoparticles of poly(epsilon-caprolactone), poly(D, L-lactide) and poly (D, L-lactide-co-glycolide). Biomaterials 17:2191–2197
80. Levine H, Slade L (1988) Principles of 'cryostabilization' technology from structure/property relationships of carbohydrate/water systems—a review. Cryo-Lett 9:21–63
81. Lewis D (1990) Controlled release of bioactive agents from lactide/glycolide polymers. In: Chasin M, Langer R (eds) Biodegradable polymers as drug delivery systems. Marcel Dekker, New York, pp 1–41
82. Li B, Li S, Tan Y, Stolz D, Watkins S, Block L, Huang L (2000) Lyophilization of cationic lipid-protamine-DNA (LPD) complexes. J Pharm Sci 89:355–364
83. Linghua Z, Xingshan T, Fengzhen Z (2008) In vivo oral administration effects of various oligodeoxynucleotides containing synthetic immunostimulatory motifs in the immune response to pseudorabies attenuated virus vaccine in newborn piglets. Vaccine 26:224–233
84. Lloyd J (2000) Technologies for vaccine delivery in the 21st century. Department of Vaccines and Biologicals, World Health Organisation, Geneva, Switzerland
85. Luzardo-Alvarez A, Blarer N, Peter K, Romero J, Reymond C, Corradin G, Gander B (2005) Biodegradable microspheres alone do not stimulate murine macrophages in vitro, but prolong antigen presentation by macrophages in vitro and stimulate a solid immune response in mice. J Control Release 109:62–76
86. Mandal B, Kempf M, Merkle H, Walter E (2004) Immobilisation of GM-CSF onto particulate vaccine carrier systems. Int J Pharm 269:259–265
87. Manning M, Patel K, Borchardt R (1989) Stability of protein pharmaceuticals. Pharm Res 6:903–918
88. McCluskie M, Weeratna R, Krieg A, Davis H (2000) CpG DNA is an effective oral adjuvant to protein antigens in mice. Vaccine 19:950–957
89. Miyajima K, Tomita K, Nakagaki M (1986) Effect of saccharides on the freezing and thawing of liposome dispersion. Chem Pharm Bull 34:2689–2697
90. Mohammed A, Bramwell V, Coombes A, Perrie Y (2006) Lyophilisation and sterilisation of liposomal vaccines to produce stable and sterile products. Methods 40:30–38

91. Mohammed A, Coombes A, Perrie Y (2007) Amino acids as cryoprotectants for liposomal delivery systems. Eur J Pharm Sci 30:406–413
92. Mollenkopf H, Dietrich G, Fensterle J, Grode L, Diehl K, Knapp B, Singh M, O'Hagan D, Ulmer J, Kaufmann S (2004) Enhanced protective efficacy of a tuberculosis DNA vaccine by adsorption onto cationic PLG microparticles. Vaccine 22:2690–2695
93. Mori T, Okumura M, Matsuura M, Ueno K, Tokura S, Okamoto Y, Minami S, Fujinaga T (1997) Effects of chitin and its derivatives on the proliferation and cytokine production of fibroblasts in vitro. Biomaterials 18:947–951
94. Morokata T, Ishikawaa J, Yamada T (2000) Antigen dose defines T helper 1 and T helper 2 responses in the lungs of C57BL/6 and BALB/c mice independently of splenic responses. Immunol Lett 72:119–126
95. Moschos S, Bramwell V, Somavarapu S, Alpar H (2004) Adjuvant synergy: the effects of nasal coadministration of adjuvants. Immunol Cell Biol 82:628–637
96. Mosmann T, Sad S (1996) The expanding universe of T-cell subsets: Th1, Th2 and more. Immunol Today 17:138–146
97. Myschik J, Lendemans D, McBurney W, Demana P, Hook S, Rades T (2006) On the preparation, microscopic investigation and application of ISCOMs. Micron 37:724–734
98. Nishimura K, Nishimura S, Seo H, Nishi N, Tokura S, Azuma I (1987) Effect of multiporous microspheres derived from chitin and partially deacetylated chitin on the activation of mouse peritoneal macrophages. Vaccine 5:136–140
99. Nykamp G, Carstensen U, Muller B (2002) Jet milling a new technique for microparticle preparation. Int J Pharm 242:79–86
100. Ogawa Y, Yamamoto M, Okada H, Yashiki T, Shimamoto T (1988) A new technique to efficiently entrap leuprolide acetate into microcapsules of polylactic acid or copoly(lactic/glycolic) acid. Chem Pharm Bull 36:1095–1103
101. O'Hagan D, MacKichan M, Singh M (2001) Recent developments in adjuvants for vaccines against infectious diseases. Biomol Eng 18:69–85
102. O'Hagan D, Rahman D, McGee J, Jeffery H, Davies M, Williams P, Davis S, Challacombe S (1991) Biodegradable microparticles as controlled release antigen delivery systems. Immunology 73:239–242
103. O'Hagan D, Singh M, Dong C, Ugozzoli M, Berger K, Glazer E, Selby M, Wininger M, Ng P, Crawford K, Paliard X, Coates S, Houghton M (2004) Cationic microparticles are a potent delivery system for a HCV DNA vaccine. Vaccine 23:672–680
104. Olds G, Chedid L, Lederer E, Mahmoud A (1980) Induction of resistance to Schistosoma-mansoni by natural cord factor and synthetic lower homologs. J Infect Dis 141:473–478
105. Ozaki K, Hayashi M (1998) Effect of cycloinulohexaose with additives on the freeze-drying of liposome. Int J Pharm 160:219–227
106. Patel V, Patel M, Patel R (2005) Chitosan: a unique pharmaceutical excipient. Drug Deliv Technol 5:30–40
107. Peluso G, Petillo O, Ranieri M, Santin M, Ambrosic L, Calabro D, Avallone B, Balsamo G (1994) Chitosan-mediated stimulation of macrophage function. Biomaterials 15:1215–1220
108. Perrie Y, Kirby D, Bramwell V, Mohammed A (2007) Recent developments in particulate-based vaccines. Recent Pat Drug Deliv Formul 1:117–130
109. Perrin D, English J (1997) Polyglycolide and polylactide. In: Domb A, Kost J, Wiseman D (eds) Handbook of biodegradable polymers. Harwood Academic Publishers, Amsterdam, pp 3–28
110. Petaja T, Keranen H, Karppa T, Kawa A, Lantela S, Siitari-Mattila M, Levanen H, Tocklin T, Godeaux O, Lehtinen M, Dubin G (2009) Immunogenicity and safety of human papillomavirus (HPV)-16/18 AS04-adjuvanted vaccine in healthy boys aged 10-18 years. J Adolesc Health 44:33–40
111. Peyre M, Fleck R, Hockley D, Gander B, Sesardic D (2004) In vivo uptake of an experimental microencapsulated diphtheria vaccine following sub-cutaneous immunisation. Vaccine 22:2430–2437

112. Pimm M, Baldwin R, Polonsky J, Lederer E (1979) Immunotherapy of an ascitic rat hepatoma with cord factor (trehalose-6, 6′-dimycolate) and synthetic analogs. Int J Cancer 24:780–785
113. Playfair J, Bancroft G (2004) Infection and immunity, 2nd edn. Oxford University Press, Oxford
114. Preis I, Langer R (1979) A single-step immunization by sustained antigen release. J Immunol Methods 28:193–197
115. Quaglia F, De R, Granata E, Ungaro F, Fattal E, Immacolata La Rotonda M (2003) Feeding liquid, non-ionic surfactant and cyclodextrin affect the properties of insulin-loaded poly (lactide-co-glycolide) microspheres prepared by spray-drying. J Control Release 86:267–278
116. Rafati H, Coombes A, Adler J, Holland J, Davis S (1997) Protein-loaded poly(-lactide-co-glycolide) microparticles for oral administration: formulation, structural and release characteristics. J Control Release 43:89–102
117. Ravi Kumar M, Bakowsky U, Lehr C (2004) Preparation and characterization of cationic PLGA nanospheres as DNA carriers. Biomaterials 25:1771–1777
118. Ren J, Hong H, Song J, Ren T (2005) Particle size and distribution of biodegradable poly-D, L-lactide-co-poly(ethylene glycol) block polymer nanoparticles prepared by nanoprecipitation. J Appl Poly Sci 98:1884–1890
119. Roman B, Irache J, Gomez S, Tsapis N, Gamazo C, Espuelas M (2008) Co-encapsulation of an antigen and CpG oligonucleotides into PLGA microparticles by TROMS technology. Eur J Pharm Biopharm 70:98–108
120. Rosas J, Pedraz J, Hernandez R, Gascon A, Igartua M, Guzman F, Rodriguez R, Cortes J, Patarroyo M (2002) Remarkably high antibody levels and protection against P. falciparum malaria in Aotus monkeys after a single immunisation of SPf66 encapsulated in PLGA microspheres. Vaccine 20:1707–1710
121. Rosenkrands I, Agger E, Olsen A, Korsholm K, Andersen C, Jensen K, Andersen P (2005) Cationic liposomes containing mycobacterial lipids—a new powerful Th1 adjuvant system. Infect Immun 73:5817–5826
122. Roy D, Guillon X, Lescure F, Couvreur P, Bru N, Breton P (1997) On shelf stability of freeze-dried poly(methylidene malonate 2.1.2) nanoparticles. Int J Pharm 148:165–175
123. Saez A, Guzman M, Molpeceres J, Aberturas M (2000) Freeze-drying of polycaprolactone and poly(D, L-lactic-glycolic) nanoparticles induce minor particle size changes affecting the oral pharmacokinetics of loaded drugs. Eur J Pharm Biopharm 50:379–387
124. Sarti F, Perera G, Hintzen F, Kotti K, Karageorgiou V, Kammona O, Kiparissides C, Bernkop-Schnurch A (2011) In vivo evidence of oral vaccination with PLGA nanoparticles containing the immunostimulant monophosphoryl. Biomaterials 32:4052–4057
125. Sartia F, Pereraa G, Hintzena F, Kottib K, Karageorgioub V, Kammonab O, Kiparissidesb C, Bernkop-Schnurcha A (2011) In vivo evidence of oral vaccination with PLGA nanoparticles containing the immunostimulant monophosphoryl lipid A. Biomaterials 32:4052–4057
126. Schoenen H, Bodendorfer B, Hitchens K, Manzanero S, Werninghaus K, Nimmerjahn F, Agger E, Stenger S, Andersen P, Ruland J, Brown G, Wells C, Lang R (2010) Cutting edge: mincle is essential for recognition and adjuvanticity of the mycobacterial cord factor and its synthetic analog trehalose-dibehenate. J Immunol 184:2756–2760
127. Schondorf I, Banzhoff A, Nicolay U, Diaz-Mitoma F (2007) Overcoming the need for a cold chain with conjugated meningococcal Group C vaccine: a controlled, randomized, double-blind study in toddlers on the safety and immunogenicity of Menjugate, stored at room temperature for 6 months. Vaccine 25:1175–1182
128. Seville P, Kellaway I, Birchall J (2002) Preparation of dry powder dispersions for non-viral gene delivery by freeze-drying and spray-drying. J Gene Med 4:428–437
129. Singh A, Kasinath B, Lewis E (1992) Interaction of polycations with cell-surface negative charges of epithelial cells. Biochim Biophys Acta 1120:337–342
130. Sinha V, Trehan A (2003) Biodegradable microspheres for protein delivery. J Control Release 90:261–280

131. Smith Korsholm K, Agger E, Foged C, Christensen D, Dietrich J, Andersen C, Geisler C, Andersen P (2007) The adjuvant mechanism of cationic dimethyldioctadecylammonium liposomes. Immunology 121:216–226
132. Storni T, Kundig T, Senti G, Johansen P (2005) Immunity in response to particulate antigen-delivery systems. Adv Drug Deliv Rev 57:333–355
133. Strong P, Clark H, Reid K (2002) Intranasal application of chitin microparticles down-regulates symptoms of allergic hypersensitivity to Dermatophagoides pteronyssinus and Aspergillus fumigatus in murine models of allergy. Clin Exp Allergy 32:1794–1800
134. Sun W, Leopold A, Crowe L, Crowe J (1996) Stability of dry liposomes in sugar glasses. Biophys J 70:1769–1776
135. Tabata Y, Ikada Y (1988) Effect of the size and surface charge of polymer microspheres on their phagocytosis by macrophage. Biomaterials 9:356–362
136. Tabata Y, Ikada Y (1988) Macrophage phagocytosis of biodegradable microspheres composed of L-lactic acid/glycolic acid homo- and copolymers. J Biomed Mater Res 22:837–858
137. Tamber H, Johansen P, Merkle H, Gander B (2005) Formulation aspects of biodegradable polymeric microspheres for antigen delivery. Adv Drug Deliv Rev 57:357–376
138. Tice T, Cowsar DB (1984) Biodegradable controlled-release parenteral systems. J Pharm Technol 8:26–31
139. Vangala A, Bramwell V, McNeil S, Christensen D, Agger E, Perrie Y (2007) Comparison of vesicle based antigen delivery systems for delivery of hepatitis B surface antigen. J Control Release 119:102–110
140. Vila A, Sanchez A, Tobio M, Calvo P, Alonso M (2002) Design of biodegradable particles for protein delivery. J Control Release 78:15–24
141. Vrancken M, Claeys D (1970) Method for encapsulating water and compounds in aqueous phase by extraction. US Patent 3523907
142. Werninghaus K, Babiak A, Groß O, Holscher C, Dietrich H, Agger E, Mages J, Mocsai A, Schoenen H, Finger K, Nimmerjahn F, Brown G, Kirschning C, Heit A, Andersen P, Wagner H, Ruland J, Lang R (2009) Adjuvanticity of a synthetic cord factor analogue for subunit Mycobacterium tuberculosis vaccination requires FcRγ-Syk-Card9-dependent innate immune activation. J Exp Med 206:89–97
143. Wischke C, Borchert H, Zimmermann J, Siebenbrodt I, Lorenzen D (2006) Stable cationic microparticles for enhanced model antigen delivery to dendritic cells. J Control Release 114:359–368
144. Ahsan, F., Rivas, I.P., Khan, M.A., Torres Suarez, A.I. (2002) Targeting to macrophages: role of physicochemical properties of particulate carriers–liposomes and microspheres–on the phagocytosis by macrophages. J. Control Release, 79, 29–40
145. Alpar, H.O., Somavarapu, S., Atuah, K.N., Bramwell, V.W. (2005) Biodegradable mucoadhesive particulates for nasal and pulmonary antigen and DNA delivery. Advanced Drug Delivery Reviews, 57, 411–430
146. Brunner, R., Jensen-Jarolim, E., Pali-Schöll, I. (2010) The ABC of clinical and experimental adjuvants—A brief overview. Immunology Letters, 128(1), 29–35
147. Brandt, L., Elhay, M., Rosenkrands, I., Lindblad, E.B., Andersen, P. (2000) ESAT-6 subunit vaccination against Mycobacterium tuberculosis. Infect. Immun., 68, 791–795
148. Crowe, J.H., Leslie, S.B., Crowe, L.M. (1994a) Is vitrification sufficient to preserve liposomes during freeze-drying? Cryobiology, 31, 355–366
149. Davis, H.L., Weeratna, R., Waldschmidt, T.J., Tygrett, L., Schorr, J., Krieg, A.M. (1998) CpG DNA is a potent enhancer of specific immunity in mice immunized with recombinant hepatitis B surface antigen. J. Immunol., 160, 870–876
150. Hamdy, S., Haddadi, A., Somayaji, V., Ruan, D., Samuel, J. (2007) Pharmaceutical analysis of synthetic lipid A-based vaccine adjuvants in poly (d,l-lactic-co-glycolic acid) nanoparticle formulations. Journal of Pharmaceutical and Biomedical Analysis, 44(4), 914–92
151. Holten-Andersen, L., Doherty, T.M., Korsholm, K.S., Andersen, P. (2004) Combination of the cationic surfactant dimethyl dioctadecyl ammonium bromide and synthetic mycobacterial

cord factor as an efficient adjuvant for tuberculosis subunit vaccines. Infect. Immun., 72, 1608–1617
152. Illum, L., Farraj, N.F., Davis, S.S. (1994) Chitosan as a Novel Nasal Delivery System for Peptide Drugs. Pharmaceutical Research, 11, 1186–1189
153. Klinguer, C., Beck, A., De-Lys, P., Bussat, M.C., Blaecke, A., Derouet, F., Bonnefoy, J.Y., Nguyen, T.N., Corvaia, N., Velin, D. (2001) Lipophilic quaternary ammonium salt acts as a mucosal adjuvant when co-administered by the nasal route with vaccine antigens. Vaccine, 19, 4236–4244
154. Lindblad, E.B., Elhay, M.J., Silva, R., Appelberg, R., Andersen, P. (1997) Adjuvant modulation of immune responses to tuberculosis subunit vaccines. Infect. Immun., 65, 623–629
155. McCluskie, M.J., Davis, H.L. (1998) CpG DNA is a potent enhancer of systemic and mucosal immune responses against hepatitis B surface antigen with intranasal administration to mice. J. Immunol., 161, 4463–4466
156. Singh, M., Ugozzoli, M., Briones, M., Kazzaz, J., Soenawan, E., O'Hagan, D.T. (2003) The effect of CTAB concentration in cationic PLG microparticles on DNA adsorption and in vivo performance. Pharm. Res., 20, 247–251
157. Snippe, H., de Reuver, M.J., Beunder, J.W., van der Meer, J.B., van Wichen, D.F., Willers, J. M. (1982) Delayed-type hypersensitivity in rabbits. Comparison of the adjuvants dimethyl dioctadecyl ammonium bromide and Freund's complete adjuvant. Int. Arch. Allergy Appl. Immunol., 67, 139–144
158. Ulrich, J.T., Myers, K.R. (1995) Monophosphoryl lipid A as an adjuvant. Past experiences and new directions. Pharm. Biotechnol., 6, 495–524

Chapter 14
Powder Vaccines for Pulmonary Delivery

Tom Jin and Eric Tsao

Abstract Spray drying represents an elegant one-step process for generating powder products with unique particle characteristics. Respiratory delivery of powder vaccines for the prevention of infectious diseases has shown great promise. Pulmonary delivery using powder vaccine aerosols is an approach to immunization that offers advantages over the use of injection in terms of both delivery technology and vaccine formulation. Powder vaccines for needle-free delivery have been successfully produced during the past decade. The essential elements for the preparation of a powder vaccine through spray drying are reviewed in this chapter. For example, the screening of formulations, the spray dryers from laboratory scale to aseptic manufacturing facilities, and the selection of dry powder inhalers (DPIs) for pulmonary delivery. The advantages and challenges of manufacturing powder vaccines are also discussed.

14.1 Introduction

Current vaccines are generally administered via the intramuscular (i.m.) or subcutaneous (s.c) route using needles and syringes. Despite its common use, needle-based immunization has several disadvantages. In the developing world, there are major challenges of disease transmission through reuse of needles. Not limited to hepatitis B and C, human immunodeficiency virus, or other viruses, the infections through the needle penetration injuries increase the economic burden on health care systems. The World Health Organization (WHO) claims that up to 30 % of regular needle injections are considered unsafe [1]. Organizations such as the WHO, The Centers for Disease Control (CDC), and groups such as The Gates Foundation have supported the development of needle-free alternatives, particularly for vaccine

T. Jin (✉)
Aeras, Rockville, MD, USA
e-mail: zjin@aeras.org

D.R. Flower and Y. Perrie (eds.), *Immunomic Discovery of Adjuvants and Candidate Subunit Vaccines*, Immunomics Reviews: 5, DOI 10.1007/978-1-4614-5070-2_14,

delivery. The search for the methods of vaccine delivery not requiring a needle and syringe has been accelerated by recent concerns regarding pandemic disease, bioterrorism, and disease eradication campaigns. Needle-free vaccine delivery could aid in mass vaccinations by increasing the ease of use, speed of delivery, and by offering improved safety, compliance, decreased costs, and reduced pain associated with vaccinations.

Over the past decade, numerous vaccine delivery technologies have emerged, of which several are powder-based methods. These include microspheres for long-acting delivery, fine powders for pulmonary delivery, and biopharmaceutical/vaccine powders for intradermal delivery. Pulmonary delivery using powder vaccine aerosols is an approach to immunization that offers advantages over injection in terms of both delivery technology and vaccine formulation. The technology advantages include increased safety and ease of administration. The formulation advantages when using dry powders are the potential reduction of refrigeration requirements, and increased stability during transport and administration, thereby facilitating mass vaccination. Additionally, there is a potential for enhanced biological efficacy since pulmonary delivery may produce mucosal immunity superior to that which is produced after parenteral vaccine administration.

Spray drying, the process wherein a liquid feed is rapidly transformed into a dried particulate form by atomizing into a hot drying medium (air, nitrogen, or CO_2 gas), is a common method for preparing solids in the chemical, food, and pharmaceutical industries. It has been recommended as an alternative to freeze drying for the preparation of inhalation products, as it represents an elegant one-step process for producing biopharmaceutical formulations with unique particle characteristics. Spray drying has the additional advantage of being a faster and more cost-effective dehydration process than freeze drying. Vaccine powder formulations suitable for needle-free injection can be successfully produced by spray drying [2–4].

Pulmonary delivery of spray dried pharmaceutical products became the route of choice after the introduction in 1967 of dry powder inhalers (DPIs) to treat patients with asthma [5]. The spray drying technique being applied in vaccine development is relatively new compared to freezing drying technology. Published studies of powder vaccines are listed in Table 14.1 [6–11]. Respiratory delivery of powder vaccines for prevention of infectious diseases has shown great promise. Klas et al. reported that a single immunization with a dry powder anthrax vaccine could protect rabbits against lethal aerosol challenge. The Rhesus Macaques test showed that a dry powder measles vaccine induced robust measles virus-specific humoral and T-cell responses, without adverse effects, which completely protected the macaques from infection with wild-type virus more than one year later [6]. A clinical trial of measles vaccine is in development in India [12].

Although powder formed vaccines have shown many benefits compared to liquid forms, including increased safety of administration, storage stability, and biological efficacy, the development of methods for production of powder vaccines are still in their infancy. Several practical challenges need to be addressed before powder vaccine production can be scaled up, ultimately to meet the needs of mass vaccination. For example, optimization of formulations to generate less

Table 14.1 Current status of spray dried vaccines

Vaccines	Classification	Development status	References
Measles	Live attenuated	Preclinical	[6]
BCG	Live attenuated	Preclinical	[2]
Influenza	Subunit	Preclinical	[7]
	Split	Clinical phase I	[8]
	Whole inactivated	Preclinical	[9]
Anthrax	Subunit (*r*PA + conjugated peptide)	Preclinical	[10]
Plague	Subunit (F1-V)	Preclinical	[11]

hygroscopic particles with a more suitable size range (usually 1–5 μm) for pulmonary delivery and powder filling, and development of economic DPIs.

14.2 Formulations

The most commonly used method to stabilize biological ingredients, such as proteins, vaccines, and gene delivery systems, is to convert them to dry cakes or powders. The stability of dried formulations is believed to be related to lack of mobility of the biopharmaceutical components in the dried form, and the absence or reduction of certain degradation pathways such as hydrolysis. However, depending on the drying method, freezing and/or drying stresses may affect the structural integrity and/or activity of a dry powder vaccine. Accordingly, drying formulations using appropriate stabilizers are required for preservation of these properties. Unfortunately there is no definitive formulation that can be applied to all products. The most common excipients in formulation screening studies are classified as follows: (1) Carbohydrates, such as trehalose, mannitol, dextrans, sucrose, and myo-inositol; (2) Amino acids, such as leucine, histidine, and arginine; (3) Proteins, such as human serum albumin; (4) Polymers, such as polyvinylpyrrolidone (PVP); and (5) Buffer agents, such as PBS and histidine. Formulation screening of a powder vaccine can be time-and-labor consuming, and typically follows a trial and error process. Fortunately, there are various modern instruments that can be used to accelerate this process, such as differential scanning calorimetry (DSC), scanning electron microscopy (SEM), X-ray diffraction, and laser diffraction.

Disaccharides are amongst the most frequently used excipients, with trehalose being a particularly common selection. Trehalose has been shown to have the ability to protect active ingredients during the spray drying process and to result in improved stability in long-term storage [13–19]. However, trehalose and sucrose-based powders are more hygroscopic than other excipients, absorbing moisture during handling in the laboratory environment leading to degradation in physical properties of the powder and reduction in the ease of dispersion [4]. The sensitivity of powders to moisture uptake is important because the aerosol physical properties of inhalable dry powders are strongly dependent on moisture content; too much water can cause particle agglomeration, leading to reduced respirability. One compromise is to combine trehalose with other less hygroscopic components, such as mannitol and leucine. Sievers et al. reported a dry powder vaccine of Alum-HBsAb containing sufficient amounts of stabilizing trehalose. The powder did not lose potency after it was stored for 43 days at either −20 °C or 66 °C, and testing in mice showed full retention of immunogenicity [20].

Leucine- and mannitol-based formulations are less hygroscopic and have been used for TB powder vaccine [2, 4]. Mannitol is stable as a powder and resists moisture resorption at relatively high humidities. These characteristics make it an ideal substance to encapsulate biopharmaceuticals for inhalation, for diagnostic and therapeutic purposes. The inhalation of dry powder mannitol alone has been shown to cause a marked increase in MCC (mucociliary clearance) in the whole right lung and in all lung regions, in both asthmatic and healthy subjects. Inhalation of dry powder mannitol was well tolerated by all subjects and induced only a mild cough which was reproduced on the control day [21–26]. This increases the advantage of using a mannitol-based spray drying formulation in the development of powder form vaccines. Jin et al. reported that a TB vaccine prepared with mannitol-based formulations, which also contained small and high molecular weight sugar stabilizers (trehalose and two dextrans), successfully resisted water absorption. The spray-dried TB vaccine could be stored at 4 °C and 25 °C for 12 months without any significant change in vaccine potency. After storage at 37 °C for 5 weeks, the loss of virus activity was only 0.12 log [4]. The combination of excipients achieved optimization of viral processing and storage stability, while mitigating the negative particle forming properties of trehalose.

Immobilization of the labile materials in amorphous glass is believed to be advantageous to maintain the activity of the incorporated molecules [27]. Resistance to crystallization can be evaluated by measuring the glass transition temperature (T_g), which is the temperature at which the transition from a glassy to a rubbery state or from a low molecular mobility to a high molecular mobility (and therefore, higher risk of crystallization) occurs. PVP and albumins are known to increase T_g, which means that formulations containing these can be exposed to higher ambient temperatures before the glass transition occurs [15, 28, 29]. However, PVP alone as a stabilizer in a formulation of attenuated live Newcastle disease vaccine virus did not appear to prevent loss of virus activity during the spray drying process, and required the use of other stabilizers, such as trehalose and albumin [16].

Dextrans have a long history of being used as excipients in vaccine formulations. They have been shown to prevent crystallization during the spray drying or freeze drying processes [30, 31]. Lung delivery of aerosolized dextran is well tolerated and has potential therapeutic benefit in the treatment of cystic fibrosis [32]. Dextran has a high T_g value of −9 °C. A formulation containing dextrans has been shown to increase the T_g of trehalose from 50.55 to 97.09 °C. The formulation also generates a dry powder that inhibits recrystallization of stabilizing sugars, preventing inactivation of incorporated labile materials [4]. In formulations with a T_g occurring at about 50 °C and higher, the powders and microparticles should be physically stable at temperatures up to about 40 °C, as long as the powders are protected from moisture ingress. A higher T_g value of a formulation usually suggests enhanced long-term thermostability.

Formulation development is essential for a powder vaccine. Jin et al. showed that powder formulation helped stabilize an adenovirus 35-vectored tuberculosis (TB) vaccine so that variations in temperature did not negatively impact its effectiveness or shelf life [4]. They demonstrated that it is possible to produce a stable dry powder formulation of a TB vaccine suitable for mass vaccination in a one-step drying process. The process of identifying and optimizing key excipients directly relates to the recovery of active ingredients, the yield of powder product, and stability during storage. The following properties could be used to evaluate formulation development during or post-spray drying activities: (1) High recovery for both active ingredient and powder; (2) Formulation has relatively high T_g for good stability during storage; (3) Less hygroscopic powder could benefit both vaccine stability and powder filling process; (4) Narrow size distribution (2–5 μm) and good aerosolization characteristics of final product provide easy delivery to the deep lung parenchyma by DPIs.

14.3 Spray Drying: From Concept to cGMP Products

One of the oldest forms of industrial drying is spray drying. A patent from 1872 by Percy gives probably one of the first detailed descriptions of drying of sprays [33]. With the advancement of science and technology, pulmonary delivery of drugs has become the route of choice after the introduction of the DPI in 1967 [5]. The application of spray drying in vaccine development has only occurred in the last decade (Table 14.1). Different types of powder vaccine are in the preclinical and clinical phases. As previously mentioned, the first needle-free measles vaccine clinical trial is going to be initiated in India, using the measles powder vaccine developed by Dr. Sievers of the University of Colorado.

Spray dryers designed for cGMP vaccine production have not been fully developed. The requirements for this process are that it needs to be inexpensive, scalable, GMP-compliant, and capable of sterile manufacturing from beginning to end. Most researchers in the early stages use the Mini Spray dryer B-290 (Büchi, Switzerland) in their laboratory scale processes. The sources for "real" aseptic cGMP spray dryers are limited. The manufacturers SPX Anhydro and GEA Niro claimed that they had developed spray dryers for cGMP manufacturing of powder vaccine. One of these cGMP spray dryers, the MS-35 (SPX Anhydro), was set up in the facility of Aeras. It was custom designed by Anhydro for manufacturing of TB vaccines and other powder form products. The MS-35 meets the FDA requirement of the aseptic concept for the manufacturing of human vaccines. When the optimum parameters were selected, the output of MS-35 could reach 180 ~ 250 g of powder within 4 h (Table 14.2). The differences in output between the Büchi B-290 and MS-35 are listed in Table 14.3. The scaled up process using the MS-35 increased recovery by 20 % points, with a fourfold increase in powder yield in the final product.

Table 14.2 Output of MS-35 (Anhydro) cGMP spray dryer

Vaccine	Spray drying period/lot	Yield* (g)	Dosages/lot (10 mg/dosage)
Bacteria/virus (Live)	2~4 hr	180	18,000
Protein/peptide	2~4 hr	250	25,000

*Yield is the powder mass collected at the end of each run.

Table 14.3 Process comparison between laboratory and cGMP spray drying

	Recovery (%)	Particle size (μm)	Feeding rate (mL/min)	Yield (g/hr)
B-290 (Büchi)	50~65	3~4	3~5	15
MS-35 (Anhydro)	70~85	2~3	10~12	60

Table 14.4 Comparison of cost-effectiveness between spray drying and lyophilization

	Process time	Labor	Materials	Consumables (process gases/ electricity/cooling water)	Equipment	Output dosages* (250g solid)
Spray drying (MS-35)	2~4 h	Comparable	Comparable	$300	Comparable	10,000
Lyophilizer (Shelf area in 40 SF)	2~72 h	Comparable	Comparable	$300	Comparable	10,000

*25mg/dose or vial; 0.5 ml filling for lyo vial; 25 mg for powder product.

The smaller particle size with the MS-35 might be caused by the more effective and even evaporation with this spray dryer. A comparison of the cost-effectiveness of spray drying vs. lyophilization showed promising results: tenfold shorter processing cycle and larger evaporative capability than traditional lyophilization (Table 14.4). They are comparable in other factors relating to cost-effectiveness between the MS-35 and the lyophilizer (40 SF shelf area). Although spray drying has been successfully used in the production of food and biochemical products, use of the technology in the manufacture of human vaccines needs to consider the following additional challenges: (1) Low inlet temperature is required to avoid denaturation or inactivation of proteins or live active ingredients during the drying process, which will compromise the output of final products caused by reduced feeding rate; (2) Aseptic design for the spray dryer used in powder vaccine production is strictly required by FDA, which usually is not a concern in food, biochemical, and pharmaceutical industrials; (3) Requirement for large scale and accurate powder filling, and (4) Effective and economic DPIs need to be developed and marketed.

14.4 Dry Powder Inhalers

There are two major types of DPIs: unit-dose devices and reservoir-type multiple-dose devices. Powder vaccine could only employ a single dosage device for individual subjects, even in mass population vaccinations. Since the inception of the first DPI Spinhaler® (Aventis), device technology has continued to grow and a lot of devices are now currently available on the market, such as Aerolizer®, Diskus®, Flexhaler®, Handihaler®, Rotahaler®, Turbuhaler® and Twishaler®.

The airborne product generated by a powder inhaler should contain a significant proportion of particles less than 5 μm in size. In order for a powder to be suitable for pulmonary delivery, the aerodynamic size requirements are that particles must be in the 1–5 μm range (Fig. 14.1). PuffHaler, a dry powder device from ActivDry (Fig. 14.2), has been applied in the measles powder immunization and challenge study in rhesus macaques reported by Dr. Griffin [6]. The device consists of three components: the vaccine formulation held in an aluminum foil blister, the reservoir, and the dispersion mechanism to generate aerosols. When the PuffHaler squeeze bulb is compressed to 2 psi, the silicone rubber burst valve pops open. The air rushes into the disperser through the powder in the aluminum foil blister and the aerosol cloud fills a collapsed plastic bag reservoir. The aerosol-filled bag is detached and affixed to a facemask from which the subject is allowed to breathe for 30 s to become vaccinated. As a control, a dry powder device of BD Solovent (BD Technologies) (Fig. 14.3) was also evaluated in this study. The syringe of the BD Solovent device is used to pressurize the capsule containing the powder vaccine. As the pressure rises, the thin films sealing the capsule abruptly rupture, and the powder is expelled and captured in the disposable spacer for delivery through a silicone facemask. The study demonstrated that both the PuffHaler and Solovent devices efficiently delivered the vaccine to the deep lung, resulting in more robust antibody and T-cell responses than nasal delivery or s.c. injection of the live attenuated measles vaccine.

The inhalation route offers an enormous absorptive surface area, in the range 35–140 m^2, of thin (0.2 μm) and highly vascularized epithelium, which leads to high bioavailability. Direct delivery of drug into the deep lungs utilizing the patient's respiration is increasingly being explored as a mechanism for the delivery of systemic drugs. Successful delivery of vaccines into the deep lungs depends on the integration between powder formulations and the device performance [34, 35]. Licensing and marketing approval requires that current DPIs demonstrate in vitro performance and in vivo efficacy and reliability. However, the mass of vaccine delivered and the aerodynamic particle size can change, depending on the characteristics of inhalation. Hence, one approach to developing successful DPIs is to decrease the dependence of these devices solely on the subject's inhalation.

Among aerosol generation systems, DPIs present several advantages. They are propellant-free, portable, easy to operate, and low-cost devices with improved stability of the formulation as a result of the dry state. The challenge of any

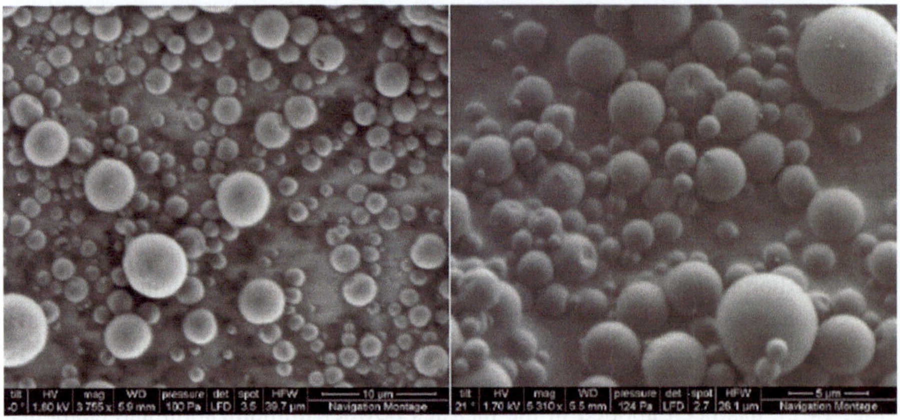

Fig. 14.1 The SEM images of Aeras 402 powder vaccine

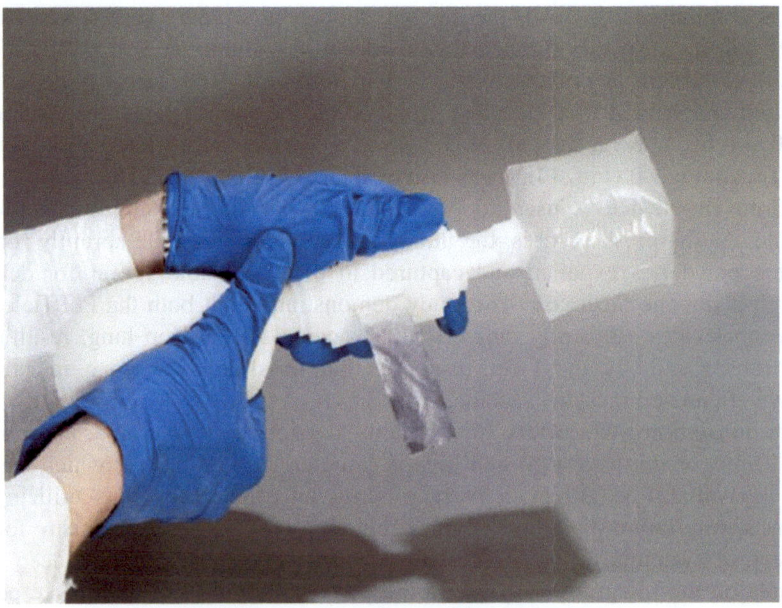

Fig. 14.2 A dry powder device, PuffHaler, from ActivDry

inhalation delivery system is, however, to generate particles with an adequate range of particle sizes. In the case of dry powders, this is greatly impeded by particle aggregation which lowers the fraction that is respirable, i.e., the fraction of particles (and particle aggregates) with an aerodynamic diameter ≤5 μm.

Efficient delivery of vaccines from DPIs depends not only on the device, but also on drug formulation and the production of suitable powders for effective respiratory

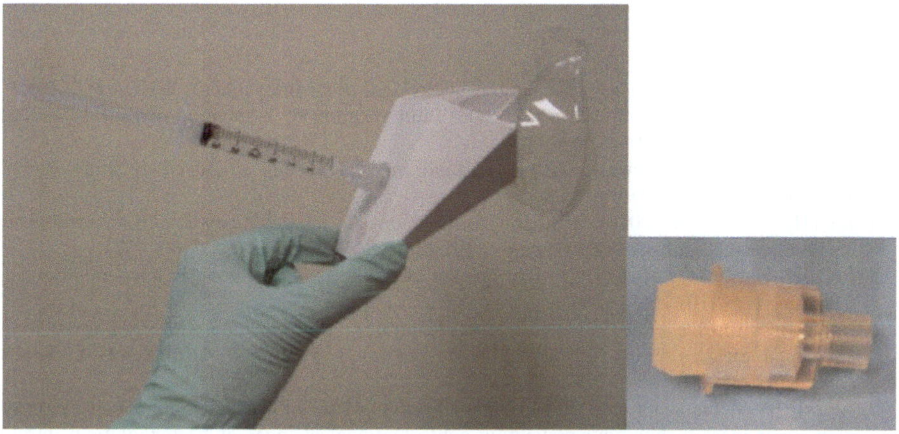

Fig. 14.3 A dry powder device, Solovent, from BD Technologies. The right figure is the enlarged photo of capsule containing powder vaccine, sealed by thin film at two ends

deposition as well as formulation of powders with or without excipients. To realize the full potential of DPIs, at the lowest cost to both vaccine companies and the recipient populations, innovation of new devices with enhanced lung deposition and reliability will play important roles in the future.

14.5 Conclusions

In conclusion, spray drying as a new technology being applied in vaccine development has shown promising results. Needle-free pulmonary vaccine delivery could aid in mass vaccinations by increasing ease and speed of delivery, and by offering improved safety and compliance, decreased costs, and reduced pain associated with vaccinations. In addition, aerosol delivery of powder vaccine has the potential for increased protection by direct stimulation of immunity in the lung compared to vaccines delivered by the parenteral route. There are three essential aspects that need to be fully investigated for the application of spray drying to vaccine development: (1) Optimum formulation for each individual vaccine, which is closely related to good stability, less hygroscopicity, and prompt powder filling of final product; (2) Aseptic design in a cGMP spray dryer; and (3) Economic and efficient DPIs to permit mass vaccinations.

Acknowledgments The authors appreciate Barbara Shepherd for her critical review of the manuscript and thoughtful suggestions. This publication was supported by the Bill & Melinda Gates Foundation.

References

1. WHO (2010) Best practices for injections and related procedures toolkit. WHO/EHT/10.02
2. Garcia-Contreras L, Wong YL et al (2008) Immunization by a bacterial aerosol. Proc Natl Acad Sci U S A 105(12):4656–4660
3. Ohtake S, Martin RA et al (2010) Heat-stable measles vaccine produced by spray drying. Vaccine 28(5):1275–1284
4. Jin TH, Tsao E et al (2010) Stabilizing formulations for inhalable powders of an adenovirus 35-vectored tuberculosis (TB) vaccine (AERAS-402). Vaccine 28(27):4369–4375
5. Bell JH, Hartley PS et al (1971) Dry powder aerosols. I. A new powder inhalation device. J Pharm Sci 60(10):1559–1564
6. Lin WJ, Griffin DE et al (2011) Successful respiratory immunization with dry powder live-attenuated measles virus vaccine in rhesus macaques. Proc Natl Acad Sci U S A 108 (7):2987–2992
7. Amorij JP, Meulenaar J et al (2007) Rational design of an influenza subunit vaccine powder with sugar glass technology: preventing conformational changes of haemagglutinin during freezing and freeze-drying. Vaccine 25(35):6447–6457
8. Chen D, Dean H et al (2003) Pre-clinical and clinical studies of epidermal powder immunization with an influenza vaccine. Int Congr Ser 1263:555–558
9. Garmise RJ, Staats HF et al (2007) Novel dry powder preparations of whole inactivated influenza virus for nasal vaccination. AAPS PharmSciTech 8(4):2–10
10. Klas SD, Petrie CR et al (2008) A single immunization with a dry powder anthrax vaccine protects rabbits against lethal aerosol challenge. Vaccine 26(43):5494–5502
11. Huang J, D'Souza AJ et al (2009) Protective immunity in mice achieved with dry powder formulation and alternative delivery of plage F1-V vaccine. Clin Vaccine Immunol 16 (5):719–725
12. Tim Parsons (2011) Researchers test inhalable measles vaccine. JH Pub Health News. http://www.jhsph.edu/publichealthnews/press_releases/2011/griffin_measles_vaccine.html. Accessed 31 Jan 2011
13. Maa YF, Nguyen PA et al (1999) Protein inhalation powder: spray drying vs. spray drying. Pharm Res 16(2):249–254
14. Tzannis ST, Prestrelski SJ (2000) Moisture effects on protein—excipient interactions in spray-dried powders. Nature of destabilizing effects of sucrose. J Pharm Sci 88(3):360–370
15. Burger JL, Cape SP et al (2008) Stabilizing formulations for inhalable powders of live-attenuated measles virus vaccine. J Aerosol Med Pulm Drug Deliv 21(1):25–34
16. Corbanie EA, Remon JP et al (2007) Spray drying of an attenuated live Newcastle disease vaccine virus intended for respiratory mass vaccination of poultry. Vaccine 25(49):8306–8317
17. Broadhead J, Rouan SK et al (1994) The effect of process and formulation variables on the properties of spray-dried beta-galactosidase. J Pharm Pharmacol 46(6):458–467
18. Labrude P, Rasolomanana M et al (1989) Protective effect of sucrose on spray drying of oxyhemoglobin. J Pharm Sci 78(3):223–239
19. Bosquillon C, Lombry C et al (2001) Comparison of particle sizing techniques in the case of inhalation dry powders. J Pharm Sci 90(12):2032–2041
20. Sievers RE, Quinn SP et al (2007) Near-critical fluid micronization of stabilized vaccines, antibiotics and anti-virals. J Supercrit Fluids 42(3):385–391
21. Glover W, Chan HK et al (2006) Lung deposition of mannitol powder aerosol in healthy subjects. J Aerosol Med 19(4):522–532
22. Daviskas E, Anderson SD et al (1997) Inhalation of dry-powder mannitol increases mucociliary clearance. Eur Respir J 10(11):2449–2454
23. Daviskas E, Anderson SD et al (1999) Inhalation of dry powder mannitol improves clearance of mucus in patients with bronchiectasis. Am J Respir Crit Care Med 159(6):1843–1848
24. Daviskas E, Anderson SD et al (2001) The 24-h Effect of mannitol on the clearance of mucus in patients with bronchiectasis. Chest 119(2):414–421

25. Daviskas E, Anderson SD et al (2005) Inhaled mannitol for the treatment of mucociliary dysfunction in patients with bronchiectasis—effect on lung function. Respirology 10(1):46–56
26. Anderson SD, Brannan J et al (1997) A new method for bronchial provocation testing in asthmatic subjects using a dry powder of mannitol. Am J Respir Crit Care Med 156 (3):758–765
27. Imamura K, Iwai M et al (2001) Evaluation of hydration states of protein in freeze-dried amorphous sugar matrix. J Pharm Sci 90(12):1955–1963
28. Mahlin D, Berggren J et al (2006) The influence of PVP incorporation on moisture-induced surface crystallization of amorphous spray-dried lactose particles. Int J Pharm 321(1–2):78–85
29. Zhang J, Zografi G (2001) Water vapor absorption into amorphous sucrose-poly(vinyl pyrrolidone) and trehalose-poly(vinyl pyrrolidone) mixtures. J Pharm Sci 90(9):1375–1385
30. Chen D, Maa YF et al (2002) Needle-free epidermal powder immunization. Expert Rev Vaccines 1(3):265–276
31. Rochelle C, Lee G (2007) Dextran or hydroxyethyl starch in spray-freeze-dried trehalose/ mannitol microparticles intended as ballistic particulate carriers for proteins. J Pharm Sci 96 (9):2296–2309
32. Finlay WH, Lange CF (2000) Lung delivery of aerosolized dextran. Am J Respir Crit Care Med 161(1):91–97
33. Percy SR (1872) US Patent 125 406
34. Cryan SA (2005) Carrier-based strategies for targeting protein and peptide drugs to the lungs. AAPS J 7(1):E20–41
35. Islam N, Gladki E (2008) Dry powder inhalers (DPIs)—a review of device reliability and innovation. Int J Pharm 360(1–2):1–11

About the Author

Dr. Darren R. Flower is an interdisciplinary scientist, with special interest in bioinformatics, computational chemistry, and cheminformatics, Dr. Flower has wide-ranging experience of the preclinical research environment in both academia and the pharmaceutical industry. Before joining Aston University as a Reader, Dr. Flower was a Jenner Research Fellow and Principal Investigator at the University of Oxford; and formerly a Senior Group Leader managing a large research group at The Edward Jenner Institute for Vaccine Research. Before that, Dr. Flower was a drug discovery scientist in the Pharmaceutical industry. Dr. Flower is a Fellow of the Royal Society of Chemistry, and the author of over 150 research papers and reviews, and seven Books, including the monograph: *Bioinformatics for Vaccinology*.

Professor Yvonne Perrie is a Pharmacist whose research focuses on the development on delivery systems for drugs and vaccines. Prof. Perrie is currently Head of Pharmacy and Chair in Drug Delivery within Aston University. Prof. Perrie received her Ph.D. from the University of London, UK where she investigated the use of liposomes for gene delivery under the supervision of Professor Gregory Gregoriadis. Prof. Perrie then joined a newly established Drug Delivery Company, Lipoxen Technologies Ltd., prior to taking her post at Aston University. Prof. Perrie is currently Chair of the UK and Ireland Controlled Release Society and has approximately 100 research papers and reviews focusing on the research and development of drug delivery systems.

D.R. Flower and Y. Perrie (eds.), *Immunomic Discovery of Adjuvants and Candidate Subunit Vaccines*, Immunomics Reviews: 5, DOI 10.1007/978-1-4614-5070-2,

Index

D.R. Flower and Y. Perrie (eds.), *Immunomic Discovery of Adjuvants and Candidate Subunit Vaccines*, Immunomics Reviews: 5, DOI 10.1007/978-1-4614-5070-2,

MIX
Papier aus verantwortungsvollen Quellen
Paper from responsible sources
FSC® C105338

If you have any concerns about our products,
you can contact us on
ProductSafety@springernature.com

In case Publisher is established outside the EU,
the EU authorized representative is:
Springer Nature Customer Service Center GmbH
Europaplatz 3, 69115 Heidelberg, Germany

Printed by Libri Plureos GmbH
in Hamburg, Germany